# Social Aspects of HIV

Volume 4

Since the start of the epidemic, HIV and AIDS have fired the imaginations of social as well as medical and public health scientists. This innovative series of books offers a setting in which to publish the very best of social scientific thinking and research. The Social Aspects of HIV series of books offers readers authoritative introductions and overviews, together with summaries of enduring and cutting edge concerns. The series is international and multidisciplinary in focus, including contributions from psychology, sociology, anthropology, education, economic, political and social theory, and international development. Individual volumes offer scholarly overviews of key topics and concerns but also address 'big issues' relevant to HIV prevention, treatment and care. Sexual and drug-related practices; adherence; disclosure; and stigma and discrimination are among topics focused upon, alongside broader cultural, political and social responses to the epidemic, including globalisation and internationalisation. The political economy of AIDS, links to broader questions of sexual health and rights, and the progressive biomedicalisation of the response, will also be among key issues examined.The series will appeal to those working in public health, health psychology, medical sociology, medical anthropology, health promotion, social work and international development. Individual volumes will be relevant to students, teachers, researchers and practitioners within each of these disciplines as well as program developers and managers working across a variety of contexts.

More information about this series at http://www.springer.com/series/11922

Deanna Kerrigan • Clare Barrington
Editors

# Structural Dynamics of HIV

## Risk, Resilience and Response

Springer

*Editors*
Deanna Kerrigan
Johns Hopkins Bloomberg School of Public Health
Baltimore, MD, USA

Clare Barrington
University of North Carolina (UNC) Gillings School of Global Public Health
Chapel Hill, NC, USA

ISSN 2509-6559 ISSN 2509-6567 (electronic)
Social Aspects of HIV
ISBN 978-3-319-63521-7 ISBN 978-3-319-63522-4 (eBook)
DOI 10.1007/978-3-319-63522-4

Library of Congress Control Number: 2017941081



Printed on acid-free paper

This Springer imprint is published by Springer Nature
The registered company is Springer International Publishing AG
The registered company address is: Gewerbestrasse 11, 6330 Cham, Switzerland

# Foreword

Over nearly four decades of the history of the HIV epidemic, understanding of the ways in which structural factors shape the epidemic and condition possible responses to it has changed dramatically. While the earliest perceptions of AIDS focused primarily on behavioral factors associated with HIV transmission, and on the need for behavior change as the primary form of HIV prevention, as the global response to the epidemic began to take shape, growing awareness of the importance of a range of structural forces influencing the epidemic gradually began to emerge.

By the late 1980s, following the creation of the Global Programme on AIDS at the World Health Organization, attention began to focus on what was described as "the third epidemic" (following on the heels of HIV infection and diagnosed cases of AIDS) – an epidemic of social responses to HIV and AIDS, characterized almost always by levels of stigma, discrimination, and denial that created serious structural barriers to effective policies and programs necessary to address a growing global pandemic. As research and analysis on these dimensions of the epidemic grew in the early to mid-1990s, greater understanding developed of factors that might be understood as social determinants of HIV infection itself and of the ways in which infection evolved into disease progression in different populations. Concepts such as "social vulnerability" and "structural violence" were adapted in order to analyze how factors such as social class and economic exclusion, racial and ethnic discrimination, gender power differences, and sexual oppression, among other similar social structural forces, shaped the path of the epidemic – just as they conditioned the kinds of responses that different communities and polities developed in response to HIV.

Awareness and concern with such issues came to a head in the late 1990s and the early 2000s, as clinically effective treatments for HIV infection finally emerged, becoming the harbinger of interventions that finally might make control of the epidemic a realistic possibility, only to collide with the reality of a global political economy that imposed barriers to the inclusion of those living with HIV who were unlucky enough to live in the poorer countries of the Global South (or, for that matter, in the poorest sectors of society in the Global North). The international treatment access movement came ultimately to be driven by this understanding of the ways in which political and economic structures created barriers to treatment access, threatening to determine who would live and who would die under the conditions of globalized capitalism that had emerged as almost universal by the end of the twentieth century.

As the response to the global epidemic entered the new millennium, the struggle for treatment access – understood fundamentally as a struggle for social justice played out on a global stage – began to carry the day in moral debates about policies that should drive the global response to the epidemic, and an important "scale-up" of programs aimed at guaranteeing prevention and treatment access gradually began to become a reality, promising the hope of real breakthroughs in relation to the goal of ultimately controlling an epidemic that had once seemed almost unstoppable.

If this history of roughly the first 25 years of the AIDS epidemic thus seemed to be one of growing awareness of structural factors shaping HIV and AIDS, at almost exactly the same time that global scale-up of HIV programs reached a kind of zenith in the late 2000s, two very different trends began to take place. On the one hand, an extended global financial crisis constrained previously expanding budgets for the global HIV response and for global health more generally. On the other hand, in what can only be seen in retrospect as somewhat misplaced optimism, enthusiasm about the growth of treatment access around the world, and excitement about the potential of "treatment as prevention," "test-and-treat" programs, the "HIV treatment cascade and care continuum," and new biomedical approaches to HIV prevention began to draw attention away from concern with structural issues, reigniting hope for the discovery of biomedical magic bullets that had seemed impossible since the earliest days of the AIDS response. By the early 2010s, this optimism had turned to misplaced triumphalism on the part of many United Nations and bilateral development aid agencies, with promises of "the end of AIDS" (or the arrival of "an AIDS-free generation") in the near future (seemingly oblivious to the contradictory reality that more than 20 years after the availability of effective treatment for HIV, still only roughly half of the people in the world who needed access to such treatment actually had it).

It is within this context that this volume in the Social Aspects of HIV series of books takes on special importance. *Structural Dynamics of HIV: Risk, Resilience, and Response*, edited by Deanna Kerrigan and Clare Barrington, brings together a cutting-edge collection of analyses by leading figures working on the structural dimensions of the HIV epidemic. It highlights the need for renewed attention to the structural dynamics of risk and resilience among key affected populations and communities, including sex workers, people who inject drugs, women and girls, transgender women, gay and other men who have sex with men, migrants, and people living with HIV. It also documents the ways in which structural factors have been confronted in different national settings as diverse as Brazil, South Africa, Ukraine, and the USA.

Together, the chapters in this volume provide a vivid account of the structural forces that shape vulnerability to HIV across such highly diverse populations and the ways in which communities have mobilized and become empowered to respond to HIV and AIDS – as well as the positive and negative ways in which governments support (or fail to support) these efforts. Chapters highlight the difficult challenge of sustaining effective responses – and, indeed, what might be described as the vulnerability of the AIDS response itself in the face of political backsliding and conservative political movements. At a time when it is increasingly clear that promises of an imminent end of the epidemic have been exaggerated, and that what is needed to sustain the global HIV response is greater realism, critical analysis, and long-term commitment to confronting the structural factors that have shaped the epidemic in the first place, this volume on the *Structural Dynamics of HIV* provides a major contribution to the research literature on the social aspects of HIV. It offers an important corrective to the recent tendency to imagine that biomedical innovations or technocratic interventions can somehow serve as magic bullets capable of escaping or circumventing the social, political, and economic structures that create global inequalities in health – and highlights the long-term commitment that will be required if we are ever to achieve real progress toward the goal of a world without AIDS.

Columbia University Mailman
School of Public Health, New York, USA
Richard G. Parker

Centre for Social Research in Health,
UNSW Sydney, Australia
Peter Aggleton

# Acknowledgments

We would like to start by thanking Richard G. Parker and Peter Aggleton for inviting us to serve as editors of this book, which is part of the Social Aspects of HIV series marking the contributions of the social sciences to the global response to HIV. Working with and learning from them in this process has been a distinct honor and privilege.

Next, we would like to extend our gratitude to all of the chapter authors that took time and care to share their work, drawing on years of field experience in many cases. These contributions provide unique insights into how to conceptualize and respond to HIV using innovations in social theory and methods. Their work, which often crosses disciplinary boundaries throughout the chapters, stimulates new opportunities for more equitable public health policies and programs and collective action for social change.

None of this work would be possible without those on the front lines, which includes members of the diverse populations discussed in this book, as well as research teams, nongovernmental organizations, intervention staff, government officials, and activist colleagues across the globe advocating for a rights-based response to HIV.

We would also like to thank colleagues who helped us organize, coordinate, format, and copyedit this volume particularly Paige Hammond, Wendy Davis, and Andrea Mantsios from the Johns Hopkins University and Bernadette Deelen-Mans and Evelien Bakker from Springer. We are grateful for the contributions of these Springer staff and the support of Springer for this special work that commemorates the role of the social sciences in public health.

# Contents

# About the Authors

**Peter Aggleton** is Scientia Professor in Education and Health in the Centre for Social Research in Health at UNSW Sydney. He has worked internationally on sexual health for over 25 years and is well known for his work on the social aspects of the HIV epidemic. Peter has worked as a senior advisor on HIV to numerous international agencies and is the editor-in-chief of several journals including *Culture, Health & Sexuality* and *Sex Education*. He is a visiting professor at the UCL Institute of Education in London and at the University of Sussex. He is an adjunct professor in the Australian Research Centre for Sex, Health and Society at La Trobe University in Melbourne.

**José Manuel Aguilar-Martínez** is an epidemiologist with a master's degree in public health who conducts quantitative and qualitative research with men who have sex with men, transgender women, sex workers, and people living with HIV. He worked at the Universidad del Valle de Guatemala as technical director of behavioral surveys in Central America. He was also the Central American coordinator for the sexually transmitted infection and HIV surveillance clinics (known as VICITS in Spanish). He is community advisor to the community-based gay rights and health organization, Colectivo Amigos Contra el SIDA (CAS), where he has also been the president of the board of directors for the last 4 years.

**Clare Barrington** is associate professor of health behavior at the University of North Carolina (UNC) Gillings School of Global Public Health. She is also the Latin American projects director for the UNC Institute for Global Health and Infectious Diseases and a fellow at the Carolina Population Center. Dr. Barrington conducts mixed-methods research to examine social network and structural influences on health and health behaviors, with a focus on HIV prevention, care, and treatment among female sex workers and their male partners, men who have sex with men, and transgender women in Latin America. She has worked in the Dominican Republic since the mid-1990s and also has current projects in Central America and with Latinos in North Carolina. Dr. Barrington also leads the qualitative component of several mixed-methods HIV studies and impact evaluations of social cash transfer programs. She teaches graduate-level courses in qualitative data analysis and writing and global health.

**Monica R. Biradavolu** is the CEO and founder of QualAnalytics and is scholar-in-residence at American University. She holds a PhD in sociology from Duke University. She studies the implementation of development projects globally with a sociological lens. Her research projects have been on HIV interventions with sex workers in India; multisector nutrition programming in Nepal; living conditions of Syrian refugees in Lebanon, Jordan, and Kurdistan region of Iraq; education interventions to improve teacher attendance in Haiti; and barriers to HIV services for the severely mentally ill in Washington DC. She advocates for mixed-methods evaluations, integrating rigorous qualitative methods with quantitative surveys. Her publications have appeared in *Social Science and Medicine*, *the Journal of Epidemiology and Community Health*, *AIDS*, *Global Health*, *AIDS Care*, *Psychosomatics*, *AIDS Patient Care and STDs*, and *Public Health Reports*.

**Kim M. Blankenship** is professor of community health and prevention in the Dornsife School of Public Health at Drexel University. Her research focuses on the social determinants of health and structural interventions to address them. More specifically, she has analyzed how structures and processes of race, class, and/or gender inequality intersect to affect HIV-related risk and disparities. Through this lens, she has focused attention on community mobilization as a strategy for addressing power imbalances that give rise to sex worker risk for HIV and on analyzing how mass incarceration in the USA impacts HIV risk in general and race disparities in risk in particular. Her research has been funded by the National Institute of Mental Health, the National Institute on Drug Abuse, the Bill & Melinda Gates Foundation, and the U.S. Centers for Disease Control and Prevention.

**Jane Brown** has over 20 years' experience in health and development communication and production, with an emphasis on gender, adolescent reproductive health, malaria, maternal and child health, HIV, and AIDS. She was one of the principal innovators of the evaluated *African Transformation* program, which enables women and men to explore the underlying gender barriers and facilitators to practice positive health behaviors and develop realistic solutions, and *Go Girls!*, a multileveled, regional intervention addressing girls' vulnerability to HIV. She has provided technical leadership on many regional social and behavior change communication projects and over a dozen country projects. Most recently she was the project director for a regional initiative helping to restore trust in and create demand for reproductive, maternal, newborn, and child health (RMNCH) services in a post-Ebola context in Sierra Leone, Guinea, and Liberia.

**Maria Carrasco** is a behavioral scientist originally from Ecuador. Prior to joining the Office of HIV at the US Agency for International Development (USAID), where she currently works, Maria worked on designing, implementing, and evaluating social and behavioral interventions with the Johns Hopkins Center for

Communication Programs, the World Bank, the United Nations Population Fund, AED, and Pact. She has worked in Peru, Malawi, Mozambique, Kenya, the Dominican Republic, Mexico, South Africa, and Ecuador, and she speaks Spanish and Portuguese fluently. In her current role at USAID, Maria provides technical support to HIV prevention, treatment, and care programs implemented primarily in Africa and Central America. Maria holds a master's degree in public policy from Duke University and a PhD in behavioral sciences and a master's degree in public health from the Johns Hopkins Bloomberg School of Public Health.

**Nimesh Dhungana** holds an MA in international development and social change from Clark University. He is currently pursuing his PhD in the Department of Methodology in the London School of Economics, where he is examining the practices of rights-based, community-centric accountability as part of the recovery and reconstruction efforts in post-earthquake Nepal. His research interests span areas of international development, the interplay of disaster and development, and structural interventions in health and development. He has been involved in a mixed-methods study that examines the processes and impacts of community mobilization interventions among female sex workers in southern India. He has also been part of an HIV impact evaluation project that involves generating innovative methodological approaches to compiling, synthesizing, and analyzing HIV-related data from India.

**Yeycy Donastorg** is a Dominican medical doctor with a master's degree in public health and population studies, who has been conducting community-based and clinical research in the Dominican Republic for nearly two decades, including demographics studies, HIV preventive vaccine trial, ART clinical trials, behavioral studies, and several qualitative research studies. She has been the research coordinator of the Unidad de Vacunas at *Instituto Dermatológico y Cirugía de la Piel* (IDCP) for the last 12 years. She was one of the lead investigators on the original Abriendo Puertas intervention research project focused on female sex workers living with HIV.

**Olga Filippova** is associate professor at V.N. Karazin Kharkiv National University in Ukraine. Her educational background combines knowledge and methodological tools of analysis in history (master's degree, Kharkiv National University), sociology (candidate of science, Kharkiv National University), and sociocultural anthropology (advanced courses throughout the projects of SeFReS, France, and a Fulbright scholarship). She takes multidisciplinary approaches in her research, drawing on methodologies from sociology and anthropology and grounding her theoretical perspective in history, political science, gender studies, and cultural studies.

**César Galindo Arandi** is trained as an environmental and population sciences teacher. He has worked on HIV research, programming, and policy for 25 years in a wide range of capacities. He is currently the executive director of Colectivo Amigos Contra el SIDA (CAS), a community-based gay rights and health organization in Guatemala City. Mr. Galindo Arandi has also worked for the Universidad del Valle de Guatemala as coordinator of the sexually transmitted infections sentinel surveillance strategy for Central America, for Family Health International as the Guatemala country director, for UNAIDS as a policy analyst, for Doctors Without Borders as the Central American advisor, and for the US Agency for International Development (USAID)/Program for Strengthening the Central American Response to HIV/AIDS as program manager. He has been the lead author on several global reports for UNAIDS and the Pan American Health Organization. He has also conducted qualitative research on HIV among key populations and bullying related to sexual orientation, among other topics. He has written over 20 school texts about how to talk about sexuality and HIV in the school environment.

**Annie George** is an independent qualitative researcher who works on the intersecting themes of sex work, violence against women, trafficking, and HIV prevention. She served as the India research manager for Project Parivartan, the Bill & Melinda Gates Foundation-sponsored project analyzing the implementation and impact of a community mobilization intervention in Andhra Pradesh, India, to address HIV risk among female sex workers.

**Hoisex Gomez** is an expert in human behavior at *Instituto Dermatológico y Cirugía de la Piel* (IDCP) in the Dominican Republic with more than 20 years of experience in the field of health education and communication for behavior change. Since 2005, she has been part of the research team in the Unidad de Vacunas at *Instituto Dermatológico y Cirugía de la Piel* (IDCP). She is in charge of coordination of community education and the liaison with the community advisory committee. She was part of the team working on design, capacity building, and evaluation of the counseling component for the Abriendo Puertas intervention focused on improving HIV outcomes for female sex workers.

**Jennifer S. Hirsch** is a professor and deputy chair for doctoral studies in sociomedical sciences at Columbia University's Mailman School of Public Health, as well as co-director of the Columbia Population Research Center. A 2012 Guggenheim fellow, Professor Hirsch's research explores gender, sexuality, and reproductive health, the comparative anthropology of love, US-Mexico migration and migrant health, and the applications of anthropological theory and methods to public health research and policies. Her books include *A Courtship After Marriage: Sexuality and Love in Mexican Transnational Families* (University of California Press, 2003) and the award-winning *The Secret: Love, Marriage, and HIV* (Vanderbilt University Press, 2010).

**David R. Holtgrave** is a professor and the founding chair of the Department of Health, Behavior and Society at the Johns Hopkins Bloomberg School of Public Health and holds joint appointments in the Johns Hopkins Schools of Medicine and Nursing. He previously served as vice-chair of the Presidential Advisory Council on

HIV/AIDS, which advises the secretary of the US Department of Health and Human Services on HIV/AIDS research, programs, and policies. Dr. Holtgrave's research has focused on the effectiveness and cost-effectiveness of HIV prevention interventions and the translation of those findings to HIV prevention policy. Among his prior roles, he was a professor at the Rollins School of Public Health at Emory University; he served as director of the Division of HIV/AIDS Prevention – Intervention Research and Support at the US Centers for Disease Control and Prevention (CDC); and he was on the faculty at the Center for AIDS Intervention Research at the Medical College of Wisconsin.

**Pamela Kaduri** is an addiction psychiatrist at the Department of Psychiatry and Mental Health, Muhimbili National Hospital, Tanzania, and a clinician researcher and honorary lecturer with the Muhimbili University of Health and Allied Sciences. Dr. Kaduri completed her clinical and research fellowships in addiction psychiatry and the social aetiology of mental illness with the Department of Psychiatry at the University of Toronto and the Centre for Addiction and Mental Health, Toronto, Canada. Over the last 12 years, she has been actively involved in research, clinical, training, and policy development in mental health and/or addictions. She has conducted tobacco and alcohol interventions and worked in areas of injection drug use and HIV and drug dependence treatment. She has peer-reviewed publications on public health, policy, and treatment in substance use.

**Deanna Kerrigan** is associate professor of health, behavior, and society and international health at the Johns Hopkins Bloomberg School of Public Health. Her research focuses on the social and structural factors affecting the health of underserved populations. Much of her work has focused on developing and evaluating effective HIV prevention interventions among marginalized groups in Latin America and the Caribbean and sub-Saharan Africa such as female sex workers and people living with HIV. She is the co-director of the Prevention Core of the Johns Hopkins University Center for AIDS Research (CFAR). She previously directed the global HIV prevention research program, Project SEARCH: Research to Prevention (R2P), funded by the US Agency for International Development. She also worked as a program officer for the Ford Foundation, coordinating the sexuality and reproductive health and rights portfolio in Brazil.

**Barrot H. Lambdin** is a senior implementation scientist within the behavioral and urban health program in RTI International's behavioral health and criminal justice research division. He is also an assistant adjunct professor within the Department of Epidemiology and Biostatistics at the University of California, San Francisco, and an affiliate assistant professor within the Department of Global Health at the University of Washington. Over the last decade, he has led implementation science initiatives that have supported and strengthened health systems to more efficiently deliver evidence-based interventions. Much of his research has focused on HIV prevention and treatment in Tanzania, Zambia, Mozambique, and Zimbabwe and opioid overdose mortality prevention in the USA.

**Tim Lane** is associate professor at the University of California-San Francisco's Center for AIDS Prevention Studies. His research has focused on the intersection of sexuality with health, human rights, and social movements. Since 2005, he has conducted HIV surveillance studies and prevention and treatment intervention research with key populations of men who have sex with men and sex workers in southern Africa, including the Soweto Men's Study (2008), Mozambique Men's Study (2012), and Mpumalanga Men's Study (2012–2014) and two multisite South African Health Monitoring Surveys with both female sex workers (2013–2014) and men who have sex with men (2015–2017). He has also worked to support sexual rights and human rights activists around the world, including OutRight Action International, an international LGBTIQ human rights defense organization based in New York City. He lives in Oakland, California, with his husband and their dog.

**Anna M. Leddy** is a doctoral candidate in the Department of Health, Behavior and Society at the Johns Hopkins Bloomberg School of Public Health. Her research seeks to understand and intervene upon social and structural factors that contribute to gender-based violence and limit engagement along the HIV prevention to care continuum. Most of this work is conducted in sub-Saharan Africa and involves vulnerable populations including women, young people, and female sex workers. Recently, she has worked on a community mobilization intervention with female sex workers in Tanzania to prevent gender-based violence and improve HIV prevention and engagement in HIV care and treatment. Her research is informed by social and behavioral theory and employs both qualitative and quantitative methods to gain a more nuanced understanding of the dynamics that increase risk for gender-based violence and HIV.

**Andrea Mantsios** is assistant scientist of health, behavior, and society at the Johns Hopkins Bloomberg School of Public Health. Her research focuses on the role of social and structural factors contributing to HIV risk and impeding access to HIV treatment and care among marginalized groups. She has a specific interest in community empowerment and economic strengthening approaches as structural interventions among female sex workers and other women at heightened risk for HIV.

**Catherine H. Maulsby** is associate scientist of health, behavior, and society at the Johns Hopkins Bloomberg School of Public Health. Her research aims to understand and eliminate disparities in access to HIV care among underserved populations with a focus on social determinants of health. She has expertise in HIV prevention, retention in HIV care, and program evaluation in real-world settings. She has authored or co-authored dozens of articles in leading peer-reviewed journals and most recently authored a book on retention in HIV care titled *Improving Access to HIV Care: Lessons from Five US Sites* (Johns Hopkins University Press, 2015).

**Jessie Mbwambo** is principal mental health specialist and senior researcher with Muhimbili National Hospital/Muhimbili University of Health and Allied Sciences.

Over the last 25 years, she has conducted HIV prevention research on people who use drugs with funding support from the US National Institutes of Health and the US Centers for Disease Control and Prevention. Her work focuses on research and programming for recovery, relapse, and reintegration of heroin users in Dar es Salaam, Tanzania. She has published widely on HIV prevention and treatment for the general population as well as for people with high vulnerabilities to HIV acquisition.

**Sheryl A. McCurdy** a historical anthropologist, is an associate professor at the University of Texas Health Science Center at Houston in the School of Public Health. Over the last 25 years, she has conducted Social Science Research Council and National Institutes of Health-funded research as well as US Centers for Disease Control and Prevention (CDC)-funded harm reduction programming in Tanzania. In addition to her 15 years of harm reduction and HIV prevention research, as a member of the H3 Africa Consortium and Human Microbiome Consortium, she has conducted research on the ethical, legal, and social implications (ELSI) of genomic research in African settings and microbiome research in the USA. She is currently conducting a Fulbright-funded ethnography of recovery, relapse, and reintegration among heroin users in Dar es Salaam, Tanzania. Her publications are in public health, medicine, ethics, and African studies journals and books.

**William M. Miller** is an epidemiologist at the Measure Evaluation Project, part of the Carolina Population Center and University of North Carolina at Chapel Hill. He conducts quantitative research on HIV and other sexually transmitted infections among key populations in Latin America and sub-Saharan Africa. His studies focus on burden of disease, social and contextual vulnerability and the relation to HIV infection, population size estimates, and access to HIV prevention and treatment services. He specializes in sampling methodologies for hard-to-reach populations such as respondent-driven sampling (RDS) and venue-based strategies including Priorities for Local AIDS Control Efforts (PLACE) and time-location sampling (TLS). Most recently, he has implemented studies in Angola and Mozambique.

**Laura Murray** is a postdoctoral fellow at the Institute of Social Medicine at the State University of Rio de Janeiro (IMS/UERJ) where she conducts ethnographic research on activism, state bureaucracy, and prostitution in addition to teaching courses on activism, HIV and AIDS, migration, gender, and sexuality. She graduated from Wellesley College with a degree in political science and women's studies and has a master's degree in international health from the Johns Hopkins Bloomberg School of Public Health, a certificate in women's studies from the Institute for Research on Women and Gender at Columbia University, and a PhD in sociomedical sciences from Columbia University. Laura is a collaborator of the sex worker rights collective Davida and the Brazilian Network of Prostitutes and an executive researcher with the Prostitution Policy Watch (Observatório da Prostituição) at the Federal University of Rio de Janeiro. A filmmaker, she directed the documentary, "A Kiss for Gabriela," about Gabriela Leite (2013).

**Jill Owczarzak** is assistant professor of health, behavior, and society at Johns Hopkins Bloomberg School of Public Health in Baltimore, Maryland. She received her PhD in anthropology from the University of Kentucky in 2007. She works in both the USA and Eastern Europe on issues related to HIV prevention intervention development and implementation, how to improve the uptake and effectiveness of evidence-based HIV prevention programs, and the role of nongovernmental organizations in HIV prevention efforts.

**Vera Paiva** is a professor in the Department of Social Psychology at the University of São Paulo. She also teaches and supervises dissertations and theses at the preventive medicine program and public health graduate programs. She has served as co-coordinator of the Interdisciplinary Group for Aids Prevention (NEPAIDS-USP) since its foundation in 1991. Her research and publications focus on the psychosocial dimensions of inequality in daily life, on sexuality, and on the development of human rights-based approaches to health promotion and care, especially in relation to the AIDS response in Brazil. From 2014 to 2016, Paiva coordinated the Human Rights Commission of the Brazilian Federal Council of Psychology and represented civil society in the National Human Rights Commission. She has been a MacArthur Foundation Individual Grantee for Leadership recipient, a Fogarty scholar at the Center for AIDS Prevention Studies at the University of California-San Francisco/University of California-Berkeley, and a visiting scholar at Columbia University's Mailman School of Public Health.

**Richard G. Parker** is Professor Emeritus of Sociomedical Sciences and Anthropology as well as Special Lecturer and Special Research Scientist at Columbia University in New York City, USA. Since 1998, he has also served as the Director and President of the Brazilian Interdisciplinary AIDS Association (ABIA), one of the leading nongovernmental AIDS organizations in Brazil (http://www.abiaids.org.br), as well as the founder and co-chair of Sexuality Policy Watch, a global coalition of researchers, policymakers, and activists from a wide range of countries and regions with secretariat offices in Rio de Janeiro and New York City (http://www.sxpolitics.org), and the founder and chair of Global AIDS Policy Watch (http://www.gapwatch.org), a knowledge network and policy watchdog initiative focusing on the global HIV epidemic. He is the editor-in-chief for the journal, *Global Public Health* (http://www.tandfonline.com/loi/rgph20/current), published by Routledge, and is the author of more than 200 scholarly publications.

**Martha Perez** is a Dominican psychologist with a master's degree in clinical intervention who has been conducting community-based research in the Dominican Republic for more than a decade. She has been responsible for regulatory issues, recruitment, retention, and navigation in the Unidad de Vacunas at *Instituto Dermatológico y Cirugía de la Piel* (IDCP). She was the coordinator of the original Abriendo Puertas intervention research project for female sex workers living with HIV and currently coordinates the adaptation process of this model for use in routine HIV services and with transgender persons.

**Morgan M. Philbin** is currently assistant professor of sociomedical sciences at Columbia University's Mailman School of Public Health. Her work explores how social-structural factors impact health outcomes for vulnerable populations. Her current research includes a National Institute on Drug Abuse (NIDA)-funded K01 that examines how state-level policies impact sexual health and substance use risk for sexual minority youth. She is also a co-investigator on a Eunice Kennedy Shriver National Institute of Child Health and Human Development (NICHD)-funded project through the Adolescent Trials Network that examines how HIV-infected youth transition to adult care and has conducted ethnographic research on the uptake of HIV biomedical prevention technologies among adolescents and their care providers.

**Sarah D. Phillips** is professor of anthropology at Indiana University and director of Indiana University's Russian and East European Institute. She received her PhD in anthropology in 2002 from the University of Illinois at Urbana-Champaign. She has conducted research in Ukraine since 1995 and focuses on HIV prevention, the evolution of the disability rights movement in the former Soviet Union, women's roles in contemporary East European social movements, and community responses to the threats to health and welfare caused by the 1986 Chernobyl nuclear disaster.

**Haneefa T. Saleem** is assistant professor of international health at the Johns Hopkins University Bloomberg School of Public Health. Her work focuses on social and behavioral aspects of HIV prevention, care, and treatment, reproductive health, and substance use globally and in the USA. She has conducted implementation science research on substance abuse and methadone treatment in Tanzania and published articles on the intersections of HIV and substance abuse in sub-Saharan Africa.

**Hilary Schwandt** is assistant professor at Fairhaven College at Western Washington University in Bellingham, Washington. She earned her master's and doctoral degrees from the Johns Hopkins Bloomberg School of Public Health. Her research focuses on reproductive health in sub-Saharan Africa. Just prior to joining Fairhaven College, she worked in the research division at the Johns Hopkins Center for Communication Programs (CCP). At CCP, she worked on numerous projects, such as the Go Girls! Initiative, a project that aimed to reduce girls' vulnerability to HIV in Botswana, Malawi, and Mozambique, and the Nigerian Urban Reproductive Health Initiative, a project that aims to reduce the barriers to family planning use among the urban poor. More recently, she is the co-principal investigator on a grant from the National Science Foundation to conduct research with undergraduates in Rwanda on their successful family planning program.

**Daniel Jordan Smith** is currently professor and chair of the Anthropology Department and director of the Africa Initiative at the Watson Institute for International and Public Affairs at Brown University. He conducts research in Nigeria focusing on a range of issues, including HIV, social change, political culture, kinship, and masculinity. He won the 2008 Margaret Mead Award for his first book, *A Culture of Corruption: Everyday Deception and Popular Discontent in Nigeria* (Princeton University Press, 2007). His second book, *AIDS Doesn't Show Its Face: Inequality, Morality, and Social Change in Nigeria* (University of Chicago Press, 2014), won the 2015 Elliott P. Skinner Award from the Association for Africanist Anthropology. His most recent book, *To Be a Man Is Not a One-Day Job: Masculinity, Money, and Intimacy in Nigeria*, is forthcoming in 2017 with the University of Chicago Press.

**Nehanda Tankasala** is interested in the intersection of health, food, and agriculture in the Global South. She is particularly interested in using interdisciplinary and mixed-methods approaches to understanding the impact of the links between food traditions and agricultural practices on health. She served as a research assistant for Project Parivartan, the Bill & Melinda Gates Foundation-sponsored project analyzing the implementation and impact of a community mobilization intervention in Andhra Pradesh, India, to address HIV risk among female sex workers.

**Carol Underwood** is assistant professor in the Department of Health, Behavior and Society and senior research advisor at the Center for Communication Programs at the Johns Hopkins Bloomberg School of Public Health. Dr. Underwood has conducted research and worked in the area of international development and health communication for over 25 years. She developed the conceptual frameworks for *Arab Women Speak Out*™, *African Transformation*™, and Go Girls! ™, all programs designed to enable greater gender equity and improve health, economic well-being, and social justice among participants and in their communities. She has also contributed to research and practice on women's agency in the Arab world, gender normative change and collective action for health in sub-Saharan Africa, HIV prevention among adolescents in sub-Saharan Africa, Muslim religious leaders' views on family planning, and Islam and health policy, among others.

**Ronald O. Valdiserri** is senior research associate and distinguished scholar in the Department of Health, Behavior and Society at the Johns Hopkins Bloomberg School of Public Health. Prior to his academic appointment in February 2016, he served as the deputy assistant secretary for health and infectious diseases in the US Department of Health and Human Services. His public health career spans 26 years serving in leadership positions at the US Centers for Disease Control and Prevention and the US Department of Veterans Affairs where he developed policies and programs to control HIV, other sexually transmitted infections, tuberculosis, and viral hepatitis. He has published numerous scholarly articles on public health policy and practice and has authored/edited four academic texts. His contributions to the field of public health have been recognized by a number of awards including two Presidential Rank Awards for Meritorious Service (2000 and 2006).

**Daniel M. Woznica** is a PhD student in the Department of Health, Behavior and Society at the Johns Hopkins Bloomberg School of Public Health. His dissertation research focuses on structural factors associated with HIV and violence in South Africa. He is especially interested in HIV and violence prevention through community mobilization and health communication. He served for 3 years as a Peace Corps volunteer in South Africa, where he worked with a local municipality in KZN as well as a health communication organization in Pretoria. He participated in the women, gender, and sexuality studies program at Washington University in St. Louis and studied international perspectives on sexuality and gender at the School for International Training in Amsterdam.

# Introduction

Since the beginning of the HIV epidemic, approximately 78 million people have been infected with HIV globally, and 35 million have died from AIDS-related illnesses (Joint United Nations Programme on HIV/AIDS [UNAIDS] 2016). At the time of writing, it is estimated that 36.7 million people are living with HIV, with the majority (~70%) of those people living in sub-Saharan Africa (World Health Organization [WHO] 2016a). Approximately two million people have been infected with HIV each year since 2010, with no significant declines in the rate of new infections, globally, from that time to the present date (UNAIDS 2016).

As a result of growing access to antiretroviral therapy (ART), with 18.2 million people receiving treatment for HIV in 2016, AIDS-related mortality has declined to 45 % since 2005 (UNAIDS 2016). Yet, in 2015 alone, approximately 1.1 million individuals died of AIDS-related illnesses (UNAIDS 2016), highlighting major ongoing gaps in HIV prevention, treatment, and care for people living with HIV. Additionally, less than half (46%) of people who are in need of HIV treatment are currently receiving it (WHO 2016b), limiting both critical individual health benefits and the significant population-level impact of viral suppression resulting from optimal ART use or treatment as prevention.

Other important advances, such as pre-exposure prophylaxis (PrEP), have also begun to reshape the HIV landscape for those at higher risk in some settings, but for most of the world, PrEP remains largely inaccessible for those most in need. Moreover, fears and concerns regarding the prioritization of biomedical interventions such as PrEP or "test and treat" over more comprehensive, rights-based responses to HIV have emerged, creating debate regarding how to best bring together biomedical, behavioral, and structural approaches.

In the midst of these trends, statistics, and debates, HIV prevalence among populations such as female sex workers (Shannon et al. 2015), men who have sex with men (Beyrer et al. 2012), transgender women (Poteat et al. 2016), and people who use drugs (Mathers et al. 2008) is still staggeringly high, reaching or surpassing 50 % prevalence in many settings. HIV prevalence in these groups, which are often criminalized and marginalized, is often more than 10–15 times greater than the overall population in a given country (UNAIDS 2012). Other groups, such as young women and girls, migrants, and transport and fishing industry workers, while not generally criminalized, also face significantly increased HIV risk due to the socio-economic inequalities that they face. These issues underscore how the toll of the HIV epidemic is not only still profound, but that specific populations continue to experience highly disproportionate risk of infection, as well as poorer treatment outcomes, as a result of the socio-structural context in which they live and/or work.

These "higher-risk" populations have been characterized in different ways over the course of the global response to HIV, including initial epidemiologic language that was found to be stigmatizing, such as "core transmitters" and "vectors of disease." Language such as "vulnerable populations," "most-at-risk populations," and "key populations," has now generally taken the place of this initial epidemiologic terminology to describe groups at heightened risk for HIV infection and has begun to acknowledge the social and contextual nature of risk. More recently, this emphasis on context has come to produce its own set of related terminology such as the "risk environment," implying the potential primacy of place over a given "population" or the interplay between the two.

In parallel to these notable changes in terminology, other important conceptual shifts have taken place. The initial, nearly exclusive focus on changing individual risk behaviors associated with HIV transmission has been broadened to include attention to understanding and addressing the sociocultural contexts that shape risk and more recently the structural production of HIV risk (Parker et al. 2000; Sumartojo 2000). It is now more generally accepted that the risks faced by members of "key populations" do not occur in a socio-structural vacuum and that heightened vulnerability for HIV acquisition is largely the product of the larger environments and structures in which individual behaviors take place (Auerbach 2009; Blankenship et al. 2006; Gupta et al. 2008).

However, the ways in which "structural factors" are defined are still quite varied, with differing implications regarding the nature of appropriate interventions or responses. For example, for some, structural factors may refer to social norms and the need to shift or reshape public opinion or attitudes regarding appropriate sexual behavior, whereas for others, structural factors refer to power dynamics and socio-structural inequalities that constrain the possibilities to adopt or sustain HIV protective behaviors and to access HIV prevention, treatment, and care interventions, resources, and services (Evans et al. 2010). The distinction between these two understandings is critical, in that the former implies a reshaping of attitudes, whereas the latter implies challenging power dynamics. Of additional importance is the need to examine the intersection between individual and structural factors or attention to the interconnections between "structure *and* agency" (Kippax et al. 2013), given the interplay between shifts in individual perspectives and practices and engagement in and the impact of broader social change that influences HIV behaviors and outcomes.

For populations such as sex workers, men who have sex with men, transgender persons, and people who inject drugs, as well as young women and girls and migrant workers, the environments and socio-structural contexts that shape their HIV risk across settings, while diverse and dynamic in important ways, are often characterized by similar and long-standing constraints including legal constraints, poverty, gender inequality, and stigma, discrimination, and violence related to HIV status and the negative moral charge of "deviant behaviors" associated with group membership. This deeply ingrained paradigm of what constitutes "good behavior" and "good people" feeds and facilitates the production and reproduction of the aforementioned structural constraints.

A growing body of literature has contributed to our understanding of how the HIV risk of these populations cannot be separated from structural dynamics, including the material and social processes of "othering," that marginalize and exclude their members from the benefits of full citizenship such as access to resources to promote, protect, and fulfill their human rights, including the right to health and the right to HIV prevention, treatment, and care (Goffman 1963; Link and Phelan 2001; Terrence Higgins Trust 2001). Recent literature has also begun to demonstrate how these various forms of "othering" and social stigma intersect in complex manners, to intensify the risk of groups that cross or transgress multiple societal boundaries associated with gender, sexuality, race/ethnicity, class, occupation, and/or substance use (Deacon et al. 2005; Herek 1999; Parker and Aggleton 2003).

Given the significant and ongoing challenges facing the global response to HIV today, further critical exploration regarding how these structural factors play out, as well as documentation of the innovative strategies being employed to challenge and modify these factors to reduce HIV risk and improve outcomes in diverse populations and settings, continues to be urgent. *Structural Dynamics of HIV: Risk, Resilience, and Response* aims to depict, interrogate, and problematize social and structural factors related to the heightened HIV-related vulnerability of key populations due to their marginalization from society and exclusion from access to interventions and services, with an eye toward reframing and/or strengthening public health and social policies, programs, and responses.

This book not only seeks to describe and examine how distinct socio-structural contexts shape and drive higher risk for HIV infection but also works to document how affected populations have responded to these contextual forces through community-driven approaches building upon rights-based frameworks. The book also explores how national governmental responses to HIV have or have not attended to the needs and realities of key populations historically and the implications of these varied responses on the current state of the HIV epidemic across geographic settings.

The first section of the book, entitled *Risk*, includes a set of chapters that focus on the structural dynamics of HIV risk among key populations such as transgender women in Guatemala; migrant workers in Vietnam, Mexico, and Nigeria; and injection drug users in Tanzania. In these chapters, we are reminded that the patterns of HIV risk observed within key populations are consistently and strongly culturally, economically, and sociopolitically constructed. In essence, the nature of their risk is structured by dynamics of power related to group-level access to resources or the lack thereof. These chapters also serve to advance our understanding of how these social and structural determinants shape and affect the behaviors that are the shared proximal determinants of HIV risk across populations regardless of their social and structural positioning.

A second set of chapters provides examples of community-driven, structural, and multilevel HIV responses including examples among female sex workers in India and the Dominican Republic and young women and girls in three sub-Saharan African countries (Botswana, Malawi, and Mozambique). Despite the challenges posed by social and structural inequity, the chapters in the *Resilience* section demonstrate that communities of resistance can and must form and use their voice and collective agency to challenge the current power structures that limit their access to health and human rights. These chapters again highlight how processes of collective action can occur across distinct settings, as well as the challenges and difficulties inherent to promoting and achieving sustainable social change.

In a third set of chapters, *Response,* the authors explore how national governments have responded to the heightened HIV burden of key populations in Brazil, the USA, Ukraine, and South Africa with particular attention to men who have sex with men, sex workers, and people who inject drugs. In this last set of chapters, the contributors force us to question the "appropriate" role of government in the HIV response as it relates to marginalized populations. We are confronted with questions surrounding the state's role and responsibility to recognize, conceptualize, fund, implement, and/or partner to make possible social and public health actions that reduce the dramatically heightened risk for HIV infection among key populations.

Ultimately, the book seeks to share insights from multilevel efforts and actions to characterize and respond to the structural nature of HIV in a diverse set of populations and sociopolitical and economic contexts; to identify gaps in understanding for future research related to the structural production of HIV risk, outcomes, and the uptake of interventions and services; and to inspire continued solidarity and social change. The complexity of the structural forces described here reinforces the need for holistic thinking and multi-sectoral action and make clear that there is no magic bullet or one intervention, biomedical or otherwise, likely to curb the global HIV epidemic.

Ongoing efforts therefore must continue to focus on the elimination of the root causes of risk, which in many cases are linked to intersecting social inequalities and forms of stigma. These efforts to advance equitable and just social change must continue in close communication with biomedical research to end AIDS. Ultimately, only when cutting-edge social science and biomedical science work together can the quest to eliminate the negative health impacts of HIV become a reality.

Johns Hopkins Bloomberg School of Public Health Baltimore, MD, USA — Deanna Kerrigan

University of North Carolina (UNC) Gillings School of Global Public Health Chapel Hill, NC, USA — Clare Barrington

## References


Auerbach, J. (2009). Transforming social structures and environments to help in HIV prevention. *Health Affairs, 28*(6), 1655–1665. doi:10.1377/hlthaff.28.6.1655.

Beyrer, C., Baral, S. D., Van Griensven, F., Goodreau, S. M., Chariyalertsak, S., Wirtz, A. L., & Brookmeyer, R. (2012). Global epidemiology of HIV infection in men who have sex with men. *The Lancet, 380*(9839), 367–377. doi:10.1016/s0140-6736(12)60821-6.

Blankenship, K. M., Friedman, S. R., Dworkin, S., & Mantell, J. E. (2006). Structural interventions: Concepts, challenges and opportunities for research. *Journal of Urban Health, 83*(1), 59–72. doi:10.1007/s11524-005-9007-4.

Deacon, H., Stephney, I., & Prosalendis, S. (2005). *Understanding HIV/AIDS stigma: A theoretical and methodological analysis*. Cape Town: HSRC Press.

Evans, C., Jana, S., & Lambert, H. (2010). What makes a structural intervention? Reducing vulnerability to HIV in community settings, with particular reference to sex work. *Global Public Health, 5*(5), 449–461. doi:10.1080/17441690902942472.

Goffman, E. (1963). *Stigma: Notes on the management of spoiled identity*. New York: Simon and Schuster.

Gupta, G. R., Parkhurst, J. O., Ogden, J. A., Aggleton, P., Mahal, A. (2008). Structural approaches to HIV prevention. *The Lancet, 372*(9640), 764–775. doi:10.1016/s0140-6736(08)60887-9.

Herek, G. M. (1999). AIDS and stigma. *American Behavioral Scientist, 42*(7), 1106–1116. doi:10.1177/0002764299042007004.

Kippax, S., Stephenson, N., Parker, R. G., & Aggleton, P. (2013). Between individual agency and structure in HIV prevention: Understanding the middle ground of social practice. *American Journal of Public Health, 103*(8), 1367–1375. doi:10.2105/ajph.2013.301301.

Link, B. G., & Phelan, J. C. (2001). Conceptualizing stigma. *Annual Review of Sociology, 27*(1), 363–385. doi:10.1146/annurev.soc.27.1.363.

Mathers, B. M., Degenhardt, L., Phillips, B., Wiessing, L., Hickman, M., Strathdee, S. A., Panda, S., Tyndall, M., Toufik, A., Mattick, R. P., & for the 2001 Reference Group to the UN on HIV and Injecting Drug Use. (2008). Global epidemiology of injecting drug use and HIV among people who inject drugs: A systematic review. *The Lancet, 372*(9651), 1733–1745. doi:10.1016/s0140-6736(08)61311-2.

Parker, R., & Aggleton, P. (2003). HIV and AIDS-related stigma and discrimination: A conceptual framework and implications for action. *Social Science & Medicine, 57*(1), 13–24. doi:10.1016/s0277-9536(02)00304-0.

Parker, R., Easton, D., & Klein, C. (2000). Structural barriers and facilitators in HIV prevention: A review of international research. *AIDS, 14*(Suppl 1), S22–S32. doi:10.1097/00002030-200,006,001-00004.

Poteat, T., Scheim, A., Xavier, J., Reisner, S., & Baral, S. (2016). Global epidemiology of HIV infection and related syndemics affecting transgender people. *Journal of Acquired Immune Deficiency Syndromes (1999), 72*(Suppl 3), S210. doi:10.1097/qai.0000000000001087.

Shannon, K., Strathdee, S. A., Goldenberg, S. M., Duff, P., Mwangi, P., Rusakova, M., Reza-Paul, S., Lau, J., Deering, K., Pickles, M., & Boily, M. C. (2015). Global epidemiology of HIV among female sex workers: Influence of structural determinants. *The Lancet, 385*(9962), 55–71. doi:10.1016/s0140-6736(14)60931-4.

Sumartojo, E. (2000). Structural factors in HIV prevention: Concepts, examples, and implications for research. *Aids, 14*, S3–S10. doi:10.1097/00002030-200006001-00002.

Terrence Higgins Trust. (2001). *Social exclusion and HIV: A report*. London: Terrence Higgins Trust.

UNAIDS. (2012). Report on the global AIDS epidemic, 2012. http://www.unaids.org/sites/default/files/media_asset/20121120_UNAIDS_Global_Report_2012_with_annexes_en_1.pdf. Accessed 28 May 2017.

UNAIDS. (2016). Fact sheet. http://www.unaids.org/en/resources/fact-sheet. Accessed 27 Apr 2017.

World Health Organization (WHO). (2016a). Global Health Observatory (GHO) data: HIV/AIDS. http://www.who.int/gho/hiv/en/. Accessed 27 Apr 2017.

World Health Organization (WHO). (2016b). HIV/AIDS fact sheet. http://www.who.int/mediacentre/factsheets/fs360/en/. Accessed 27 Apr 2017.

# Part I
# Risk

# Chapter 1
# Understanding HIV Disparities Among Transgender Women in Guatemala: Linking Social and Structural Factors to HIV Vulnerability

**Clare Barrington, César Galindo Arandi, José Manuel Aguilar-Martínez, and William M. Miller**

## 1.1 Introduction

Transgender women across the globe experience dramatic HIV disparities. In Guatemala, HIV prevalence among transgender women is 23.8% compared to 0.8% national adult prevalence (Morales-Miranda et al. 2013). Understanding and addressing this disparity requires a holistic perspective that recognizes the role of social and structural factors over the life course. We analyzed qualitative in-depth interviews with transgender women in Guatemala City to explore how social and structural factors, in particular family rejection and violence, create a context of heightened HIV vulnerability. Grounded in participants' narratives of social exclusion, stigma, discrimination, and poverty we consider the pathways through which they are disproportionately exposed to HIV.

### *1.1.1 HIV Disparities Among Transgender Women*

One historical limitation of much HIV surveillance data and research has been the classification of transgender women as a sub-group of the epidemiological category of 'men who have sex with men' (MSM), which leads to a lack of specificity and precision in the knowledge about distinct populations (Baral et al. 2013; Barrington 2016; Poteat et al. 2016; Pollock et al. 2016). Increasingly, data are being collected

C. Barrington (✉) • W.M. Miller
University of North Carolina (UNC) Gillings School of Global Public Health, Chapel Hill, NC 27599, USA
e-mail: cbarring@email.unc.edu

C. Galindo Arandi • J.M. Aguilar-Martínez
Colectivo Amigos Contra el SIDA (CAS), Guatemala City, Guatemala



D. Kerrigan, C. Barrington (eds.), *Structural Dynamics of HIV*, Social Aspects of HIV 4, DOI 10.1007/978-3-319-63522-4_1

with greater attention to the fluidity of identities related to both sexual orientation and gender. Despite the messiness of categories and potential bias in sampling transgender women for surveillance (Baral et al. 2013; Reisner et al. 2016), compelling empirical data exist documenting a substantial and disproportionate HIV burden among transgender women across the globe. Baral et al. (2013) conducted a meta-analysis documenting a global HIV prevalence of 19% among transgender women. Additionally, these authors found that transgender women in low and middle income countries have 50 times the risk of HIV infection as compared to non-transgender adults of reproductive age. In the Latin American and Caribbean region, HIV prevalence among transgender women is estimated to be 17.7% (García et al. 2014). There is a small but growing literature suggesting that transgender women living with HIV also experience sub-optimal care and treatment outcomes compared to other populations (Baguso et al. 2016; Chow et al. 2016; Melendez et al. 2006; Mizuno et al. 2015). Individual behaviors alone cannot explain the HIV prevention, care and treatment disparities experienced by transgender women nor can behavioral interventions fully address these disparities, which are the products of broader social and structural forces.

### *1.1.2 Theoretical Frameworks for Understanding HIV Disparities Among Transgender Women*

The anthropological concept of syndemics has been used to frame and measure HIV vulnerability among transgender women (Brennan et al. 2012; Operario and Nemoto 2010). Singer refers to a syndemic as, 'a set of enmeshed and mutually enhancing health problems that, working together in a context of deleterious social and physical conditions that increase vulnerability, significantly affect the overall disease status of a population' (Singer 2010: 15). A critical component of Singer's definition that is relevant for understanding HIV vulnerability among transgender women is the recognition of the 'context of deleterious social and physical conditions'. Multiple, overlapping health problems do not occur in isolation but rather are the products of the context and conditions in which people live (Operario and Nemoto 2010). Of note, the concept of syndemics has been applied to both the health outcomes as well as the determinants that drive those outcomes. In the application of the concept of syndemics to transgender health, overlapping health problems such as HIV, mental health, substance use, and violence are directly connected to overlapping social and structural determinants such as stigma and discrimination, poverty, and social exclusion (Brennan et al. 2012; Operario and Nemoto 2010; Poteat et al. 2016; Reisner et al. 2016). Embedded within both applications of the concept is recognition and appreciation that any attempt to address syndemics – whether outcomes or determinants – requires research and intervention at multiple levels.

Brennan et al. (2012) created a syndemic index for young transgender women in two cities in the US based on four factors including: self-esteem; polysubstance use; victimization; and intimate partner violence. These authors report an additive relationship between the syndemic index and both HIV infection and unprotected sex whereby the associations become stronger with the addition of each factor. In a recent study in India, Chakrapani et al. (2017) also used an additive measure of three syndemic psychosocial factors including alcohol use, depression and victimization. They found that over half of their sample (55%, n = 300) experienced two or three of these factors and, like Brennan, that the factors were additively associated with sexual risk behaviors. One critique of these additive measures is that they do not capture the synergistic interactions of the determinants, which has been interpreted as the intention of syndemic theory (Tsai and Burns 2015; Tsai and Venkataramani 2016). There is also still limited understanding of the *processes* that create such extremely heightened HIV vulnerability within this population.

Highlighting current gaps in the understanding of the synergistic determinants of health disparities, including HIV, among transgender women, Reisner and colleagues state:

> *For transgender people, health inequities are hypothesized to arise from systematic exposure to multiple, intersecting social stressors, including legal and other structural factors that are a result of being part of a socially marginalized group.[140] Social and economic exclusion are therefore conceptualised as causal pathways to adverse health—however, we found very few studies actually linking these social stressors to health indicators.* (Reisner et al. 2016: 17)

To further advance a contextualized understanding of the synergistic determinants and mechanisms of transgender health disparities, including but not limited to HIV, Hughto et al. (2015) propose a multilevel framework of transgender stigma to guide the identification of the determinants and mechanisms of influence of health outcomes among transgender women. In this framework, they consider stigma experienced at the individual (e.g. internalized stigma), interpersonal (e.g. family rejection; healthcare discrimination) and structural levels (e.g. economic equality; inadequate provider training). These authors call for studies to 'simultaneously and interactively' examine transgender stigma at these multiple levels in order to improve understanding of transgender health disparities (Hughto et al. 2015: 228).

The purpose of this chapter is to contribute to the theoretical and empirical literature on social and structural determinants of HIV vulnerability among transgender women. Specifically, we aim to identify mechanisms of influence, including both mediators, or the factors through which influence occurs, and moderators, or the factors that affect the strength of influence, between interpersonal stigma and HIV vulnerability.

### 1.1.3 Transgender Women and HIV in Guatemala

Transgender women in Guatemala are consistently denied basic human rights and experience disproportionate levels of violence in an already extremely violent society (Merlo and Murali 2012). Violence against transgender women and general transphobia are rampant (HIVOS 2012; Merlo and Murali 2012). Only recently have targeted HIV surveillance data been collected to document the burden of HIV specifically among individuals who identify as transgender. While the national HIV prevalence among adults is estimated to be less than 1.0% (CNE 2012), the most recent prevalence estimates among MSM and transgender women are 8.9% and 23.8% respectively (Morales-Miranda et al. 2013).

In the only quantitative study of social determinants of HIV among transgender women in Guatemala City, Miller (2016) compared syndemic factors among transgender sex workers (n = 122), cisgender male sex workers (n = 280) and cisgender MSM who had not engaged in sex work in the last 12 months (n = 649) recruited using both respondent driven sampling and time location sampling. This study included a behavioral survey of syndemic factors including: discrimination related to sexual orientation, physical abuse (being hit, punched kicked), forced sex, all in the last 12 months, and family rejection (ever). They also measured substance use, including illicit drug use in the last 12 months and binge drinking in the last 7 days. Of note, a total of 142 transgender women were recruited for the study and 86% (n = 122) reported sex work in the last year.

Overall, transgender sex workers experienced disproportionate levels of all syndemic factors. In the case of substance use, they were significantly more likely to use illicit drugs (aPR = 2.7, 95% CI: 2.0–3.5) and engage in binge drinking (aPR = 1.6, 95% CI: 1.2–2.1) than non-sex worker MSM counterparts. Drug and alcohol levels were not significantly different between transgender women sex workers and male sex workers, suggesting heightened use of substances in the context of sex work regardless of gender identity or expression. Transgender women experienced higher levels of violence, discrimination, and forced sex than both non-sex worker MSM and cisgender male sex workers. Transgender women were over two times more likely to be discriminated against (aPR = 2.6, 95% CI: 2.2–3.2), over seven times more likely to be physically abused (aPR = 7.5, 95% CI: 4.4–12.7) and over seven times more likely to be forced to have sex (aPR = 7.5, 95% CI: 3.1–18.2) than non-sex worker cisgender male counterparts. Compared to cisgender male sex workers, transgender women continued to experience more discrimination (aPR = 2.0, 95% CI: 1.7–2.4), family rejection (aPR = 1.8, 95% CI: 1.3–2.3) and physical abuse (aPR = 4.3, 95% CI: 2.7–6.9). Transgender sex workers were equally as likely as male sex workers to have experienced forced sex. These findings provide a descriptive foundation of the syndemics of discrimination, violence (physical and sexual), substance use, and family exclusion. We seek to extend this work by considering potential mechanisms, both mediators and moderators, to explain how the social and structural context influences HIV vulnerability.

To this end, we analyzed in-depth interviews conducted with transgender women (n = 8) in Guatemala City in 2010 as part of a qualitative, comparative study on the social and sexual networks and sexual healthcare experiences of sexual and gender minorities funded by a developmental award from the Center for AIDS Research at the University of North Carolina, a program funded by the National Institutes of Health (P30 AI50410). In this study, we found that compared to both gay identifying (n = 13) and non-gay identifying (n = 8) cisgender men, transgender women had the smallest social networks and the least amount of social support (Tucker et al. 2014). We also found that transgender women experience discrimination in sexual health services, even in clinics that are intended to be 'friendly' (Boyce et al. 2012).

Several participants described sexually transmitted infection staff refusing to use their preferred female names. One transgender participant relayed the following conversation with the staff member, for example:

> *'Look, I don't like being called Juan; I like to be called Berta because I feel like I'm Berta'. She [The secretary] doesn't understand. She [the secretary] said, 'But your papers say that your name is Juan and to me you are Juan because you are a man.'* (Berta, transgender, 37 years old) (Boyce et al. 2012: 6)

Once inside the doctor's office, transgender participants expressed embarrassment about being examined by a doctor. Participants also discussed how removing the physical expressions of their femininity while disrobing for a physical exam made them feel vulnerable and embarrassed.

These prior analyses improved our understanding of the context in which transgender women negotiate HIV vulnerability. For this chapter, we re-analyzed the interviews with transgender women to further deepen our understanding of the pathways of influence between what Hughto et al. (2015) refer to as interpersonal transgender stigma and HIV vulnerability. To this end, we reviewed the transcripts and the previous analytic products (codebook, outputs, matrices, network summaries) to gain a holistic sense of the data. In this review, we identified narratives and processes that could further improve our understanding of *how* social and structural factors influence HIV. Building on the previous thematic work, we use a case presentation of our data, focusing on examples from specific participants, rather than themes across participants, to provide a more in-depth and holistic account (Maxwell and Miller 2008). We were informed by the findings from Miller's 2016 study of syndemic factors to focus on narratives related to family exclusion and violence.

In Table 1.1, we present the key characteristics of participants. Participants ranged from 20 to 59 years of age (mean 29 years). Two participants identified as transgender, one as *trans* and the rest as *travesti*, which one participant defined as 'man during the day, woman at night'. One participant was a college graduate and one had graduated from secondary school; the other six had left school during their primary education. All but one participant was single at the time of the interview.

We first look at how participants experienced social exclusion, especially in the form of family rejection starting early in life. We also consider how in response to this exclusion, participants generated new social structures and reciprocal systems of support. We then describe experiences of violence, in the context of families, intimate partnerships and from clients and consider how they contribute to HIV vulnerability in this context.

### *1.1.4 Trajectories of Rejection and Social Exclusion*

Lydia, 59, was born to a middle class, educated family in Guatemala City. Her parents were both deceased at the time of the interview and she lived in her family's home; her siblings were successful professionals who had moved out of the family

**Table 1.1** Study participant characteristics (n = 8)

| Pseudonym | Age | Education | Self identification | Relationship status | Current or past sex work |
|---|---|---|---|---|---|
| Karla | 25 | 6th grade primary | *Transgenero* | Single | Yes |
| Carlos | 26 | 2nd grade primary | *Transformista, Travesti* | Single | Yes |
| Josefina | 37 | 6th grade primary | *Trans* | Single | Yes |
| Rubi | 21 | Secondary school | *Travesti* | Single | No |
| Emily | 21 | 3rd grade primary | *Travesti* | In a relationship | Yes |
| Manuela | 20 | 3rd grade primary | *Transvesti* | Single | Yes |
| Karina | 22 | 3rd grade primary | *Gay Travesti* | Single | Yes |
| Lydia | 59 | College graduate | *Transgenero* | Single/separated from wife | Yes |

home. They gathered a few times a year but had minimal contact most of the time. Lydia had a college degree and diverse work experience. Lydia lived her life as a man for 47 years and transitioned following the death of her parents. She had married twice to cisgender women and had two daughters. At the time of the interview, she indicated having a beauty salon and doing freelance work as an editor. She also had a small amount of income from a garage apartment she rented out.

Lydia described experiencing a desire to wear her mother's clothes starting when she was a young child:

> *I always observed...and I knew where the faja (girdle) was kept. And I was dying to put it on. Eight years old, so, I was still pre-pubescent. So, the point is that the moment arrived and I was able to grab the girdle from where my mother kept it.*

Lydia loved wearing the *faja* and used it until it was 'filthy', hiding it in her clothes without washing it to avoid being discovered. Upon finding that Lydia had been using the *faja*, her mother reacted with violence:

> *Look, of all the beatings I got, this was the best. A spectacular beating to the extreme that at the age of 8 years, I made a promise to myself at that moment, that I wouldn't do it [dress as a girl] again, until I could. I had to wait until my mother died. So, for 47 years of my life, I lived my life as a man because my parents didn't accept my...inclination...towards femininity.*

Lydia emphasizes the impact of this childhood experience of violence on her life trajectory, continuing to live as a man for nearly four decades. Just as the beating from her mother was a key turning point in her childhood, her mother's death when she was 47 was another critical turning point that allowed her to begin living her life openly as a woman:

*As soon as my mother died, and she was the last [of her parents] to die, I basically made the decision to live the life I wanted to live, because I was tired of the lies, 47 years of lies, both words and actions. As a person of faith, this was really hard for me. In my heart, in my soul, in my mind....it was not uncommon for me to cry, almost every night...due to the frustration I felt and everything else. You see, I live, act and dress as a woman because I see myself this way and I like myself this way.*

While she lived so much of her life suppressing her gender identity and struggling with the emotional burden of this suppression, Lydia recognized that this, along with her family's stable, middle-class economic position, allowed her to gain more education and experience less discrimination than other transgender women in Guatemala.

*Those who are kicked out of their houses as kids for being gay, many haven't even finished middle school. In the best scenario, they have finished primary. And then they have to face a society that discriminates, that pushes them out.... that denies them work. So, they have always had to paddle against the current.*

While she had her basic needs covered and was able to complete her education, after transitioning Lydia lacked a strong social support network and felt socially isolated, as she maintained only functional relationships with her siblings and saw her own children only once a year. As a response, she was committed to speaking out to raise awareness about the trans community:

*...however, one of the other things I do is give talks in schools. There is an obligation to offer, to provide holistic sex education so that people can know and see in real life a person who is not 'normal' [in quotes]. And I am not embarrassed about it. I mean, what I protest, basically, is the discrimination, the discrimination I am a target of, for no reason.*

Despite her strong educational background and stable housing situation, Lydia could not escape the impact of trans discrimination and, at the time of the interview, was considering engaging in sex work in order to address her economic needs, something she had done only once before:

*No, this was the only, the only time. But I am seriously thinking about it, in light of the hunger I am experiencing and all of it, due to the same discrimination and all of that. Yes, I am thinking about prostituting myself.*

Lydia makes the direct link between the discrimination she experiences as a transgender woman and her lack of sufficient food and subsequent 'hunger'. Her reference to hunger is important in the Guatemalan context, a country with dramatic income inequality resulting in a paradox of fairly stable and positive overall economic indicators along with pervasive chronic malnutrition (Loewenberg 2009). While Lydia had lived a 'normal life' for nearly 50 years, after transitioning, she was exposed to the social exclusion and limited economic opportunities that ultimately led her to experience extreme poverty and hunger and heightened exposure to HIV. As a result of family rejection, in a context of societal stigma towards transgender women in Guatemala, all but one participant ultimately relied on sex work at some point in their lives as their only viable income-generating opportunity. Sex work was mostly street-based with participants meeting clients at designated areas for transgender women. Participants might wait for clients together with other transgender sex workers but there was no formal social structure nor safety mechanism, creating a context of vulnerability and violence, as we discuss in the section below.

Similar to Lydia, nearly all of the other participants in this study had been rejected by their families due to their gender identity and/or sexual orientation. In their social network inventories, few participants mentioned any family members as important people in their lives; those who did include a family member usually conditioned this on the fact that they had experienced rejection from this person at some time and received minimal support in any form. In contrast to Lydia, most of these rejections resulted in participants being kicked out of their houses at a young age, which frequently led to leaving school and assuming adult responsibilities when they were still very young, as described by this participant who was forced out of her home at age 13:

> *But, as a result of this [transgender stigma], I had to leave my house, right? At an early age. And I started to suffer, you know? Because when you are thirteen and you leave your house, things are not the same. You have to value yourself and take care of yourself, right? There are a lot of things... [she gets quiet as she says this last phrase].*

Notably, such family rejection was experienced by participants identifying along a range of gender expressions and identities. Carlos identified as *transformista* and *travesti:*

> *Ay... look... Let me tell you, as I said, I am transformista. I am, I consider myself.... well, I am a man during the day, also for my work. Then at night, weekends.... if I am invited to give a show, I dress as a woman. [Or] if I am going out to drink with my friend Santo, we dress as women. Or sometimes we go out with other friends if we feel like it and I go out as a woman. I consider myself, I don't consider myself transgender because if you can tell, I have a beard. In other words, I am almost like a man, when I am dressed, right? If I considered myself transgender, I would have dressed as a woman and I would have considered myself a woman, and I wouldn't have said 'man'. So, I consider myself a transformista, a travesti.... which is logical, right, to say travesti, man by day, woman by night.*

Carlos lived with his mother and two sisters and while he identified his mother as one of the most important people in his social network, when probed to explain how he and his mother supported each other, he lowered his voice and responded:

> *OK, between us, please. It's just that you can see, I mean, the relationship with my mother is very different. Right now she is the most important person for me. Well, what I receive from her is shelter. On the other hand, if we start to talk about topics related to sex or partners or other topics, I can't [talk to her] because she still doesn't accept that her first son is gay.*

While Carlos was not physically forced to leave his home or violently attacked, his mother's rejection due to her lack of acceptance of his sexual orientation was more implicit. Her violence was not physical but emotional through her rejection of his sexual orientation but his need for shelter forced Carlos to accept it. As he elaborated on the dynamic of his support exchange with his mother, it was clear that the nature of their relationship is more instrumentally supportive than emotionally supportive.

A distinct outcome of these dynamics of implicit and explicit family rejection was a process of generating new forms of social connection to replace what was lost from their families. The generation of these social assets reflects an important example of resilience in response to family rejection. Josefina had been rejected by her family and kicked out of her house and ultimately migrated to Guatemala City on her own. In her social network inventory, she identified a friend who played a critical support role for her in that transition:

> *...[she] is a person I met here in the capital.... when I was basically kicked out of my house. I didn't have anywhere to go and I had nothing to eat. She was the first person who gave me food, I mean, she helped me get ahead. She motivated me to keep me going and to see things in the future. And during all this time that she was helping me, giving me food, she never asked me for money. And she always gave me advice, that I should accept myself as I was and that everything happens for a reason.*

Josefina received both instrumental support in the form of shelter and food as well as emotional support and advice from her friend, including encouragement to accept herself.

In addition to receiving such critical support during her transition to the capital, Josefina also provided support to younger women in the transgender sex work community. Describing her dynamic with one of the younger friends she included in her social network, she said:

| | |
|---|---|
| *Josefina:* | *...we are colleagues, but I feel that we identify with each other because she has suffered since she was young in the same way I suffered and she is just now starting [to know] the transgender context. So, eh.... I feel some trust, talking to her, because I feel as though we identify with each other because of our life situations. My family rejected me from the beginning. Her family has not, they don't discriminate against her...while they support her, there is a lack of love.* |
| *Interviewer:* | *Hmmmhh* |
| *Josefina:* | *Not me...I basically didn't live with my family but I also have a lack of love.* |
| *Interviewer:* | *OK. So, you feel a connection because of this [lack of love].* |
| *Josefina:* | *Exactly, because she has suffered lack of cariño (affection) from her parents and since I have also suffered this, I feel like we identify around it.... She is 17, I am 37, so I give her advice about the path she is starting to take. I have a little more experience.* |

Josefina was able to share her experience and also receive support through the connection she created with her younger friend. As reflected at the end of this quote, this social connection, grounded in the shared experience of family rejection, also transcended into support related to managing the vulnerability and risks of the environments in which they work.

Beyond their immediate social support networks, some participants identified receiving support in response to social exclusion from non-governmental organizations focused on the trans community. Karla, a transgender identifying participant who had been rejected by her family but was living with her mother, brother and step-father at the time of the interview, described how she received support related to self-acceptance and self-esteem through involvement at an NGO:

> *...A person's self-esteem...when a person doesn't accept themselves as they are or when the family [doesn't accept] ... .it really affects that person. We get from this [activity at an NGO], that we have the power to make a new world. This is what they have taught us.*

Family exclusion also created extreme poverty, which led to involvement in street-based sex work among nearly all participants. While Lydia was essentially shielded from the poverty described by others who were forced to leave their homes and school at a young age, she was confronting these issues of poverty and hunger at a later age due to a combination of transgender stigma and her age. In contrast to Lydia's unique story, the more common trajectory was family rejection and expulsion early in life, which lead to limited opportunities and support, social exclusion, and vulnerability, especially through involvement in sex work and related violence, which is described below. Understanding these trajectories aids in shifting the focus away from individual behaviors to the social processes which produce the environments in which such behaviors proliferate. These stories of implicit and explicit social rejection reflect an important pathway from transgender stigma to HIV vulnerability.

### *1.1.5 Violence*

Violence was a critical factor in Lydia's life trajectory; the beating from her mother as a child forced her to live as a man for nearly five decades. Across other partici pants' narratives, violence was a consistent source of interpersonal stigma that created HIV vulnerability. Violence was perpetrated across settings and types of partners but ultimately had some connection to trans identity. Karla described violent relationships with her clients as well as her friends 'with benefits'. Her first experience with a client evolved into a volatile violent night. Rather than going to a hotel, the client, who she noted as being high, took her to an abandoned house with no electricity in a remote part of the city:

> *And, that is where I started to get scared.... we went into the bedroom. The house was practically empty. Eh...he began to take off his clothes and take off my clothes and we began to have sex. But then I realize that he is using drugs and getting high. That is when I freaked out and I got even more scared. And then he didn't want to let me leave. He locked the door... and threw the key out the window. So, I didn't know how to get out, I was a prisoner in the house. And the guy wanted to have sex constantly and then he started to attack me, beat me, pull my hair, he began to insult me... and I started to yell but no one came. So...the only thing I could do was to be quiet and stay calm. Because I said if I don't stay quiet then this guy...is going to kill me here inside. So, I stayed quiet. He didn't let me know until 4:30 in the morning. Totally abandoned, without a cent. He didn't pay me.*

In contrast to this anonymous client who took Karla to a remote area and used violence to control her, she also experienced violence from a partner who was a friend 'with benefits' and became violent in response to jealousy.

> *One time I experienced violence with him. Because he saw me talking to a really close friend who hugged me and put his hands on my waist. But he is just a friend. I wasn't going to tell him [the friend] to stop.... So, when my friend left, he [friend with benefits] comes to me and says 'look, why were you with him?' and he wanted to physically attack me. Basically, I got away as I could. But, yes, I had various physical aggressions from him.*

Karla's 'friend' engaged in a public expression of jealousy, while again using violence to control her. While the scenario with the client created a more explicit form of HIV vulnerability by taking away her control of the sexual encounter, her 'friend' with benefits exerted a more extended attack on her personal safety through a series of physical aggressions that could ultimately limit her control of their sexual encounters and her overall wellbeing.

In contrast to Karla, whose gender non-conforming identity and presentation as '*transgenero*' greatly limited her employment opportunities and created a total reliance on sex work, Carlos had a gender-conforming presentation as a man during the day and had a daytime job with a perfume distributor. While Carlos had a job other than sex work at the time of the interview, he had experienced rape, violence and sexually transmitted infections in the context of his street-based sex work and other intimate partnerships. Carlos identified a partner in his sexual network inventory who he initially referred to as '*divino*' (divine). They met at a disco, where Carlos went dressed as a woman, and the first time they had sex, it was a group orgy. The second time Carlos was extremely drunk and the partner raped him. Carlos' voice softened as he shared his experience:

> *Rape. I mean, I consider it that because I was under the effects of a lot of alcohol and my body was essentially unconscious. What I do remember feeling is when he was taking my clothes off, and I couldn't do anything because I was really, really drunk. And, how do you say, the only thing I remember is when he penetrated me and I don't remember anything else. I do remember resisting a bit but I was under the influence of alcohol. I mean, he did it without my consent and I think that is a rape. I think.*

While he initially described this partner as 'divine', after sharing this story he indicated that he had no desire to see or know anything about him since this incident. Carlos prefaced this difficult story by saying:

> *[Embarrassed laugh] Mmm. Well, I think that everyone has, I think this has happened to the majority of people, I think, getting raped. I am not the first person who has been raped when they were drunk. [silence]*

This preface served to normalize this traumatic experience but also served as an indicator of the pervasiveness of violence experienced by trans populations in Guatemala in a broader context of widespread violence across Guatemalan society. With regard to HIV prevention, there were no condoms used during this rape. While he did not get exposed to an STI during that incident, Carlos had previously been diagnosed with an STI at his local health center following an unprotected sex act.

In addition to his experience with rape, Carlos also experienced violence with his clients in the context of street-based sex work, or what he called being a '*talonera*', which literally translates to 'heel', reflecting that transgender women frequently use high heels. These experiences included having clients pulling out guns when they were with him, being physically and sexually aggressive, and even the extreme of having a client want him to go commit suicide together. Again, Carlos considered this part of the job of being a *travesti talonera*, working in the street. He also directly linked this violence to transgender stigma:

> *Interviewer: Why does violence exist in these situations?*

*Carlos: Ay, I don't know. One, for homophobia. Two for transphobia. Three, the client who wanted to kill himself with me didn't want to live any longer. He had a lot going on in his life and I was the first to get in his car and he wanted to kill himself with me.*

Through Carlos's narratives we can see how violence was another critical pathway between transgender stigma and HIV risk behaviors, such as unprotected sex.

## 1.2 Conclusions

We analyzed the narratives of family exclusion and violence among transgender and *travesti* women in Guatemala City to improve understanding of the pathways between transgender stigma and HIV vulnerability (Hughto et al. 2015; Poteat et al. 2016; Reisner et al. 2016). Grounded in our analysis, we developed a conceptual model to visualize these potential pathways of influence that help to answer the question of how stigma influences HIV vulnerability (Fig. 1.1). In participants' narratives, they clearly depicted a context in which transgender stigma is a ubiquitous part of their daily lives. One of the most destructive manifestations of this stigma was family exclusion, which led to young trans women living in extreme poverty and having limited economic opportunities, and, subsequently, a high concentration of trans women being involved in sex work. Violence also appears to potentially be a mediator between stigma and unprotected sex, by serving as the mechanism through which stigma impacts behavior, such as unprotected sex. We also found that violence can serve as an effect modifier, increasing the possibility of trans women having unprotected sex, with clients and other partners.

Our model aims to recognize exclusion and violence not just as additive or cumulative but as synergistic (Tsai and Burns 2015). An additional synergistic factor we saw in the case of Carlos was substance use, which impeded his ability to defend himself against forced sex or to use condoms. Future research, both qualitative and quantitative, should continue to explore the mediators and moderators

**Fig. 1.1** Conceptual model of pathways of influence between transgender stigma and unprotected sex

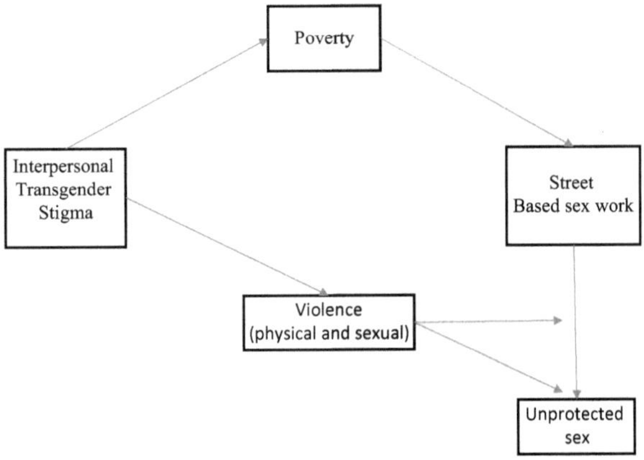

between interpersonal transgender stigma and HIV vulnerability across diverse settings. It is also important to identify how these pathways affect outcomes along the HIV continuum of care, especially in light of data suggesting that transgender women living with HIV experience sub-optimal outcomes (Baguso et al. 2016; Chow et al. 2016; Melendez et al. 2006; Mizuno et al. 2015).

Addressing these pathways will require using a life-course, family-based approach given that so much of the initial impact of expressing a non-conforming gender identity is the rejection from the family. A life course perspective aids in obtaining a fuller understanding of the cumulative nature of social and structural factors and the accumulated HIV vulnerability among transgender women (Nuttbrock et al. 2010). We also found examples of trans women's resilience in the face of social exclusion, creating new social support networks when they lost the support of their families, which has been described elsewhere (Chakrapani et al. 2017). The importance of social cohesion has been well documented in the case of HIV prevention, care and treatment among female sex workers in diverse settings (Carrasco et al. 2017; Kerrigan et al. 2017) and among transgender women in Peru (Perez-Brumer et al. 2017). It is important to build on the social resources that trans women develop themselves to address their social exclusion. It is also important to obtain an in-depth understanding of the dynamics of these social resources to avoid any repetition of the power and discriminatory practices that may be generated within them.

## References


Baguso, G. N., Gay, C. L., & Lee, K. A. (2016). Medication adherence among transgender women living with HIV. *AIDS Care, 28*(8), 976–981. doi:10.1080/09540121.2016.1146401.

Baral, S. D., Poteat, T., Strömdahl, S., Wirtz, A. L., Guadamuz, T. E., & Beyrer, C. (2013). Worldwide burden of HIV in transgender women: A systematic review and meta-analysis. *The Lancet Infectious Diseases, 13*(3), 214–222. doi:10.1016/S1473-3099(12)70315-8.

Barrington, C. (2016). Understanding and addressing human immunodeficiency virus and sexually transmitted disease disparities among transgender persons. *Sexually Transmitted Diseases, 43*(7), 412–413. doi:10.1097/OLQ.0000000000000485.

Boyce, S., Barrington, C., Bolaños, H., Galindo Arandi, C., & Paz-Bailey, G. (2012). Facilitating access to sexual health services for men who have sex with men and male-to-female transgender persons in Guatemala City. *Culture, Health & Sexuality, 14*(3), 313–327. doi:10.1080/13691058.2011.639393\.

Brennan, J., Kuhns, L. M., Johnson, A. K., Belzer, M., Wilson, E. C., & Garofalo, R. (2012). Syndemic theory and HIV-related risk among young transgender women: The role of multiple, co-occurring health problems and social marginalization. *American Journal of Public Health, 102*(9), 1751–1757. doi:10.2105/AJPH.2011.300433.

Carrasco, M. A., Barrington, C., Kennedy, C., Perez, M., Donastorg, Y., & Kerrigan, D. (2017). 'We talk, we do not have shame': Addressing stigma by reconstructing identity through enhancing social cohesion among female sex workers living with HIV in the Dominican Republic. *Culture, Health and Sexuality, 19*(5), 543–556. doi:10.1080/13691058.2016.1242779.

Centro Nacional de Epidemiología (CNE). (2012). Estimaciones y proyecciones del VIH y VIH avanzado Guatemala. Guatemala: Ministerio de Salud Pública y Asistencia Social de Guatemala.

http://infecciosashr.org/wp-content/uploads/2014/02/Estimaciones-y-Proyecciones-Gua2013-Sept.pdf. Accessed 19 May 2017.

Chakrapani, V., Newman, P. A., Shunmugam, M., Logie, C. H., & Samuel, M. (2017). Syndemics of depression, alcohol use, and victimisation, and their association with HIV-related sexual risk among men who have sex with men and transgender women in India. *Global Public Health, 12*(2), 250–265. doi:10.1080/17441692.2015.1091024.

Chow, J. Y., Konda, K. A., Borquez, A., Caballero, P., Silva-Santisteban, A., Klausner, J. D., & Cáceres, C. F. (2016). Peru's HIV care continuum among men who have sex with men and transgender women: Opportunities to optimize treatment and prevention. *International Journal of STD & AIDS, 27*(12), 1039–1048. doi:10.1177/0956462416645727.

García, P. J., Bayer, A., & Cárcamo, C. P. (2014). The changing face of HIV in Latin America and the Caribbean. *Current HIV/AIDS Reports, 11*(2), 146–157. doi:10.1007/s11904-014-0204-1.

HIVOS. (2012). E studio diagnóstico de stigma y discriminación hacia personas con VIH, hombres que tiene sexo con hombres (HSH) y mujeres trabajadoras sexuales (MTS) Guatemala: RP-HIVOS.

Hughto, J. M. W., Reisner, S. L., & Pachankis, J. E. (2015). Transgender stigma and health: A critical review of stigma determinants, mechanisms, and interventions. *Social Science & Medicine, 147*, 222–231. doi:10.1016/j.socscimed.2015.11.010.

Kerrigan, D., Mbwambo, J., Likindikoki, S., Beckham, S., Mwampashi, A., Shembilu, C., Montsios, A., Leddy, A., Davis, W., & Galai, N. (2017). Project Shikamana: Baseline findings from a community empowerment-based combination HIV prevention trial among female sex workers in Iringa, Tanzania. *Journal of Acquired Immune Deficiency Syndrome, 74*(Suppl 1), S60–S68. doi:10.1097/qai.0000000000001203.

Loewenberg, S. (2009). Hungry in Guatemala. The Atlantic, August issue. https://www.theatlantic.com/magazine/archive/2009/08/hungry-in-guatemala/307675/. Accessed 20 May 2017.

Maxwell, J. A., & Miller, B. (2008). Categorizing and connecting strategies in qualitative data analysis. In S. N. Hesse-Biber & P. Leavy (Eds.), *Handbook of emergent methods* (pp. 461–477). New York: The Guildford Press.

Melendez, R. M., Exner, T. A., Ehrhardt, A. A., Dodge, B., Remien, R. H., Rotheram-Borus, M. J., Lightfoot, M., & Hong, D. (2006). Health and health care among male-to-female transgender persons who are HIV positive. *American Journal of Public Health, 96*(6), 1034–1037. doi:10.2105/AJPH.2004.042010.

Merlo, T & Murali, S. (2012). Human rights violations of lesbian, gay, bisexual, and transgender (LGBT) people in Guatemala: A shadow report. (Submitted for consideration at the 104th Session of the Human Rights Committee) New York: United Nations Human Rights Committee. https://www.law.gwu.edu/sites/www.law.gwu.edu/files/downloads/LGBT%20Guatemala%20Joint%20Submission%20%28English%29%20FINAL.pdf. Accessed 20 May 2017.

Miller, W.C. (2016). Contextual factors that contribute to increased risk of HIV among transgender and MSM sex workers and recommendations for service delivery. The University of North Carolina at Chapel Hill, ProQuest Dissertations Publishing. 10119723.

Mizuno, Y., Frazier, E. L., Huang, P., & Skarbinski, J. (2015). Characteristics of transgender women living with HIV receiving medical care in the United States. *LGBT Health, 2*(3), 228–234. doi:10.1089/lgbt.2014.0099.

Morales-Miranda, S., Álvarez-Rodríguez. B. E., Arambú, N., Aguilar, J., Huamán, B., Figueroa, W., Osuna-Ramírez, I., Mendizábal, R., Rosales-Arroyo, R. P., & Castillo, A.. (2013). *Encuesta de Vigilancia de Comportamiento Sexual y Prevalencia del VIH e ITS, en poblaciones vulnerables y poblaciones clave. Guatemala 2013*. Universidad del Valle de Guatemala, MSPAS, HIVOS Inc., Publicación UVG. No.27. http://www.mcr-comisca.org/sites/all/modules/ckeditor/ckfinder/userfiles/files/Informe%20ECVC%20Guatemala%202012-2013%209%20dic%2013%20final.pdf. Accessed 24 May 2017.

Nuttbrock, L., Hwahng, S., Bockting, W., Rosenblum, A., Mason, M., Macri, M., & Becker, J. (2010). Psychiatric impact of gender-related abuse across the life course of male-to-female transgender persons. *Journal of Sex Research, 47*(1), 12–23. doi:10.1080/00224490903062258.

Operario, D., & Nemoto, T. (2010). HIV in transgender communities: Syndemic dynamics and a need for multicomponent interventions. *Journal of Acquired Immune Deficiency Syndromes, 55*(Suppl. 2), S91–S93. doi:10.1097/QAI.0b013e3181fbc9ec.

Perez-Brumer, A. G., Reisner, S. L., McLean, S. A., Silva-Santisteban, A., Huerta, L., Mayer, K. H., ... & Lama, J. R.. (2017). Leveraging social capital: Multilevel stigma, associated HIV vulnerabilities, and social resilience strategies among transgender women in Lima, Peru. *Journal of the International AIDS Society, 20*(1), 20(1), 1–8. doi: 10.7448/IAS.20.1.21462.

Pollock, L., Silva-Santisteban, A., Sevelius, J., & Salazar, X. (2016). 'You should build yourself up as a whole product': Transgender female identity in Lima, Peru. *Global Public Health, 11*(7–8), 981–993. doi:10.1080/17441692.2016.1167932.

Poteat, T., Scheim, A., Xavier, J., Reisner, S., & Baral, S. (2016). Global epidemiology of HIV infection and related syndemics affecting transgender people. *Journal of Acquired Immune Deficiency Syndromes, 72*(Suppl. 3), S210–S219. doi:10.1097/QAI.0000000000001087.

Reisner, S. L., Poteat, T., Keatley, J., Cabral, M., Mothopeng, T., Dunham, E., Holland, C. E., Max, R., & Baral, S. D. (2016). Global health burden and needs of transgender populations: A review. *The Lancet, 388*(10042), 412–436. doi:10.1016/S0140-6736(16)00684-X.

Singer, M. (2010). Pathogen-pathogen interaction: A syndemic model of complex biosocial processes in disease. *Virulence, 1*(1), 10–18. doi:10.4161/viru.1.1.9933.

Tsai, A. C., & Burns, B. F. (2015). Syndemics of psychosocial problems and HIV risk: A systematic review of empirical tests of the disease interaction concept. *Social Science & Medicine, 139*, 26–35. doi:10.1016/j.socscimed.2015.06.024.

Tsai, A. C., & Venkataramani, A. S. (2016). Syndemics and health disparities: A methodological note. *AIDS and Behavior, 20*(2), 423–430. doi:10.1007/s10461-015-1260-2.

Tucker, C., Galindo Arandi, C., Herbert Bolaño, J., Paz Bailey, G., & Barrington, C. (2014). Social networks and HIV prevention among men who have sex with men and transgender persons in Guatemala City. *Journal of Health Care for the Poor and Underserved, 25*(4), 1698–1717. doi:10.1353/hpu.2014.0163.

# Chapter 2
# From Structural Analysis to Pragmatic Action: The Meso-level Modifiable Social Determinants of HIV Vulnerability for Labor Migrants

**Jennifer S. Hirsch, Morgan M. Philbin, Daniel Jordan Smith, and Richard G. Parker**

## 2.1 Background

Despite the current emphasis on biomedical approaches to HIV prevention, many vulnerable populations have limited access to preventive health services of any kind; this is particularly true for labor migrants. In this chapter, we review the factors that produce structural vulnerability to HIV among labor migrants, and develop further the notion of the meso-level (Hirsch 2014b) as a focus of structural analysis and collective action. Through case studies focused on labor migrants from three countries (Mexico, Nigeria, and Vietnam), we examine the ways in which policies in domains such as mobility, labor rights, and access to housing and health care produce vulnerability. The core of our argument is that addressing the vulnerability-producing circumstances in which many migrants live and work offers a concrete and promising structural approach to HIV prevention.

Over the past two decades, researchers have clearly established that migrants, both within and across national borders, face an elevated risk of HIV infection (Camlin et al. 2010; Weine and Kashuba 2012). Global multilateral organizations, such as the International Labour Organization, the International Organization for Migration (IOM), the United National Programme on HIV/AIDS (UNAIDS), and the United Nations Development Program (UNDP) have all also acknowledged migration as a driver of HIV vulnerability (UNAIDS and IOM 1998). The turn towards biomedical approaches to HIV prevention raises critical questions about migrants' vulnerabilities, since they so frequently lack either the consistent access to

J.S. Hirsch (✉) • M.M. Philbin • R.G. Parker
Columbia University Mailman School of Public Health, New York, USA
e-mail: jsh2124@columbia.edu; rgp11@columbia.edu

D.J. Smith
Department of Anthropology, Brown University, Providence, RL, USA



D. Kerrigan, C. Barrington (eds.), *Structural Dynamics of HIV*, Social Aspects of HIV 4, DOI 10.1007/978-3-319-63522-4_2

primary health care through which they might access HIV pre-exposure prophylaxis or, for those who are already infected with HIV, the engagement with HIV care that could support levels of adherence to antiretroviral therapy (ART) necessary to lower viral loads and reduce ongoing transmission (Dennis et al. 2011; Levy et al. 2007).

To be sure, migration is linked to many positive health outcomes for migrants as well as their sending communities (Argeseanu Cunningham et al. 2008; Kanaiaupuni and Donato 1999). Moreover, the emphasis on structural determinants of vulnerability to HIV is not meant to diminish the importance of attending to the ways in which individual and collective action shape both the migration process and its effects (Castles 2002; Okamoto and Ebert 2010). Nevertheless, there is evidence that migration can have a detrimental impact on a wide range of health outcomes, including HIV (Preibisch and Hennebry 2011). Weine and Kashuba (2012) conducted a systematic review of the multiple drivers of vulnerability to HIV risk for labor migrants. Policy-driven determinants of risk include: structural adjustment policies that favor export-oriented development and contribute to the lack of economic opportunity in rural communities; migrants' liminal legal status and consequent barriers to accessing services; the quality of housing available to workers; the dangerous and stressful conditions under which they work; banking and language laws, which create barriers to financial and social integration; and migration policies themselves, which can contribute to prolonged absences from their country of origin (Weine and Kashuba 2012). In their review, Weine and Kashuba also synthesize work suggesting that the likelihood of engaging in HIV risk behaviors can be increased by exposure to new cultural norms, separation from families, the mental health impacts of prolonged absences, and a lack of nearby familial and social support. They synthesize research showing that individual-level factors such as substance use, stress, and depression (which may be caused by prolonged absences but also by working and living conditions or xenophobia) may also lead migrant workers to engage in sexual behaviors that put them at risk of HIV infection. Their review, as well as a great deal of other work (Hirsch et al. 2009a, b; Vasquez and Hirsch 2012), demonstrates that the social processes through which migration creates vulnerabilities to HIV infection range from the most micro-level to the broadly macro-social.

Despite identifying factors at – and far beyond – the community level, there has been only scant discussion of structural approaches that might mitigate these vulnerabilities. A limited number of community-level interventions have sought to increase access to health care services, including sexually transmitted infection (STI) testing and treatment; to protect human rights; and to increase access to education and credit (Mooney and Sarangi 2005; Williams et al. 2000) or even to make changes to working conditions, such as modifying the schedules of transport workers so that they are away from home for shorter periods of time (Lurie et al. 1995). More commonly, however, interventions for migrants reflect a structural analysis (by focusing on a population rendered vulnerable through broad social processes), but then focus implementation at the individual or interpersonal level. Such examples include interventions to increase HIV knowledge and condom use, frequently with an element of community participation or culturally-appropriate adaptation (McCoy et al. 2009; Rhodes et al. 2006; Sanchez et al. 2004). In the above-cited work, environmental-structural determinants of migration-related risk have often been seen as intractable elements of social reality instead of as potentially amenable to intervention. Recently, however, some of these same authors as well as others have begun to focus on the policy context that shapes the health of migrants and their families (Martinez et al. 2013; Potochnick et al. 2016; Rhodes et al. 2015).

This growing attention to policy as a determinant of migrants' HIV vulnerability brings migration and HIV research up to date with the now decades-old chorus calling for structural interventions to prevent HIV (Gupta et al. 2008; Sommer and Parker 2013), as well as the more recent attention to 'combination' prevention, which in theory should include at least some intervention beyond the intra- and inter-personal (Hankins and de Zalduondo 2010). The notions of both structural and combination prevention are clearly applicable to interventions focused on the migration-HIV nexus, where the multiple social and policy factors contributing to vulnerability have already been traced out in such exhaustive detail. Nevertheless, much more progress has been made in developing structural prevention approaches for people who inject drugs and sex workers than migrants (Degenhardt et al. 2010; Shannon et al. 2015).

Considering migration policy as the only policy regulating movement offers a relatively limited range of policy targets for structural interventions. Our argument, therefore, is that a much broader range of policy domains shape the daily lives, well-being, and HIV vulnerability of migrant populations, and that attending to this broader range provides an expanded set of structural strategies to reduce the vulnerability of migrant populations. To delineate this broader range, and also more generally to advance work on structural approaches to HIV prevention, we use the idea of the 'meso-level', which refers to, as we have written previously:

> ...institutions, ideologies, or social processes that are 1) neither at the micro, individual, or interpersonal level (i.e. beliefs or characteristics of interactions) nor at the macro-social level (i.e. socially-structured inequalities of race, gender, sexuality), 2) characterized by a 'sociologically-plausible' or empirically-described causal relationship to a health-relevant practice, and 3) conceivably modifiable through sustained strategically-organized collective action. (Hirsch 2014b: 38)

The first and third dimensions of the definition above suggest that this framing of the meso-level is intended to inspire an approach to HIV prevention in between despair and triviality. Without question, the most macro-level dimensions of social inequality have driven the epidemic, and yet work that only focuses on those macro-level factors is unlikely to produce results along a timeline that fits into current public health institutions and funding structures. A focus on the meso-level carries forward that structural analysis, but with action targeted at modifiable dimensions of society that are produced by and reflective of macro-level inequalities in a way that can fit more comfortably with institutionalized public health. At the same time, the perspective hews to an emphasis on population-level determinants of health, directing attention to activities that would create a health-producing context rather than working 'one penis at a time' (Hirsch 2014a: S29) on individual and group interventions that are neither sustainable nor scalable. Moreover, it expands the potential targets of action by pointing to multi-sectoral sources of HIV vulnerability. In places where the politics of migration make changes to migration laws unlikely, this provides an approach to improving the conditions in which migrants live and work.

The second dimension of the meso-level perspective as defined above reminds us that social context must get under the skin. Not every policy drives HIV vulnerability; rather, we must identify specific policies and institutions for which there are evidence, or at least plausible relationships to limited engagement with health services and high-risk sex practices and drinking and drug use which impact sex practices. In other work, we have articulated this approach to delineating the pathways through which policies related to labor, policing, health services, education, language, legal identification, and public spaces shape three crucial realms of migrants' social experiences: the relative level of hostility towards/exploitation of migrants; ease or difficulty of accessing beneficial social institutions; and contexts influenced by policy climates (Galeucia and Hirsch 2016). In the case studies that follow on Mexico, Nigeria and Vietnam, we provide examples of both what this form of meso-level analysis entails and the prevention approaches it can generate.

## 2.2 Case Studies

### *2.2.1 Mexican Migrants in the U.S.*

According to the American Community Survey (US Census Bureau 2009), there were nearly 11.5 million Mexican immigrants in the United States (U.S.) in 2012, which made them almost a third of the country's foreign-born population (Brown and Patten 2014). Recent estimates suggest that the estimated 5.6 million of those who are undocumented account for approximately half of the U.S.'s undocumented immigrants (Krogstad et al. 2016). Their geographic distribution across the country reflects increasingly diverse settlement patterns – though 37.5 % of Mexican migrants resided in California, 20.9 % in Texas, and 6 % in Illinois, steadily growing communities had developed elsewhere with 5.1 % in Arizona, 2.4 % in Florida and Georgia, another 2.1 % in North Carolina and Colorado, and 2.0 % in New York (Motel and Patten 2013). This dispersion is of substantial relevance to the policy environment since so much is determined in the U.S. at the state and local level. Despite the feminization of the Mexican migrant flows to the U.S. over time, there were at least a million more Mexican-born men than women in the U.S. in 2009. In addition to work describing sexual risk practices among Mexican immigrant men (Albarrán and Nyamathi 2011; Apostolopoulos et al. 2006; Hirsch et al. 2009a; Wilson et al. 2010), a number of other dimensions of the U.S. epidemic underline the importance of great attention to the drivers of vulnerability of migrants, including Mexican migrants. First, there is evidence of a disproportionate burden of HIV disease among the foreign-born. Although national-level data are not available for Mexican-born individuals specifically, overall foreign-born individuals bear a disproportionate burden of HIV infection in the U.S. (Prosser et al. 2012) and a substantial proportion of those infections are believed to have occurred in the U.S. as opposed to prior to migration (Wiewel et al. 2015). Second, Latinos, regardless of nativity, also account for a disproportionate share of those infected with HIV in the U.S., with the preponderance of infections among Latinos occurring among men, particularly men who have sex with men (Centers for Disease Control and Prevention 2016).

Third, Mexican and other Latino migrants increasingly settle in areas with relatively high HIV prevalence (Painter 2008). For example, the metropolitan areas that experienced the largest percent increase in foreign-born population between 2000 and 2009, including Jackson, Charlotte, Jacksonville, and Atlanta, also had some of the highest national rates of new infections by 2009 (Centers for Disease Control and Prevention 2011; Wilson and Svajlenka 2014). These trends have continued, with the South experiencing the nation's most rapid growth in the foreign-born between 2010 and 2013 (Pew Research Center 2015) and continuing to show the nation's highest rates of HIV prevalence (Centers for Disease Control and Prevention 2015). Data on late presentation for care provides further evidence of the need for more attention to prevention for Mexican migrants; although most U.S. HIV surveillance data does not report on the foreign-born separately, or else does not specify country of origin, the effect of Mexican migrants' generally limited access to health care on vulnerability to HIV is reflected in the disproportionate numbers of Mexican-origin individuals in the U.S. who, by the time they receive a diagnosis of HIV, already have reduced CD4 cell counts or even an AIDS diagnosis (Dennis et al. 2011). One study found Mexican-born individuals with HIV were almost twice as likely as U.S.-born Latinos to progress to a diagnosis of AIDS less than 12 months after learning that they were seropositive (Espinoza et al. 2008). This late presentation is associated with an increased likelihood of viral transmission and poorer therapeutic outcomes for those who receive antiretroviral therapy (ART) (Battegay et al. 2006).

The risk of HIV infection, however, ranks relatively low in the day-to-day concerns of many Mexican migrants. Before coming to the U.S., many worry about dying in transit from dehydration, snakes in the desert, or the rapaciousness of their fellow humans. Once here, they worry about how to work in places in which there is limited public transportation and in which they are unable to secure a driver's license or car insurance (Bazar 2008; Preston and Gebeloff 2010). At work, they worry about discrimination (Marín et al. 2009), exposure to toxic levels of pesticides (Villarejo 2003), fatal construction accidents (Gany et al. 2011), or being robbed of their cash wages on their way home (Abel and Amrhein 2009). During moments of rest at the end of 6-day weeks, they worry about the physical and economic well-being of loved ones back home (Familiar et al. 2011; Negi 2011). Given the limited recreational options and unbalanced sex ratios in the communities in which they frequently reside, they may drown those worries in alcohol (Loury et al. 2011) or seek solace with a sex worker (Hirsch et al. 2009a; Munoz-Laboy et al. 2009). At the heart of our argument in the succeeding paragraphs lies the idea that at least some of these abovementioned worries are shaped by specific state and municipal level policies, all of which fall within the domain of the meso-level.

Those policies and the resulting climate they create in turn shape the three proximate determinants of HIV vulnerability noted above: high-risk sexual practices, limited engagement with health- promoting institutions, including health care services, and high-risk alcohol and drug use.

#### 2.2.1.1 Labor

Labor policies can reproduce a climate of social exclusion, force impoverished workers into substandard housing or into neighborhoods with limited recreational options, contribute to stress and anxiety, and keep workers in poverty. Those factors, in turn, can limit their access to health care and other health promoting institutions and render workers more likely to turn to high-risk drug and alcohol use. Specific examples of these policies in the U.S. include the exclusion of farm work and domestic work, both of which are occupations disproportionately filled by Latino migrant workers (Burnham and Theodore 2012; Hess and Henrici 2013), from the National Labor Relations Act (NLRA). Because they are excluded from the NLRA, those workers, many of whom hail from Mexico, lack many basic protections (NLRB 2016), such as the right to collective bargaining, workers' compensation, or overtime pay. Agricultural workers in California, for example, have for decades had the right to collective bargaining, and have recently won improvements in overtime pay (Lazo 2016), but conditions vary widely across the country (U.S. Department of Labor, Employment and Training Administration 2016).

There is a great deal of variability across the U.S. in the policy environment regulating unionization; this highlights the importance of considering policies that may not even be targeted towards migrants as part of the meso-level policy context. With the exceptions of New York and Colorado, all of the states that have seen substantial recent growth in the Mexican migrant population (Arizona, Georgia, Florida, and North Carolina) feature substantial legal barriers to the growth of unions (Rust 2015). But state-level labor policies, which may be focused on workers in general rather than migrants, can also be protective. Living wage ordinances have affected all workers, including Latino migrants, in Miami, Los Angeles, and Boston, as well as at the San Francisco and Seattle airports (Thompson and Chapman 2006; UC Berkeley Labor Center 2014). And, to great acclaim, agricultural workers were included in New York State's recent increase of the minimum wage due to sustained political pressure from labor and migrants' rights advocates. Legislation that prevents employers from punishing immigrant workers for work-related complaints solely based on their legal status is also potentially protective (Shen 2013). These protective laws could lower stress and anxiety and raise wages, thereby reducing vulnerability to HIV.

#### 2.2.1.2 Policing

In 1996, the U.S. Immigration and Nationality Act (INA) provided authorization for Immigration and Customs Enforcement (the arm of the Department of Homeland Security responsible for border patrol and enforcement commonly known as ICE) to collaborate with state and local police in the enforcement of federal immigration law as part of their daily activities (ICE 2016). There has been a great deal of recent state and municipal-level legislation shaping policing practices targeted at migrants (National Council of State Legislatures 2014), with some states and cities enacting policies known as 'sanctuary city' laws, restricting local law enforcement's ability to engage in immigration enforcement (Mitnik et al. 2008), while others seek to expand police force's cooperation with ICE. In Arizona, for example, the 'Support Our Law Enforcement Safe Neighborhoods Act' (SB 1070) permits the police to detain individuals on 'reasonable suspicion' that they are in the U.S. illegally and makes failing to possess immigration documents a crime (Martinez et al. 2013). The presence of ICE in communities has been shown to be related to reduced engagement with health services (Hacker et al. 2011), immigration status-related fears, and decreased likelihood of receiving health care (Berk and Schur 2001; Martinez et al. 2013), all of which are clearly relevant both to stress and anxiety (and thus to substance use) and to health care engagement. Research with undocumented Latinos (Berk and Schur 2001), as well as with undocumented immigrants more generally (Martinez et al. 2013), has demonstrated that migrants' fears about the potential revelation of their immigration status reduces the likelihood of accessing HIV prevention services, getting tested for HIV and other cofactors, including STIs, or receiving adequate treatment if they are living with HIV. We could find no research specific to undocumented Mexican migrants on HIV testing, but there is little reason to believe that their experience in this regard would differ substantially from that of other undocumented Latino migrants.

#### 2.2.1.3 Healthcare Services

Some policies related to health have, at least conceptually, reduced vulnerability. Municipalities, including San Francisco, Los Angeles, and Massachusetts have removed documentation status as an eligibility requirement to access public services, and these policies that directly facilitate the provision of at least basic health services may create opportunities for HIV prevention (Florido 2014; Marrow 2012). For any migrant seeking pre-exposure prophylaxis (PrEP), access to primary care is critical. State-level reform in Massachusetts in 2006, which served as the model for the Patient Protection and Affordable Care Act (ACA), expanded Medicaid to all eligible low-income residents with legal documentation and granted access to basic services for individuals without legal status (Marrow and Joseph 2015; Wilson 2008). Currently, some state-funded programs provide substance abuse treatment programs and mental health services, which may reduce migrants' vulnerability to HIV by addressing substance use behaviors (Wallace et al. 2012). All of these are changes in the policy environment that fall well short of comprehensive immigration reform, and yet which might have a substantial impact on migrants' vulnerabilities.

At the national level, policy changes over the past two decades have constrained access to care. In 1996, the Personal Responsibility and Work Opportunity Reconciliation Act (PRWORA) instituted, among other restrictions, a 5-year residency requirement for legal immigrants to be eligible to receive federal public assistance (Levinson 2002). This barred unauthorized immigrants outright from receiving Medicaid and other means-tested benefits, such as the Supplemental Nutrition Assistance Program (SNAP), regardless of how many years they have lived in the U.S. (Levinson 2002). PRWORA was enacted the same year as the Illegal Immigration Reform and Immigrant Responsibility Act (IIRIRA), a policy that arguably contributed to the climate of hostility by making non-citizens subject to deportation for minor criminal offenses like traffic violations (Rabinovitz 2011). In some cases, research on the health impacts of policy change have used the more general category Latinos rather than focusing on Mexicans or Mexican immigrants; for example, the ACA, which was intended to increase overall access to health insurance, bars unauthorized immigrants from purchasing private insurance via the exchanges, and thus has actually reduced access to healthcare services for some Latino immigrants (Marrow and Joseph 2015; Wallace et al. 2012). Even for legal migrants, the residency requirement to enroll in Medicaid and the mandate to pay 2 % of their income for insurance premiums combined with language and bureaucratic barriers experienced in municipal, state, and federal health insurance programs may serve as structural barriers to enrollment (Wallace et al. 2012). Efforts to screen individuals for citizenship status during enrollment may deter individuals from seeking care (Marrow and Joseph 2015; Martinez et al. 2013). Latino migrants' access to HIV prevention services, specifically, may be further limited under the ACA, as clinics will not be reimbursed for screening for some STIs or for STI prevention counseling for adults at higher risk for HIV infection and sexually active adolescents (Martinez et al. 2013).

#### 2.2.1.4 The State-Level Policy Climate Towards LGBT Individuals

Our focus here has been on policies that affect the Mexican migrant population, or in some cases on polices that affect Latino migrants overall and thus could reasonably be understood to affect Mexican migrants as well. However, given the concentration of HIV in Latinos among men who have sex with men (MSM), it is also relevant to mention the policy environment in relation to sexual minorities and gender non-conforming individuals. Depending on where they settle, the young Latino MSM who account for a disproportionate share of new infections may also face substantial day-to-day discrimination directed towards them not just as Latinos but because of their sexual practices or gender performance or identity (Ford 2011; Hardy et al. 2012; Hatzenbuehler 2014). There is considerable variation, both across and within states, in the extent to which social policies create a hostile or welcoming environment for lesbian, gay, bisexual, and transgender individuals. One study at the state-level, for example, found a 12-year difference in life expectancy for sexual minorities in communities with high-levels of anti-gay prejudice, compared to those living in low-prejudice areas (Hatzenbuehler et al. 2014). (Without question, this raises the broader idea of intersectionality: whether in Mexico, Nigeria, or Vietnam, the policy environment relevant to an individual migrants' vulnerability to HIV is shaped not just by migration-related policies but also by the broader policy environment that differentially allocates resources and opportunities to men and women, the young and old, heterosexual and non-heterosexual, and other relevant axes of social difference.)

This is hardly a thorough list of the kinds of policies that produce (or reduce) HIV vulnerability for Mexican migrants in the U.S. Other relevant policy domains include allocation of funds for parks, libraries, English classes, and other salutary, community-building spaces; transportation policy, which can promote social interaction and reduce the anxiety related to driving without a legal license; state-authorized identification policies, which can enable undocumented migrants to open U.S. bank accounts; language policies (which can be either exclusionary, such as 'English-only' laws, or inclusionary, facilitating social integration); and education policies, which can expand opportunities for young people who migrated to the U.S. as children by enabling them to qualify for in-state college tuition (Morse 2014). The broader point here is that the relative hostility or inclusiveness of the contexts in which migrants settle is not an unchangeable social fact, but rather the product of a complex and geographically variable policy environment. Other work underlines both the cross-state variability of that policy environment and its connection to pathways relevant to HIV vulnerability. Research on an index of the state-level policy climate across four domains (immigration, race/ethnicity, language, and agricultural worker protection) showed that Latinos in states with an overall less supportive policy climate experienced more days of poor mental health, and more mental distress, than in states with more supportive policies (Hatzenbueher et al. 2017). Policymakers and advocates in regions and municipalities with substantial numbers of incident cases of HIV among Latinos, and substantial proportions of their Latino population who are foreign-born, should consider how the local policy environment may actually be contributing to those new infections.

### *2.2.2 Rural-to-Urban Internal Migrants in Nigeria*

With all the recent – and well-warranted – attention to the hardships faced by millions of international migrants, spurred by Europe's migration crisis, the fact that about three-quarters of the world's migrants are internal is easily overlooked. Indeed, official estimates suggest that the world now has 244 million international migrants (UN DESA 2015), but more than three times as many (763 million) migrants have moved within the borders of their home countries (UN DESA 2013). Further, the difficulties faced by internal migrants can be equally daunting, or worse, than those faced by international migrants. Specifically, the risk of contracting HIV is often exacerbated by the structural inequalities faced by internal migrants, which are just as much the consequence of state policies and programs (or their absence) as is the case for international migrants. In this section, we examine the case of rural-to-urban internal migrants in Nigeria, and some of the structural factors that increase their risk of contracting HIV.

Nigeria has the third largest number of people in the world living with HIV, after only South Africa and India, and an adult prevalence of 3.2 % in 2014 (UNAIDS 2016). Further, levels of internal migration in the country are high. While precise numbers are impossible to come by, Nigeria's population is now about half urban and, according to a national urbanization and migration survey in 1993, more than 20 % of rural-born people had moved to Nigeria's cities (Mberu 2005). Recent scholarship suggests that current numbers are even higher (Oyeniyi 2013). While data on HIV infection in Nigeria are not broken down by migration status, making it impossible to know the actual prevalence among this population, data broken down by age and by geographical region in Nigeria suggest that young rural-to-urban migrants are an important risk group (Mberu and White 2011).

As in most contexts, the overwhelming impetus for internal migration is the aspiration for improved socioeconomic circumstances. The desire for education, employment, higher incomes, and urban amenities attracts many migrants to Nigeria's cities, as do the hardships of rural life. But despite its allure, the reality of life in the city is often difficult and structural inequalities expose migrants to many hazards, including the risk of contracting HIV. In this section, we focus on three specific factors that fit within our meso-level approach (in between the individual and the most macro-structural level, relevant (in ways that we describe) to HIV vulnerability, and malleable through collective action): (1) political representation; (2) housing (specifically family-friendly housing); and (3) health care.

#### 2.2.2.1 Political Representation

In Nigeria, internal migrants face the unwelcome fact that they are always considered settlers, strangers, and outsiders in the places to which they migrate. This can persist over more than a generation. Even the children of migrants who are born, for example, in Lagos, Nigeria's huge commercial capital, are not considered indigenes, either legally or socially. The most basic consequence of this is that migrants – who, if one includes their offspring, often make up well more than half a city's population – do not have basic political rights. It is noteworthy that Nigeria's official policy is that people can vote where they reside, but little is done to enforce this right. The common expectation and practice is that migrants should vote (or run for office) 'at home', where they came from (that is, not where they currently reside), even if they have not ever, in their entire lives, lived at that 'home'. Many of the other problems that create the structural contexts for HIV risk devolve directly from this fundamental lack of political voice. Specifically, the lack of political influence means that migrants are marginalized economically in a political economy in which patronage ties often determine access to resources. In addition, political marginalization results in inadequate government services, including HIV-related prevention and treatment programs.

Nigeria has a three-tier system of government – federal, state, and local. Most of the basic services and infrastructural amenities for urban populations are the responsibility of state and local governments. Although there has been some push to increase migrants' representation and influence in municipal governance, and some actual progress in Lagos and Abuja (Nigeria's political capital), in most of Nigeria's cities, migrants are rarely represented in state and local administrations. Migrant marginalization is perpetuated not only by the failure to make or enforce effective policies, but also by political narratives that associate place and political representation with ethnicity or autochthony, what Nigerians call 'tribalism'. These narratives not only perpetuate political exclusion that affects the direct provision of AIDS-related services, they also contribute to stigmas that associate HIV risk with cultural 'others'.

#### 2.2.2.2 Family-Friendly Housing

The politics of internal migration affects many dimensions of human welfare in Nigeria. Two that directly increase the risk of HIV infection are in relation to housing and the provision of health services. Many of Nigeria's cities face an acute shortage of adequate housing and migrants in particular struggle to find decent accommodations. Nigeria's federal, state, and local governments have, over the years, developed various policies and programs to create more affordable housing, including some supported by World Bank loans (World Bank 2013). But the little government-sponsored housing that has been built has barely made a dent in the demand. The overwhelming majority of migrants seek housing – usually just a room or two to rent—in the private market. In most Nigerian cities, landlords expect at least a year's rent (and sometimes 2 or 3 years' rent) in advance, a prohibitive amount for most migrants.

As a result of the absolute housing shortage and burdensome lease agreements, many migrants who come to cities in search of work or business opportunities leave their families behind. This situation is exacerbated by the fact that many employers – including the government – do not provide adequate allowances (or at any at all) for people who are transferred from one location to another to bring their families. Such transfers are common in Nigeria's civil service and among many private firms. This regularly leads to family separation. A study of the marital transmission of HIV in Nigeria found that one of the most common factors leading men to engage in extramarital sexual behavior was spousal separation due to labor migration (Hirsch et al. 2009b; Smith 2007). The Nigerian government does not have the wherewithal to solve the overall housing shortage. But the fact that a few simple policies – rigorously enforced – could make a significant difference underlines the power of this emphasis on meso-level drivers of vulnerability. For example, laws or regulations could prevent landlords from charging more than 1 month's rent at a time, or require firms (and the government itself) to provide adequate allowances to move family members when an employee is transferred. Such measures could go a long way toward mitigating the structural underpinnings of HIV risk caused by migrant housing issues. Unfortunately, even relatively simple regulations are difficult to enact and implement in a country where the government is preoccupied with multiple violent insurgencies, entrenched elite interests often dictate state policy, and HIV is still a problem that most politicians do not want to talk about.

#### 2.2.2.3 Health Care Services

A third meso-level source of migrants' risk of HIV in Nigeria is the organization and provision of health care services. In theory, Nigeria has a nationwide primary health care system in which basic care is financed, organized, and provided by local government health departments, referral hospitals are administered at the state level, and specialist hospitals and tertiary care are the responsibility of the federal government. In some places, this system works reasonably well, but in most cities, the majority of migrants seek health care through Nigeria's large private medical sector (Amaghionyeodiwe 2008). This is primarily because government health services are either inaccessible or perceived to be inferior. The inadequate provision of health services, both preventive and curative, exacerbates Nigeria's HIV epidemic in myriad ways. Weak or nonexistent public prevention activities leave Nigerians, including migrants, vulnerable. Further, although treatment is much more widely available than in the past, many HIV-positive individuals are not on ART and do not benefit from either its life-saving or infection-inhibiting effects. While no specific data exists that is broken down by migrant status, the most recent estimates are that about 747,000 individuals in Nigeria are receiving antiretroviral drugs, out of an estimated 3.2 million people infected with HIV (National Agency for the Control of AIDS 2015). Based on the Nigerian government's main criterion for treatment (that people with CD4 counts below 350 should be on treatment), approximately 55 % of people who should be receiving treatment are not. Fixing, or at least improving, government health services, even if sufficient political will existed, is much easier said than done. But as previously emphasized, one of the reasons for the poor provision of state-run health care for urban migrants is their lack of local political representation, which in turn leads most migrants to avoid, as best they can, paying any local taxes – further diminishing the likelihood that local governments will address the lack of access to high quality and affordable health services.

Many other structural factors that underlie HIV risk for urban migrants in Nigeria could be identified. Arguably, most would also be more likely to be ameliorated if migrants had a greater stake in, and more influence over, local political processes. Further, the Nigerian case is a reminder that to address the structural bases for HIV risk among migrants – but for many other at-risk populations too – we need not only better policies, but also their rigorous implementation and enforcement. In Nigeria, the link between political voice and HIV risk can be directly traced through housing policies and government priorities about where to provide high-quality public health services. Most of the country's rural-to-urban internal migrants recognize their political marginalization. Concrete demands for better housing policies and health services may stimulate changes that would affect not only HIV risk, but migrants' underlying structural vulnerability.

### 2.2.3 Rural-to-Urban and Interprovincial Migration in Vietnam

Vietnam provides a complementary example of how migration can intersect with rapid economic change and a very strong central government to generate structural vulnerability to HIV. The distribution of wealth in Vietnam has shifted over the last half century and is now firmly rooted in its urban centers. The market reforms of the 1980s, Doi Moi, resulted in urban-based employment opportunities around export-related manufacturing, trade, and services; many rural areas in Vietnam must contend with land shortages, price fluctuations on agricultural goods, and lack of financial credit (Thao 2003). These reforms also led to the elimination or reduction of welfare and social subsidies such as healthcare, childcare and educational support (Phinney 2008). This gap between the increasingly wealthy cities and poorer rural areas led to a surge in migration, particularly among young people (Pham and Hill 2008). The most recent national census in 2009 reported a total of 6.7 million internal migrants (~7 % of the total population) of whom half were interprovincial migrants (Anh et al. 2012). Women constituted 55 % of rural-to-urban migrants and 61 % of rural-to-rural migrants (Anh et al. 2012). The majority of these migrants do not cross international borders and Vietnam's relatively small size means that the frequency of home visits is much greater than amongst migrants in other countries (e.g., some migrants reported returning home monthly or even every 2 weeks) (Nguyen et al. 2011).

There are currently 250,000 HIV-infected people in Vietnam (an overall prevalence of 0.5 %), with the epidemic concentrated among people who inject drugs, sex workers, and men who have sex with men (Asian Development Bank 2013). There are potential overlaps between these sub-populations and migrants. Studies conducted in 12 provinces with high HIV rates and mobile populations found that one third of male migrants reported having sex with a female sex worker in the previous year, half of whom reported inconsistent condom use with sex workers (Nguyen et al. 2008). One study among drug users showed that men who reported selling sex were more likely to be migrants than those who did not sell sex (Clatts et al. 2007). A hospital-based prospective study found that half of HIV-infected pregnant women reported their primary partner as employed in the informal sector, most commonly as a migrant laborer or long distance truck driver (Nguyen et al. 2008).

There are three primary meso-level factors in Vietnam that constrain migrant workers' behaviors and shape their HIV risk: registration policies, the labor market, and housing availability.

#### 2.2.3.1 Registration Policies

In striking contrast to the Nigerian case, where internal migrants' 'foreignness' is a matter of culture, it is the Vietnamese state that renders internal migrants outsiders. Vietnam's household registration system creates a structural-level barrier for migrants, limiting migrants' ability to access government services outside the region in which they are registered. The 'Ho Khau' household registration system has four categories (K1–K4): K1 are officially registered permanent residents who can access all types of social services; K2 are individuals who have registered in an area other than their location of birth but who maintain full rights; K3 are migrants who stay in a destination less than a month and have limited access to services; and K4 are 'floating' migrants who are not registered in their area of destination, cannot own land, and have the least access to rights within this hierarchy (Haughton 2010; UNFPA 2010). These limitations mean that migrants in the K3 and K4 categories are often excluded from receiving healthcare, schooling, and social services in their district of residence; they are also often excluded from jobs and financial and poverty reduction services (Haughton 2010).

While originally designed for population management, the Ho Khau system exacerbates inequities between permanent residents and migrants and has direct implications for HIV risk. Migrants who live within a region where they are not registered may not be targeted by outreach and education programs, and may be excluded from HIV prevention, care, and treatment because they cannot access general medical care. Unregistered migrants are also less likely to seek professional care when ill and are less likely to have health insurance (Haughton 2010). While research has yet to measure the impact of such policies on biomedical HIV outcomes, existing data demonstrate that their impact can increase HIV vulnerability and risk (Haughton 2010). These registration policies exist even though they are often in direct conflict with migrants' rights as citizens under Vietnam's constitution. While some steps have been made (most notably the new 'Law of Residence' in 2007), additional changes are needed to decrease migrant-specific vulnerabilities.

#### 2.2.3.2 Labor Market Structures

Nearly all migrants move for economic reasons, and many experience labor market discrimination and exploitation. Migrant workers are paid lower salaries than non-migrants, particularly female and ethnic minority migrants (UNFPA 2010). This occurs for three primary reasons: (1) the jobs available to migrants are often informal, lower paid jobs; (2) migrants are rarely offered contracts and are easily replaced; and (3) employers use the household registration system as an excuse (though they are not legally permitted to do so) to exclude migrants from certain positions, or to pay them less than permanent residents (Guest 1998). As a result of these structural factors, migrants often feel unable to defend themselves against unfair and unsafe labor practices (Asian Development Bank 2014).

The jobs available to migrants can also increase HIV risk due to unsafe working conditions. Job opportunities for young female migrants have increased in the urban informal sector, including domestic housekeepers, restaurant employees, karaoke bar workers, and street traders (Anh et al. 2012; International Labour Organization 2002). The process of migration exposes women in particular to situations where they are vulnerable to sexual exploitation as result of limited economic opportunities and poor working conditions; migrant women also report higher levels of sex work than non-migrants (International Labour Organization 2002; Rushing et al. 2005). In contrast, men more frequently access jobs in heavy industry such as iron and steel processing, mining, chemical processing, and electronic assembly (Anh 2006). Coalmines in Quang Ninh province provide an example of how migration, occupation, and HIV risk intersect (Tuan 2010). Coal mines employ nearly one-third of the province's workforce, nearly all of whom are migrant men under the age of 30. Research suggests that migrants in coal mines use sex as a way to affirm masculinity and strengthen social networks; miners challenged each other to produce a higher output of coal in order to earn more money so that they could afford the more expensive sex workers with a goal of 'high income, high consumption' (Tuan 2010). Miners affirmed their group membership through sharing sexual experiences and described the importance of being able to ejaculate, which often led to condomless sex. As a result of working in an all-male environment, miners often reported sex workers as confidantes and the only people with whom they could share frustrations, stress, or sorrow (Tuan 2010).

In addition to increased HIV vulnerability as a result of the jobs and working conditions available to migrants, they also lack access to healthcare and social services that could mitigate HIV risk. Quang Ninh province, for example, has the highest reported HIV prevalence in Vietnam, with migrants excluded both from HIV surveillance and from local healthcare and social services (Tuan 2010). They are also left out of prevention, with provincial public health authorities targeting only local residents for intervention and treatment services and excluding migrants (Tuan 2010).

#### 2.2.3.3 Housing Policies

Finding a place to live is hampered by the household registration system; UNFPA described the housing crisis in Vietnamese cities as the most salient challenge for migrants (UNFPA 2010). Increasing urbanization has challenged existing infrastructure such as water and sanitation, transportation, schooling, and the provision of adequate housing (UNFPA 2010). Housing prices in Ho Chi Minh City (HCMC) have grown exponentially, yet comparatively low wages and a restrictive registration system limit migrants' ability to participate in the housing market (UNFPA 2010). In addition, migrants often lack access to formal financial services, which limits their ability to secure more stable housing.

A common example of available housing, 'boarding houses,' are located close to industrial zones, are generally built using cheap materials, lack electricity and sewage systems, and are overcrowded and overpriced; drug abuse and sex work are common (Noltze 2008). Areas around these boarding houses also now include squatter and slum settlements. The Vietnamese 2009 census found that only 24 % of interprovincial migrants lived in permanent houses with concrete roofs while 49 % lived in semi-permanent houses with tile or tin roofs, and 29 % lived in simple houses with leaf or straw-oil paper roofs (Anh et al. 2012). Estimates suggest that over 40 % of urban households lack sustainable housing or access to safe water or sanitation facilities. Migrants are often forced to spend the majority of their money on unsafe housing, which limits their ability to pay for food or healthcare. These instabilities make migrants more susceptible to health risks, particularly HIV risk, and limit migrants' ability to address health challenges that arise.

## 2.3 Policy Implications and Conclusion

One theme that emerges across all three cases is the health vulnerabilities produced by the differential valuation of people according to place of origin. Those distinctions may be driven by policy (as in the Vietnamese case) or have cultural roots (as in the Nigerian case), or can be a combination of the intertwining of policy and culture, as in the U.S. state of Arizona, in which strongly anti-immigrant sentiment both reflects and reproduces discriminatory and health-damaging policies. Across all three settings, the deck is stacked against migrants in terms of accessing housing and health care and the organization of the labor market in ways that produce HIV vulnerability. This framing of immigrant vulnerability in relation to the meso-level, however, moves us away from gesturing vaguely towards a discriminatory context, and provides concrete policy targets for change. In some cases, those targets may be widespread social attitudes, and in other places they may be specific laws or policies. The point is that they are specific, potentially modifiable, meso-level social determinants. Just as importantly, these examples underline that the inequalities faced by migrants reside not in one policy but in many, and thus that there are many possible strategies to mitigating those inequalities.

Another theme across all three cases is that the challenges faced by migrants are compounded by multiple other forms of social inequality – to which, it is important to emphasize, this notion of the meso-level is equally applicable. Whether it is discrimination against non-Khin migrants in Vietnam, anti-LGBTQ policies in North Carolina, or what Nigerians call 'tribalism', people face socially-organized inequalities along multiple dimensions. These challenges remind us of the multiple lines of work needed, perhaps necessarily simultaneously, to reduce their vulnerability.

There are also important differences across the three cases. The Vietnamese example, in which there is a very strong state and the majority of the inequalities stem from the 'Ho Khau' system at the federal level, suggests that in some cases an emphasis on the meso-level may be of limited utility. Improved regulation of the informal sector, a loosening of restrictions on health service provision to migrants, or new zoning policies for industrial centers, might contribute to improvements in the lives of the floating population, addressing some of the symptoms of the underlying social inequality, but it is hard to see those changes as fraying a strand of the rope that binds migrants' hands. Until the constitutional guarantee that all citizens have *'equal rights in all fields – political, economic, cultural and social'* is actually extended to those living outside of the area of their birth, substantial changes in their living and working conditions, and thus their vulnerability to HIV, seem unlikely. There may even be additional vulnerabilities in relation to specific policies or contexts that are invisible; because migration status/natality is unevenly included in the collection of health data, greater attention to measurement of migration status in health research in all three countries, as well as in other settings, might reveal a great deal more about how specific elements of the meso-level context drive vulnerability.

The Vietnamese case, then, reveals an important empirical question about a focus on the meso-level, which is whether changes in a particular social institution, whether they are laws, the labor market, the family, or schools, will actually refract back to address broader social inequality, rather than just mitigating its effects. In the case of access to driver's licenses for undocumented immigrants in the United States, there is a great deal of evidence that this one policy factor is related to anxiety, limited access to health care, and limits on physical mobility, which can have both social and economic impacts, and so it seems probable that a single legal change might have positive economic and social ripple effects that would improve migrants' lives more generally. The Vietnamese case reminds us that some meso-level factors may be more significant than others in creating persistent vulnerability; it is hard to imagine transformational change to enhance social protections for Vietnam's floating population without substantial reform to the Ho Kau system. In contrast, in both the Mexican and Nigerian contexts, the complex overlay of policies that shape migrants' lives offers many possible routes to making change that would affect a particular domain such as housing or health care, as well as, critically, the possibility that changes at that meso-level might actually address some dimension of the broader social inequality. In some ways, the lack of movement at the federal level in terms of immigration reform in the U.S. has created the country's own 'floating population', conveniently (from the point of view of employers) available to be slotted into the most dangerous and lowest-paying jobs. However, the variation in the policy context across states, with some states and cities offering highly inclusionary policies and others brimming with hostility, and many of those policies newly-created over the past decade, underlines the extent to which collective action can create change; despite their undocumented status, migrants living in contexts where they can move freely and without fear, work under better conditions and access more salubrious housing and recreational options. Evidence certainly exists that those factors affect mental health, substance use, and high-risk sexual practices, and thus it is eminently plausible that state and municipal-level efforts to chip away at the force of illegality could actually reduce vulnerability to HIV, as well as to other morbidities.

The enumeration of the ways in which the social context renders migrants vulnerable to HIV can seem, at first, like a very determinist argument, in which migrants are inevitably subject to social forces beyond their control, and thus solely a cause for despair. The complexity of the policy context described here suggests that there may even be a kind of negative synergy at work, in which multiple intersecting policies contribute to entrenched conditions of social vulnerability, to the extent that no single policy change could, by itself, reduce migrants' vulnerability to HIV. Moreover, these policies themselves have a social history, being produced at best by a lack of concern for the well-being of migrants, and, in some cases, by a deliberate animus towards them; the comment from a sponsor of Alabama's anti-immigrant omnibus legislation that his goal was to 'make their [immigrants'] lives difficult and they will deport themselves' (Fausset 2014) should remind us that powerful social coalitions produce this legislative context. Change is unlikely to come just as a result of our pointing to these and similar policy targets as root causes of health vulnerabilities for migrants.

A focus on the meso-level also, however, provides both a specific set of targets for collective action and a reminder that, as others have described (Kippax et al. 2013), the conditions that produce that collective action are themselves an important component of the response to HIV. Nigerian migrants' exclusion from local governance is both a source of vulnerability and, because collective mobilization for greater political representation could lead to better housing and improved access to health services, a potential route for intervention. While Mexican undocumented migrants may themselves be unable to vote on new legislation, in the United States the organization of political life offers possibilities to shape the outcome of elections and to change policy through civic engagement even for individuals who lack the rights of citizens (Greenhouse 2014; Tobar 2016). Our analysis provides a conceptual basis for empirical work to explore the impact of grassroots-level political engagement on migrants' vulnerability to HIV. Work in other contexts suggests that collective efficacy might be related to reduced individual HIV-related risk behaviors (Kerrigan et al. 2006); here, we add the suggestion that that collective efficacy might also contribute to the diminution of the social factors that produce those behaviors.

It is no more likely that any single program or intervention could eliminate discrimination towards migrants' or entirely improve the sometimes abject conditions in which they live and work than it is that any program or intervention would end gender inequality, racial inequality, poverty, or LGBTQ inequality. However, given all that we know about how these underlying dimensions of social inequality produce disparities in infection rates, it is vital to find a strategy to work, bit by bit, to build a more just world. And yet, as much as we might feel in our hearts that it is more valuable to fail at an audacious task than to succeed at a trivial one, failure does not beget future funding, and so it is also vital to elaborate a strategy, grounded in a structural analysis, that will enable those focused on migrants and HIV, or any population and HIV, to accomplish measurable progress at changing factors demonstrably relevant to HIV. Along those lines, the focus on the meso-level that we have articulated here provides the conceptual grounding for those seeking to address HIV among migrants to work through multi-sectoral alliances to complement efforts to promote HIV prevention in tandem with efforts to improve housing, access to primary health care, labor rights and democratic governance.

## References

Abel, J., & Amrhein, S. (2009, January 3). Hispanic workers tempting targets for robbers. *Tampa Bay Times*. http://www.tampabay.com/news/hispanic-workers-tempting-targets-for-robbers/956114. Accessed 17 Oct 2016.

Albarrán, C. R., & Nyamathi, A. (2011). HIV and Mexican migrant workers in the United States: A review applying the vulnerable populations conceptual model. *Journal of the Association of Nurses in AIDS Care, 22*(3), 173–185. doi:10.1016/j.jana.2010.08.001.

Amaghionyeodiwe, L. A. (2008). Determinants of the choice of health care provider in Nigeria. *Health Care Management Science, 11*(3), 215–227.

Anh, D. N. (2006). Sociological issues in renovation period. In *Internal migration in Viet Nam: Solutions for rural development* (pp. 351–366). Hanoi: Chinh tri Quoc gia Publisher.

Anh, L. T. K., Vu, L. H., Bonfoh, B., & Schelling, E. (2012). An analysis of interprovincial migration in Vietnam from 1989–2009. *Global Health Action, 5*(1), 9334. doi:10.3402/gha.v5i0.9334.

Apostolopoulos, Y., Sonmez, S., Kronenfeld, J., Castillo, E., McLendon, L., & Smith, D. (2006). STI/HIV risks for Mexican migrant laborers: Exploratory ethnographies. *Journal of Immigrant and Minority Health, 8*(3), 291–302. doi:10.1007/s10903-006-9334-2.

Argeseanu Cunningham, S., Ruben, J. D., & Venkat Narayan, K. M. (2008). Health of foreign-born people in the United States: A review. *Health & Place, 14*(4), 623–635. doi:10.1016/j.healthplace.2007.12.002.

Asian Development Bank. (2013). *Viet Nam: HIV/AIDS prevention among youth project*. Completion Report 3858102. http://www.adb.org/sites/default/files/project-document/79116/38581-022-vie-pcr.pdf. Accessed 28 Feb 2017.

Asian Development Bank. (2014). *Technical and ocational education and training in the Socialist Republic of Vietnam: An assessment*. Assessment ISBN 978-92-9254-462-1. Ha Noi, Vietnam. http://www.adb.org/sites/default/files/publication/59724/tvet-viet-nam-assessment.pdf. Accessed 28 Feb 2017.

Battegay, M., Fluckiger, U., Hirschel, B., & Furrer, H. (2006). Late presentation of HIV-infected individuals. *Antiviral Therapy, 12*(6), 841–851.

Bazar, E. (2008). Fewer licenses for illegal migrants: More states require legal status to drive. *USA Today*. http://usatoday30.usatoday.com/printedition/news/20080130/a_licenses30.art.htm Accessed 17 Oct 2016.

Berk, M. L., & Schur, C. L. (2001). The effect of fear on access to care among undocumented Latino immigrants. *Journal of Immigrant Health, 3*(3), 151–156. doi:10.1023/A:1011389105821.

Brown, A., & Patten, E. (2014). *Statistical portrait of the foreign-born population of the United States, 2012*. Washington, DC: Pew Research Center. http://www.pewhispanic.org/2014/04/29/statistical-portrait-of-the-foreign-born-population-in-the-united-states-2012/#report-materials. Accessed 28 Feb 2017.

Burnham, L., & Theodore, N. (2012). *Home economics: The invisible and unregulated world of domestic work*. National Domestic Workers Alliance and the Center for Urban Economic Development, University of Illinois at Chicago.

Camlin, C. S., Hosegood, V., Newell, M. L., McGrath, N., Barnighausen, T., & Snow, R. C. (2010). Gender, migration and HIV in rural KwaZulu-Natal, South Africa. *PloS One, 5*(7), e11539. doi:10.1371/journal.pone.0011539.

Castles, S. (2002). Migration and community formation under conditions of globalization. *International Migration Review, 36*(4), 1143–1168. doi:10.1111/j.1747-7379.2002.tb00121.x.

Centers for Disease Control and Prevention. (2011). *HIV surveillance report 2009*. http://www.cdc.gov/hiv/pdf/statistics_2009_hiv_surveillance_report_vol_21.pdf. Accessed 28 Feb 2017.

Centers for Disease Control and Prevention. (2015). *HIV surveillance report: Diagnoses of HIV infection in the United States and dependent areas, 2014*. Volume 26. http://www.cdc.gov/hiv/pdf/library/reports/surveillance/cdc-hiv-surveillance-report-us.pdf. Accessed 28 Feb 2017.

Centers for Disease Control and Prevention. (2016). *Fact sheet: New HIV infections in the United States*. Atlanta: National Center for HIV/AIDS, Viral Hepatitis, STD and TB Prevention. http://www.cdc.gov/nchhstp/newsroom/docs/factsheets/new-hiv-infections-508.pdf. Accessed 28 Feb 2017.

Clatts, M. C., Giang, L. M., Goldsamt, L. A., & Yi, H. (2007). Male sex work and HIV risk among young heroin users in Hanoi, Vietnam. *Sexual Health, 4*(4), 261–267. doi:10.1071/sh07018.

Degenhardt, L., Mathers, B., Vickerman, P., Rhodes, T., Latkin, C., & Hickman, M. (2010). Prevention of HIV infection for people who inject drugs: Why individual, structural, and combination approaches are needed. *The Lancet, 376*(9737), 285–301. doi:10.1016/s0140-6736(10)60742-8.

Dennis, A. M., Napravnik, S., Seña, A. C., & Eron, J. J. (2011). Late entry to HIV care among Latinos compared with non-Latinos in a Southeastern US cohort. *Clinical Infectious Diseases, 53*(5), 480–487. doi:10.1093/cid/cir434.

Espinoza, L., Hall, H. I., Selik, R. M., & Hu, X. (2008). Characteristics of HIV infection among Hispanics, United States 2003–2006. *JAIDS Journal of Acquired Immune Deficiency Syndromes, 49*(1), 94–101. doi:10.1097/qai.0b013e3181820129.

Familiar, I., Borges, G., Orozco, R., & Medina-Mora, M. E. (2011). Mexican migration experiences to the US and risk for anxiety and depressive symptoms. *Journal of Affective Disorders, 130*(1), 83–91. doi:10.1016/j.jad.2010.09.025.

Fausset, R. (2014, November 21). In Alabama town, Obama immigration move brings hope and sneers. *The New York Times*, sec. A. https://www.nytimes.com/2014/11/22/us/immigration-alabama-reaction.html. Accessed 28 Feb 2017.

Florido, A. 2014, September 30). *LA County to launch new health care program for uninsured migrants*. http://www.scpr.org/news/2014/09/30/47077/new-county-health-program-covers-uninsured-immigra/. Accessed 28 Feb 2017.

Ford, C. L. (2011). Structural racism and health inequalities. *Du Bois Review: Social Science Research on Race, 8*(01), 115–132. doi:10.1017/S1742058X11000130.

Galeucia, M., & Hirsch, J. S. (2016). State and local policies as a structural and modifiable determinant of HIV vulnerability among Latino migrants in the United States. *American Journal of Public Health, 106*(5), 800–807. doi:10.2105/AJPH.2016.303081.

Gany, F., Dobslaw, R., Ramirez, J., Tonda, J., Lobach, I., & Leng, J. (2011). Mexican urban occupational health in the US: A population at risk. *Journal of Community Health, 36*(2), 175–179. doi:10.1007/s10900-010-9295-9.

Greenhouse, S. (2014, April 24). In Florida tomato fields, a penny buys progress. *The New York Times*. http://www.nytimes.com/2014/04/25/business/in-florida-tomato-fields-a-penny-buys-progress.html. Accessed 28 Feb 2017.

Guest, P. (1998). *The dynamics of internal migration in Viet Nam*. United Nations Development Programme. Discussion Paper. Ha Noi, Vietnam.

Gupta, G. R., Parkhurst, J. O., Ogden, J. A., Aggleton, P., & Mahal, A. (2008). Structural approaches to HIV prevention. *The Lancet, 372*(9640), 764–775. doi:10.1016/S0140-6736(08)60887-9.

Hacker, K., Chu, J., Leung, C., Marra, R., Pirie, A., Brahimi, M., English, M., Beckmann, J., Acevedo-Garcia, D., & Marlin, R. P. (2011). The impact of immigration and customs enforcement on immigrant health: Perceptions of immigrants in Everett, Massachusetts, USA. *Social Science & Medicine, 73*(4), 586–594. doi:10.1016/j.socscimed.2011.06.007.

Hankins, C. A., & de Zalduondo, B. O. (2010). Combination prevention: A deeper understanding of effective HIV prevention. *AIDS, 24*(Suppl 4), S70–S80. doi:10.1097/01.aids.0000390709.04255.fd.

Hardy, L. J., Getrich, C. M., Quezada, J. C., Guay, A., Michalowski, R. J., & Henley, E. (2012). A call for further research on the impact of state-level immigration policies on public health. *American Journal of Public Health, 102*(7), 1250–1254. doi:10.2105/AJPH.2011.300541.

Hatzenbuehler, M. L. (2014). Structural stigma and the health of lesbian, gay, and bisexual populations. *Current Directions in Psychological Science, 23*(2), 127–132. doi:10.1177/0963721414523775.

Hatzenbuehler, M. L., Bellatorre, A., Lee, Y., Finch, B. K., Muennig, P., & Fiscella, K. (2014). Structural stigma and all-cause mortality in sexual minority populations. *Social Science & Medicine, 103*, 33–41. doi:10.1016/j.socscimed.2013.06.005.

Hatzenbuehler, M. L., Prins, S., Flake, M., Philbin, M., Frazer, S., Hagen, D., & Hirsch, J. S. (2017). Immigration policies and mental health morbidity among Latinos: A state-level analysis. *Social Science & Medicine, 174*, 169–178. doi:10.1016/j.socscimed.2016.11.040.

Haughton, J. (2010). *Urban poverty assessment in Ha Noi and Ho Chi Minh City*. United Nations Development Programme. Hanoi. http://www.un.org.vn/en/publications/government-agency-publications/doc_details/264-urban-poverty-assessment-in-ha-noi-and-ho-chi-minh-city.html. Accessed 28 Feb 2017.

Hess, C., & Henrici, J. (2013). *Increasing pathways to legal status for immigrant in-home care workers*. Washington, DC: Institute for Women's Policy Research. http://www.iwpr.org/publications/pubs/increasing-pathways-to-legal-status-for-immigrant-in-home-care-workers. Accessed 28 Feb 2017.

Hirsch, J. S. (2014a). Desire across borders: Markets, migration, and marital HIV risk in rural Mexico. *Culture, Health & Sexuality, 17*(S1), S20–S33. doi:http://dx.doi.org/10.1080/13691058.2014.963681.

Hirsch, J. S. (2014b). Labor migration, externalities and ethics: Theorizing the meso-level determinants of HIV vulnerability. *Social Science & Medicine, 100*, 38–45. doi:10.1016/j.socscimed.2013.10.021.

Hirsch, J. S., Muñoz-Laboy, M., Nyhus, C. M., Yount, K. M., & Bauermeister, J. A. (2009a). They 'miss more than anything their normal life back home': Masculinity and extramarital sex among Mexican migrants in Atlanta. *Perspectives on Sexual and Reproductive Health, 41*(1), 23–32. doi:10.1111/j.1931-2393.2009.4112309.

Hirsch, J. S., Wardlow, H., Smith, D. J., Phinney, H., Parikh, S., & Nathanson, C. A. (2009b). *The secret: Love, marriage, and HIV*. Nashville: Vanderbilt University Press.

Immigration and Customs Enforcement (ICE). (2016). *Delegation of Immigration Authority Section 287(g) Immigration and Nationality Act*. https://www.ice.gov/factsheets/287g. Accessed 28 Feb 2017.

International Labour Organization. (2002). *Viet Nam – children in prostitution in Hanoi, Hai Phong, Ho Chi Minh City and Can Tho: A rapid assessment, IWFCL, No 16*. Geneva: International Programme on the Elimination of Child Labour (IPEC).

Kanaiaupuni, S. M., & Donato, K. M. (1999). Migradollars and mortality: The effects of migration on infant survival in Mexico. *Demography, 36*(3), 339–353. doi:10.2307/2648057.

Kerrigan, D., Witt, S., Glass, B., Chung, S. E., & Ellen, J. (2006). Perceived neighborhood social cohesion and condom use among adolescents vulnerable to HIV/STI. *AIDS and Behavior, 10*(6), 723–729. doi:10.1007/s10461-006-9075-9.

Kippax, S., Stephenson, N., Parker, R. G., & Aggleton, P. (2013). Between individual agency and structure in HIV prevention: Understanding the middle ground of social practice. *American Journal of Public Health, 103*(8), 1367–1375. doi:10.2105/AJPH.2013.301301.

Krogstad, J. M., Passel, J. S., & Cohn, D. (2016). *5 facts about illegal immigration in the U.S.* Washington, DC: Pew Research Center. http://www.pewresearch.org/fact-tank/2016/11/03/5-facts-about-illegal-immigration-in-the-u-s/. Accessed 28 Feb 2017.

Lazo, A. (2016). California farmworkers to get overtime pay after 8 hours under new law. *The Wall Street Journal*. http://www.wsj.com/articles/california-farmworkers-to-get-overtime-pay-after-8-hours-under-new-law-1473726418. Accessed 28 Feb 2017.

Levinson, A. (2002). *Immigrants and welfare use*. Migration Policy Institute. http://www.migrationpolicy.org/article/immigrants-and-welfare-use. Accessed 28 Feb 2017.

Levy, V., Prentiss, D., Balmas, G., Chen, S., Israelski, D., Katzenstein, D., & Page-Shafer, K. (2007). Factors in the delayed HIV presentation of immigrants in northern California: Implications for voluntary counseling and testing programs. *Journal of Immigrant and Minority Health, 9*(1), 49–54. doi:10.1007/s10903-006-9015-9.

Loury, S., Jesse, E., & Wu, Q. (2011). Binge drinking among male Mexican immigrants in rural North Carolina. *Journal of Immigrant and Minority Health, 13*(4), 664–670. doi:10.1007/s10903-010-9402-0.

Lurie, P., Hintzen, P., & Lowe, R. A. (1995). Socioeconomic obstacles to HIV prevention and treatment in developing countries: The roles of the Internation Monestary Fund and the World Bank. *AIDS, 9*(6), 539–546. doi:10.1097/00002030-199506000-00002.

Marín, A. J., Grzywacz, J. G., Arcury, T. A., Carrillo, L., Coates, M. L., & Quandt, S. A. (2009). Evidence of organizational injustice in poultry processing plants: Possible effects on occupational health and safety among Latino workers in North Carolina. *American Journal of Industrial Medicine, 52*(1), 37–48. doi:10.1002/ajim.20643.

Marrow, H. B. (2012). Deserving to a point: Unauthorized immigrants in San Francisco's universal access healthcare model. *Social Science & Medicine, 74*(6), 846–854. doi:10.1016/j.socscimed.2011.08.001.

Marrow, H. B., & Joseph, T. D. (2015). Excluded and frozen out: Unauthorised immigrants' (non) access to care after US health care reform. *Journal of Ethnic and Migration Studies, 41*(14), 2253–2273. doi:10.1080/1369183X.2015.1051465.

Martinez, O., Wu, E., Sandfort, T., Dodge, B., Carballo-Dieguez, A., Pinto, R., Rhodes, S., Moya, E., & Chavez-Baray, S. (2013). Evaluating the impact of immigration policies on health status among undocumented immigrants: A systematic review. *Journal of Immigrant and Minority Health/Center for Minority Public Health, 17*(3), 947–970. doi:10.1007/s10903-013-9968-4.

Mberu, B. U. (2005). Who moves and who stays?: Rural out-migration in Nigeria. *Journal of Population Research, 22*(2), 141–161. doi:10.1007/bf03031826.

Mberu, B. U., & White, M. J. (2011). Internal migration and health: Premarital sexual initiation in Nigeria. *Social Science & Medicine, 72*(8), 1284–1293. doi:10.1016/j.socscimed.2011.02.019.

McCoy, S. I., Miller, W. C., MacDonald, P. D. M., Hurt, C. B., Leone, P. A., Eron, J. J., & Strauss, R. P. (2009). Barriers and facilitators to HIV testing and linkage to primary care: Narratives of people with advanced HIV in the Southeast. *AIDS Care, 21*(10), 1313–1320. doi:10.1080/09540120902803174.

Mitnik, P. A., Halpern-Finnerty, J., & Vidal, M. (2008). *Cities and immigration: Local policies for immigrant-friendly cities*. University of Wisconsin-Madison.. http://www.immigrationresearch-info.org/report/other/cities-and-immigration-local-policies-immigrant-friendly-cities. Accessed 25 Apr 2017.

Mooney, A., & Sarangi, S. (2005). An ecological framing of HIV preventive intervention: A case Study of non-government organizational work in the developing world. *Health, 9*(3), 275–296. doi:10.1177/1363459305052901.

Morse, A. (2014, February 9). *In-state tuition and unauthorized immigrant students*. National Council of State Legislatures. http://www.ncsl.org/research/immigration/in-state-tuition-and-unauthorized-immigrants.aspx. Accessed 28 Feb 2017.

Motel, S., & Patten, E. (2013, January 29). StatisticalpPortrait of the foreign-born population in the United States, 2011. *Pew Research Center's Hispanic Trends Project*. http://www.pewhispanic.org/2013/01/29/statistical-portrait-of-the-foreign-born-population-in-the-united-states-2011/. Accessed 28 Feb 2017.

Munoz-Laboy, M., Hirsch, J. S., & Quispe-Lazaro, A. (2009). Loneliness as a sexual risk factor for male Mexican migrant workers. *American Journal of Public Health, 99*(5), 802–810. doi:10.2105/ajph.2007.122283.

National Agency for the Control of AIDS. (2015). *Global AIDS response country progress report*. Abuja: Federal Government of Nigeria.

National Council of State Legislatures. (2014, January 20). *2013 year end report*. http://www.ncsl.org/research/immigration/2013-immigration-report.aspx. Accessed 28 Feb 2017.

National Labor Relations Board (NLRB). (2016). *National Labor Relations Act|NLRB*. https://www.nlrb.gov/resources/national-labor-relations-act. Accessed 28 Feb 2017.

Negi, N. J. (2011). Identifying psychosocial stressors of well-being and factors related to substance use among Latino day laborers. *Journal of Immigrant and Minority Health, 13*(4), 748–755. doi:10.1007/s10903-010-9413-x.

Nguyen, T. A., Oosterhoff, P., Hardon, A., Tran, H. N., Coutinho, R. A., & Wright, P. (2008). A hidden HIV epidemic among women in Vietnam. *BMC Public Health, 8*(1), 37. doi:10.1186/1471-2458-8-37.

Nguyen, H. N., Hardesty, M., & Hong, K. T. (2011). In full swing?: How do pendulum migrant labourers in Vietnam adjust their sexual perspectives to their rural-urban lives? *Culture, Health and Sexuality, 13*(10), 1193–1206. doi:10.1080/13691058.2011.609909.

Noltze, M. (2008). Backyard living – Integrative policies towards migrant workers: Housing microfinance in greater Ho Chi Minh City, Vietnam. *Austrian Journal of South-East Asian Studies, 1*(2), 19–33.

Okamoto, D., & Ebert, K. (2010). Beyond the ballot: Immigrant collective action in gateways and new destinations in the United States. *Social Problems, 57*(4), 529–558. doi:10.1525/sp.2010.57.4.529.

Oyeniyi, B. A. (2013). Internal migration in Nigeria: A positive contribution to human development. *African Caribbean Pacific Observatory on Migration Research Report.* http://publications.iom.int/system/files/pdf/nigeria.pdf. Accessed 25 Apr 2017.

Painter, T. M. (2008). Connecting the dots: When the risks of HIV/STD infection appear high but the burden of infection is not known – The case of male Latino migrants in the southern United States. *AIDS and Behavior, 12*(2), 213–226. doi:10.1007/s10461-007-9220-0.

Pew Research Center. (2015, September 28). Modern immigration wave brings 59 million to U.S., driving population growth and change through 2065. Washington, DC. http://www.pewhispanic.org/files/2015/09/2015-09-28_modern-immigration-wave_REPORT.pdf. Accessed 28 Feb 2017.

Pham, N. B., & Hill, P. S. (2008). The role of temporary migration in rural household economic strategy in a transitional period for the economy of Vietnam. *Asian Population Studies, 4*(1), 57–75. doi:10.1080/17441730801966683.

Phinney, H. M. (2008). 'Rice is essential but tiresome; you should get some noodles': Doi Moi and the political economy of men's extramarital sexual relations and marital HIV risk in Hanoi, Vietnam. *American Journal of Public Health, 98*(4), 650–660. doi:10.2105/AJPH.2007.111534.

Potochnick, S., Chen, J. H., & Perreira, P. (2016). Local-level immigration enforcement and food insecurity risk among Hispanic immigrant families with children: National-level evidence. *Journal of Immigrant and Minority Health.* doi:10.1007/s10903-016-0464-5.

Preibisch, K., & Hennebry, J. (2011). Temporary migration, chronic effects: The health of international migrant workers in Canada. *Canadian Medical Association Journal, 183*(9), 1033–1038. doi:10.1503/cmaj.090736.

Preston, J., & Gebeloff, R. (2010). Some nnlicensed drivers risk more than a fine. *The New York Times.* http://www.nytimes.com/2010/12/10/us/10license.html. Accessed 28 Feb 2017.

Prosser, A., Tang, T., & Hall, H. I. (2012). HIV in persons born outside the United States, 2007–2010. *JAMA, 308*(6), 601–607. doi:10.1001/jama.2012.9046.

Rabinovitz, J. (2011, October 20). Ending the laws that fuel mass detention and deportation. *American Civil Liberties Union.* https://www.aclu.org/blog/ending-laws-fuel-mass-detention-and-deportation. Accessed 28 Feb 2017.

Rhodes, S. D., Hergenrather, K. C., Montano, J., Remnitz, I. M., Arceo, R., Bloom, F. R., Leichliter, J. S., & Bowden, W. P. (2006). Using community-based participatory research to develop an intervention to reduce HIV and STD infections among Latino men. *AIDS Education and Prevention, 18*(5), 375–389. doi:10.1521/aeap.2006.18.5.375.

Rhodes, S. D., Mann, L., Simán, F. M., Song, E., Alonzo, J., Downs, M., Lawlor, E., et al. (2015). The impact of local immigration enforcement policies on the health of immigrant Hispanics/Latinos in the United States. *American Journal of Public Health, 105*(2), 329–337. doi:10.2105/ajph.2014.302218.

Rushing, R., Watts, C., & Rushing, S. (2005). Living the reality of forced sex work: Perspectives from young migrant women sex workers in Northern Vietnam. *Journal of Midwifery and Women's Health, 50*(4), 42–44. doi:10.1016/j.jmwh.2005.03.008.

Rust, M. (2015, September 6). ANALYSIS: What 'right-to-work' states look like. *Chicago Sun Times.* http://chicago.suntimes.com/news/analysis-what-right-to-work-states-look-like/. Accessed 28 Feb 2017.

Sanchez, M. A., Lemp, G. F., Magis-Rodríguez, C., Bravo-García, E., Carter, S., & Ruiz, S. D. (2004). The epidemiology of HIV among Mexican migrants and recent immigrants in California and Mexico. *Journal of Acquired Immune Deficiency Syndromes, 37*(Suppl 4), S204–S214. doi:10.1097/01.qai.0000141253.54217.24.

Shannon, K., Strathdee, S. A., Goldenberg, S. M., Duff, P., Mwangi, P., Rusakova, M., Reza-Paul, S., Lau, J., Deering, K., & Pickles, M. R. (2015). Global epidemiology of HIV among female sex workers: Influence of structural determinants. *The Lancet, 385*(9962), 55–71. doi:10.1016/s0140-6736(14)60931-4.

Shen A. (2013, May 1) *California bills would punish employers who take advantage of immigrant workers.* http://thinkprogress.org/immigration/2013/05/01/1946261/california-punish-immigrant-abus/. Accessed 28 Feb 2017.

Smith, D. J. (2007). Modern marriage, men's extramarital sex, and HIV risk in southeastern Nigeria. *American Journal of Public Health, 97*(6), 997–1005. doi:10.2105/ajph.2006.088583.

Sommer, M., & Parker, R. G. (2013). *Structural approaches in public health.* London: Routledge.

Thao, V. T. (2003). Making a living in rural Vietnam from (im)mobile livelihoods: A case of women's migration. *Population, Space and Place, 19*, 87–102. doi:10.1002/psp.1706.

Thompson, J., & Chapman, J. (2006). *The economic impact of local living wages.* Washington, DC: Economic Policy Institute. http://www.epi.org/publication/bp170/. Accessed 28 Feb 2017.

Tobar, H. (2016). Can Latinos swing Arizona? *The New Yorker.* http://www.newyorker.com/magazine/2016/08/01/promise-arizona-and-the-power-of-the-latino-vote. Accessed 28 Feb 2017.

Tuan, T. V. (2010). Meanings of sex, concepts of risk and sexual practices among migrant coal miners in Quang Ninh, Vietnam. *Culture, Health and Sexuality, 12*(Suppl 1), S31–S40. doi:10.1080/13691051003731296.

U.S. Census Bureau (2009). *2009 American community survey.* https://www.census.gov/programs-surveys/acs/guidance/comparing-acs-data/2009.html. Accessed 25 Apr 2017.

U.S. Department of Labor, Employment and Training Administration. (2016). *National agricultural workers survey.* Washington, DC. https://naws.jbsinternational.com/3/table2b.pdf. Accessed 5 Sept 2016.

UC Berkeley Labor Center. (2014). *Living wage and self-sufficiency resources.* http://laborcenter.berkeley.edu/livingwage/resources.shtml. Accessed 15 May 2016.

UN DESA (United Nations Department of Economic and Social Affairs). (2013). *Cross-national comparisons of internal migration: An update on global patterns and trends.* http://www.un.org/en/development/desa/population/publications/pdf/technical/TP2013-1.pdf. Accessed 25 Apr 2017.

UN DESA (United Nations Department of Economic and Social Affairs). (2015). *International migrant stock 2015.* http://www.un.org/en/development/desa/population/migration/data/estimates2/data/UN_MigrantStockTotal_2015. Accessed 28 Feb 2017.

UNAIDS. (2016). *Nigeria.* http://www.unaids.org/en/regionscountries/countries/nigeria/. Accessed 28 Feb 2017.

UNAIDS & IOM. (1998). Migration and AIDS. *International Migration, 36*(4), 445–468.

UNFPA (United Nations Population Fund). (2010). *Internal migration and socio-economic development in Viet Nam: A call to action.* Ha Noi, Vietnam. http://www.un.org.vn/en/publications/government-agency-publications/doc_details/173-internal-migration-opportunities-and-challenges-for-socio-economic-development-in-viet-nam.html. Accessed 27 June 2016.

Vasquez, E., & Hirsch, J. (2012). Mexico-U.S. migration, social exclusion, and HIV risk: Multisectoral approahces to understanding and preventing ionfection. In K. C. Organista (Ed.), *HIV prevention with Latinos: Theory, research, and practice* (pp. 103–120). Oxford: Oxford University Press.

Villarejo, D. (2003). The health of U.S. hired farm workers. *Annual Review of Public Health, 24*, 175–193. doi:10.1146/annurev.publhealth.24.100901.140901.

Wallace, S. P., Torres, J., Sadegh-Nobari, T., Pourat, N., & Brown, E. R. (2012). *Undocumented immigrants and health care reform.* Los Angeles: UCLA Center for Health Policy. http://healthpolicy.ucla.edu/publications/Documents/PDF/undocumentedreport-aug2013.pdf. Accessed 28 Feb 2017.

Weine, S. M., & Kashuba, A. B. (2012). Labor migration and HIV risk: A systematic review of the literature. *AIDS and Behavior, 16*(6), 1605–1621. doi:10.1007/s10461-012-0183-4.

Wiewel, E. W., Torian, L. V., Hanna, D. B., Bocour, A., & Shepard, C. W. (2015). Foreign-born persons diagnosed with HIV: Where are they from and where weere they infected? *AIDS and Behavior, 19*(5), 890–898. doi:10.1007/s10461-014-0954-1.

Williams, B. G., MacPhail, C., Campbell, C., Taljaard, D., Gouws, E., Moema, S., Mzaidume, Z., & Rasego, B. (2000). The Carletonville-Mothusimpilo project: Limiting transmission of HIV through community-based interventions. *South African Journal of Science, 96*(6), 351–359.

Wilson, J. F. (2008). Massachusetts health care reform is a pioneer effort, but complications remain. *Annals of Internal Medicine, 148*(6), 489–492. doi:10.7326/0003-4819-148-6-200803180-00029.

Wilson, J. H., & Svajlenka, N. P. (2014). *Immigrants continue to disperse, with fastest growth in the suburbs*. Washington, DC: The Brooking Institution. https://www.brookings.edu/research/immigrants-continue-to-disperse-with-fastest-growth-in-the-suburbs/. Accessed 28 Feb 2017.

Wilson, K. S., Eggleston, E., Diaz-Olavarrieta, C., & Garcia, S. G. (2010). HIV/STI risk among male Mexican immigrants in Dallas, Texas: Findings from a pilot study. *Journal of Immigrant and Minority Health, 12*(6), 947–951. doi:10.1007/s10903-010-9323-y.

World Bank. (2013, September 23). *The World Bank approves funds to support Nigeria's expansion of its housing finance market*. World Bank. http://www.worldbank.org/en/news/press-release/2013/09/26/world-bank-support-nigeria-expansion-housing-finance-market. Accessed 28 Feb 2017.

# Chapter 3
# Addressing the Micro- and Macro-Environmental Vulnerabilities to HIV of People Who Inject Drugs in Tanzania: A Case Study of the Muhimbili Medication-Assisted Treatment Clinic

**Jessie Mbwambo, Haneefa T. Saleem, Pamela Kaduri, Barrot H. Lambdin, and Sheryl A. McCurdy**

It is estimated that there are 30,000 people who inject drugs in mainland Tanzania, with an approximate HIV prevalence of 35% in this key population (NACP 2014). Drug use is criminalized in Tanzania and treatment options are limited. However, in February 2011, a cutting-edge medication-assisted treatment (MAT) clinic for opioid addiction offering methadone maintenance treatment was established at Muhimbili National Hospital in Dar es Salaam. The clinic, which began offering drug treatment and harm reduction services, now offers a multi-faceted array of health and social services to address the myriad of psychosocial and structural factors impacting the well-being of people who use drugs in that setting. These services include HIV counseling and testing and linkages to on-site HIV care and treatment services, screening and treatment for tuberculosis and other medical and mental

J. Mbwambo (✉) • P. Kaduri
Department of Psychiatry and Mental Health, Muhimbili National Hospital, Muhimbili University of Health and Allied Sciences, Dar es Salaam, Tanzania
e-mail: jmbwambo@gmail.com

H.T. Saleem
Department of International Health, Johns Hopkins Bloomberg School of Public Health, Baltimore, Maryland, USA

B.H. Lambdin
Behavioral Health and Criminal Justice Research Division, RTI International, San Francisco, CA, USA

Department of Epidemiology and Biostatistics, University of California, San Francisco, CA, USA

Department of Global Health, University of Washington, Seattle, WA, USA

S.A. McCurdy
School of Public Health, University of Texas Health Science Center at Houston, Houston, TX, USA



D. Kerrigan, C. Barrington (eds.), *Structural Dynamics of HIV*, Social Aspects of HIV 4, DOI 10.1007/978-3-319-63522-4_3

disorders, and access to on-site social workers and affiliated occupational therapists. Social workers at the Muhimbili MAT clinic link MAT clients to community-based organizations that provide individual counseling, 12-step programs, family group therapy, and incomegenerating skills training, among other services for people who use drugs. This chapter uses a risk environment framework to describe the microand macro-environmental factors that place people who inject drugs at increased risk of HIV and documents innovative initiatives and partnerships that have been formed to address these factors through an in-depth case study of the Muhimbili National Hospital MAT clinic.

## 3.1 A Risk Environment Framework

There has been growing attention to the need for a paradigm shift in public health from a focus on individual harm reduction models to models that acknowledge the important role that social situations and structures play in contributing to HIV risk and drug harm (Blankenship et al. 2000, 2015; Des Jarlais 2000; Rhodes et al. 2005). As a result, it is now understood that harms associated with injection drug use are situated within risk environments that contribute to heightened vulnerability to HIV (Des Jarlais 2000; Rhodes 2009).

Tim Rhodes described a risk environment framework as one that:

> ...envisages drug harms as a product of the social situations and environments in which individuals participate. It shifts the responsibility for drug harm, and the focus of harm reducing actions, from individuals alone to include the social and political institutions which have a role in harm reduction. (Rhodes 2009: 193)

The framework envisages different types of environments, including physical, social, economic, and policy environments, operating at micro- and macro-levels of influence (Rhodes et al. 2005; Rhodes 2009). It stresses how relations between individuals and the micro- and macro-environments in which they live impact the production and reduction of drug harms. Within the risk environment framework, the micro-environment is defined as the physical and social space in which a variety of proximal factors exogenous to the individual interact to produce harm or enable the reduction of harm. It encompasses the environment immediately experienced and embodied as part of everyday practices, and includes interpersonal relationships, social and group interactions, and institutional and organizational responses to drug harm, such as prisons, drug addiction treatment centers, and needle and syringe exchange programs. The macro-environment, on the other hand, comprises the social and political-economic structures that play a role in harm production but also have the potential to influence broad reductions of harm for women and men who use drugs. It includes such structures as drug trafficking routes, laws governing drug possession, gender inequalities, and economic inequities in the broader global economy. Figure 3.1 illustrates these multiple types and levels of the risk environment within the context of drug harm.

In this chapter, we describe how the interplay of micro- and macro-environmental factors contributes to the heightened HIV vulnerability of people who inject drugs

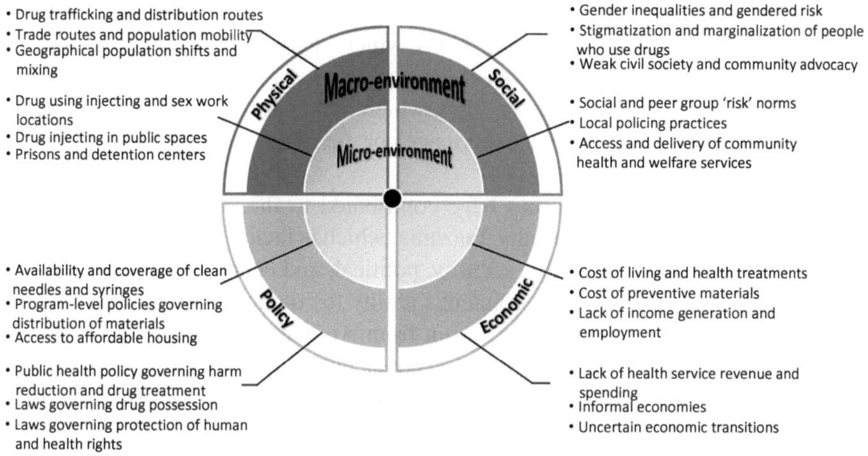


**Fig. 3.1** Risk and enabling environment framework for drug harms (Rhodes 2009)

in Tanzania. We begin by discussing how changes in the type of drugs available and accessible in Tanzania have affected injecting practices. Next, we discuss the socio-structural realities of people who inject drugs in the Tanzanian context. We move on to introduce and describe the medication assisted treatment (MAT) clinic at Muhimbili National Hospital and discuss how the clinic is responding to environmental factors that place people who inject drugs at increased risk of HIV and poor HIV prognoses. We then describe innovative initiatives within the clinic to integrate tuberculosis and HIV services, the challenges of people who inject drugs in accessing and remaining in MAT and HIV treatment services, and the positive outcomes of the MAT program to date. We end the chapter with a discussion of ways forward.

## 3.2 The Rise of Heroin Injection in Tanzania

Since the late 1990s, the injection of heroin has become widespread in Dar es Salaam, Tanzania, and is spreading throughout the country (McCurdy et al. 2005a, 2006). The rise of heroin injection in Tanzania has been precipitated by structural changes in drug trafficking within the macro-environment that have led to changes in the heroin supply in East Africa. Before the late 1990s, brown heroin, or 'brown sugar', imported predominantly from Myanmar in Southeast Asia, dominated the heroin market in the region (Beckerleg et al. 2005; McCurdy and Maruyama 2013). Brown heroin is coarse, heat stable, and has poor water solubility unless an acid is added, which makes it less suitable for injecting (Ciccarone 2009). Given brown heroin must be processed and cooked before injecting, people who use brown heroin typically smoke or chase it, which is a practice that involves heating the heroin then inhaling the vapors emitted. Processing brown heroin for injection requires time, skill, and effort, in addition to a safe place to prepare it. White heroin, on the other hand, has different physical properties that lend well to injecting. It is finer and highly water-soluble (Ciccarone 2009), which means it can be easily dissolved in water and injected directly, instead of having to cook it first. Injecting white heroin also delivers a more intense high, which makes it more desirable for those seeking to elevate their heroin experience, or for those with a higher level of dependency.

A series of geopolitical forces have contributed to the rise of heroin use and injection in East Africa, specifically Tanzania, which is facing an epidemic of heroin abuse. As a result of the unstable security, political, and economic environments in Afghanistan that limited the government's ability to counter opium production and trafficking, starting in 2000, white heroin from Afghanistan became more readily available in Tanzania (McCurdy et al. 2005a; Office of National Drug Control Policy n.d.). Additionally, as traditional overland trafficking routes through Central Asia and Iran have become less attractive heroin trafficking routes to Western Europe due to improved law enforcement in central Europe and the conflict in Syria, East Africa has become an increasingly important trans-shipment hub for heroin from Afghanistan (The Economist 2015; McCurdy and Maruyama 2013). This change in the type of heroin available (from brown heroin to white heroin) was accompanied by a rise in heroin injection. Today, there are about 30,000 people who inject drugs, mostly heroin, living in mainland Tanzania, representing 10% of the total reported drug using population in the country (NACP 2014).

## 3.3 The Socio-structural Vulnerabilities to HIV of People Who Inject Drugs

People who inject drugs in Tanzania have high rates of HIV. In Dar es Salaam, approximately 35% of people who inject drugs are living with HIV (NACP 2014), compared to 5.1% in the general adult population (United Republic of Tanzania 2014). The lives of people who inject drugs in Tanzania are fraught with the harsh realities of poverty, stigma, discrimination, strict police surveillance, and other factors that create an environment that places them at increased risk of HIV.

Within the social environment at the macro-level, people who inject drugs in Tanzania face high levels of mistrust that result in stigma and discrimination. In research conducted with Muhimbili MAT clients on their enrollment experiences, Zamudio-Haas et al. (2016) reported how clients' narratives regarding their desperate actions of stealing from family and neighbors to quell the pains of heroin withdrawal were linked to the generation of mistrust of people who inject drugs by families and communities. For instance, a female MAT client stated: 'My whole family cast me out. Wherever I went, they would close the doors, "she will just steal," they would say' (Zamudio-Haas et al. 2016: 47). The sense of loss and social isolation that was the result of being cast aside by family and community led many to seek refuge from judgment and discrimination in local drug hangout spots, where risky injecting practices are pervasive.

Even within the healthcare system, people who inject drugs report facing stigma and discrimination. A female Muhimbili MAT client reported how people who use drugs are sometimes treated by healthcare providers when seeking care:

> If people know you're a drug user, well you'll receive the same [medical] services you came for, but not without some trouble. The attitude is, 'She's a junkie. Don't bother with her.' I mean, like, if you're a thief and you got beat down trying to steal something, when you go to the hospital, they probably wouldn't assist you until everyone else has been attended to. (Zamudio-Haas 2013: 23)

Stigma and discrimination against people who inject drugs within the healthcare system can limit their access to care and increase their vulnerability to negative HIV clinical outcomes (Burke et al. 2015; Wolfe et al. 2010). In our prior research in Tanzania, we found that perceived and enacted stigma due to a history of drug addiction from family and healthcare providers deter HIV-positive MAT clients from seeking HIV care and treatment through HIV clinics that serve the general population (Saleem et al. 2016). As a social worker based at the Muhimbili MAT clinic interviewed for the study described:

> [MAT clients] are lost [to follow-up to HIV care] because some do not like to attend the same clinic with other patients from different areas due to their behaviors. Once they are [at the HIV clinic], they feel like they are thieves, lawbreakers. They feel anxious thinking that someone may see him/her as a thief. (Saleem et al. 2016: 62)

The multiple layers of stigma enacted on and experienced by people who use drugs, particularly those living with HIV, limits the availability of addiction and HIV treatment programs for this sub-population at high risk of contracting HIV and can negatively affect their ability to access any treatment that is available. An HIV-positive woman receiving methadone treatment at the Muhimbili MAT clinic who was interviewed for the same study further reported on the link between HIV stigma enacted by family and HIV care-seeking behaviors:

> There are some families that honestly accept that [HIV] is a disease, so they send her early to start treatment to be safe. But others think it is a big problem, so they stigmatize you. So, the issue of stigma and being degraded could also make someone delay [HIV] treatment. First she feels down that her family does not offer support. They discourage you, abandon you: 'She has AIDS!' (Saleem et al. 2016: 62)

The criminalization of heroin use and possession through national laws and its manifestation within the microenvironment in strict police surveillance also increase vulnerability to HIV among people who inject drugs. In 1995, the Parliament of Tanzania enacted the *Drugs and Prevention of Illicit Traffic in Drugs Act*, which prohibited and penalized drug production, trafficking, possession, and use (United Republic of Tanzania 1995). This was the beginning of Tanzania's 'War on Drugs'. The act included a provision for the establishment of a commission for the coordination of drug control (which was later officially established as the Drug Control Commission). The commission was mandated to develop national policies and implement international conventions on drug control, among other functions. And though one of the functions of the Commission outlined in the Act was to develop treatment and rehabilitation programs for people with drug addictions, the overall enforcement of the law centered on drug supply and demand reduction (Ratliff et al. 2016).

Following the rise of heroin injection in Tanzania in the early 2000s, and as part of the 'war on drugs', law enforcement officials began escalating efforts to reduce heroin trafficking and consumption. The frequency of arrests of those caught selling or using drugs increased, which contributed to an environment that fostered risky injecting practices (McCurdy et al. 2007). The price of heroin increased as a result of the reduction in heroin supply. Increased heroin costs and fear of being arrested for possession of injecting paraphrenalia forced many who use heroin to go further underground and resort to sharing needles and syringes (McCurdy et al. 2005a, b, 2007). An even more risky injecting practice, influenced by economic factors that included the increase in heroin costs coupled with a lack of income-generating prospects, is the use of *flashblood*, which was first documented in Dar es Salaam in 2005 (McCurdy et al. 2005b), and later spread to Zanzibar and up the Swahili Coast to Kenya (McNeil 2010; Njenga et al. 2012). *Flashblood* is the intended injection of blood from someone who has recently injected heroin to another person to ward off withdrawal symptoms (McCurdy et al. 2010). Women in Tanzania have been shown to be more likely to engage in the practice of *flashblood* compared to men (Mlunde et al. 2016), especially women who are unstably housed, have a history of sexual abuse, or those who may be economically dependent on their partners and who lack power within the relationship (McCurdy et al. 2010).

In Tanzania, women who use heroin are more vulnerable to sex-related HIV exposure than their male counterparts. There are several factors that place these women at higher risk of being exposed to HIV. In a study conducted by Lambdin et al. (2013) in Dar es Salaam among women and men who injected drugs who were the recipients of community outreach services and enrolled in the methadone maintenance treatment program, they found there were no significant differences in the rates of sharing needles and other injecting equipment between women and men (Lambdin et al. 2013). However, there were noted differences that increased the risk of HIV exposure among women. In Tanzania, most women who use heroin prefer to smoke it, which carries no direct risk of HIV transmission. However, dependence on heroin may increase their engagement in risky sexual behaviors (Lambdin et al. 2013; Zamudio-Haas et al. 2016). Many women who are dependent on heroin in Tanzania engage in sex work and/or trade sex for heroin (McCurdy et al. 2005a). Desperate for that next *fix*, earning money to feed one's addiction and stave off the pains of withdrawal may override any concern about using a condom to prevent disease. Women living in Dar es Salaam who use heroin have also described the heightened risks of physical and sexual violence that they experience in male-dominated drug hangout spots (McCurdy et al. 2005a; Zamudio-Haas et al. 2016). The threats of sexual and physical violence from men in drug hangout spots lead many women who use heroin to avoid these spaces altogether and isolate themselves in more hidden places, which makes it more difficult for outreach workers to reach them with HIV prevention messages and harm reduction interventions (Zamudio-Haas et al. 2016).

## 3.4 The Medication-Assisted Therapy (MAT) Clinic at the Muhimbili National Hospital

In response to the high HIV burden among people who inject drugs, in February 2011, the Government of Tanzania, with support from the US President's Emergency Plan for AIDS Relief (PEPFAR), opened the first publicly funded MAT clinic at Muhimbili National Hospital for the treatment of opioid addiction on mainland sub-Saharan Africa. The MAT clinic offers methadone maintenance treatment, a life-saving, chronic medical intervention that lowers mortality, morbidity, and illegal activities associated with opioid dependence (Fullerton et al. 2014). The World Health Organization (WHO), the United Nations Office of Drugs and Crime and the Joint United Nations Programme on HIV/AIDS (UNAIDS) recommend opioid substitution therapy, such as methadone maintenance treatment, as a key HIV prevention, care, and treatment intervention for people who inject drugs (WHO et al. 2012). It has also been shown to reduce the risk of transmission of HIV, Hepatitis C virus, and other infectious diseases by reducing injection-related and sexual risk behaviors among people who use drugs (Bruce 2010; Connock et al. 2007; Metzger et al. 1993).

The Muhimbili MAT clinic offers directly observed methadone maintenance treatment to clients who attend the clinic 7 days a week. Clients are eligible for methadone treatment if they exhibit opioid dependence, have evidence of recent drug injection, and have positive urine screening for opiates. Since Muhimbili National Hospital is a referral hospital, before enrolling in methadone treatment, potential clients must first be referred to the clinic by one of the partnering community-based organizations, funded through the Tanzania AIDS Prevention Program (TAPP). These community-based organizations were created to provide outreach to people who use drugs and as an entryway to methadone treatment. Enrollment in methadone treatment is restricted to those able to demonstrate their commitment to treatment. Providers at the MAT clinic determine a potential client's commitment to treatment through his or her completion of a series of educational sessions at a community-based organization, with topics covering the transmission and treatment of HIV and other STIs, methadone treatment adherence, and supportive services offered by the organization.[1]

To date, over 1150 clients have been enrolled in the methadone maintenance program at the Muhimbili MAT clinic. About 600 of the total clients enrolled are considered active—that is, they attend the clinic on a daily basis for methadone dosing. Almost 60% of clients at the clinic are retained in methadone treatment after being

[1] In response to a very low number of female clients enrolling into methadone treatment, another MAT clinic at Mwananyamala Regional Hospital, established in September 2012, piloted an approach, beginning in February 2013, allowing women dependent on heroin to enroll directly at the clinic rather than having to first attend the series of sessions at the CBOs. In addition, existing female clients were encouraged to recruit their peers and one day of the week was set aside for enrolling female clients only. This approach improved women's enrollment into the methadone clinic at Mwananyamala, thereby increasing the proportion of female MAT clients.

initially enrolled for at least 12 months (Lambdin et al. 2014). Clients are counseled before enrolling in the methadone maintenance program that treatment could last for 2 years. Though retention of the Muhimbili MAT clients is comparable to retention rates in other parts of the world, including Europe, Asia and North America (Anderson and Warren 2004; Booth et al. 2004; Gossop et al. 2001; Liu et al. 2009; Magura et al. 1988; Sarasvita et al. 2012; Soyka et al. 2008), additional strategies are currently being explored to further reduce attrition. Since the opening of the clinic in 2011, few clients have graduated from the program. Some have remained engaged in the program by helping clients navigate treatment. The low number of graduated clients is partly due to the relatively short period in which the clinic has been open and periodic disruption of treatment from relapse among clients.

The designation of methadone in the Tanzanian context as an HIV harm reduction tool coupled with the scarcity of resources initially restricted access to methadone treatment to people who inject heroin. Since women who use heroin in Tanzania are more likely to smoke or chase it rather than inject, the number of women enrolled in methadone maintenance treatment at the MAT clinic remains low (Lambdin et al. 2013). To address the gender inequities in treatment, clinic policies have been moving in the direction of expanding eligibility for methadone maintenance treatment to non-injecting women and their partners.

MAT clients face several challenges to remaining in the methadone maintenance treatment program. Transportation costs and the travel time required to arrive at the clinic daily leads some clients to miss methadone doses and interrupt their treatment plan. Traveling outside of Dar es Salaam for socially obligated events, such as funerals, or for work purposes also results in missed methadone doses. And though the availability of methadone maintenance treatment has expanded in Dar es Salaam and Zanzibar, traveling outside these areas often results in clients missing their methadone doses. Depending on the length of travel and one's tolerance, clients may relapse to heroin use in order to manage withdrawal symptoms. A large proportion of the MAT patient population has a history of cycling through the criminal justice system (Lambdin et al. 2014). Being arrested may cause clients to default from treatment and relapse to heroin use. Relapse is a common theme for why clients default from treatment. In addition to missing methadone doses due to transport, arrest, or travel, some clients relapse and default from methadone treatment because they are not ready to change, lack social support, have comorbid use of other drugs, or continue to be burdened by the same vulnerabilities that initially led them to heroin use. During 2015, MAT clients experienced a new challenge to their efforts to remain sober. Drug dealers started coming to the MAT clinic to promote crack use as a non-addictive alternative to heroin and methadone (McCurdy and Kaduri 2016).

MAT clients are labeled as defaulting from the program if they miss their daily dosing of methadone for 30 consecutive days. Clients who default from treatment are required to go through the community-based organization that initially referred them to receive further counseling and education. After demonstrating their commitment to re-enrolling in the program, they are referred to the MAT clinic for re-enrollment. Though the re-enrollment procedures are designed to provide defaulted clients with the additional counseling and support needed to re-initiate and remain in treatment, many have complained that the process can at times be lengthy and burdensome.

In an attempt to address some of the challenges MAT clients experience in remaining in the program, the Ministry of Health and Social Welfare (MoHSW) and the Drug Control Commission have recently begun exploring alternative methadone delivery models that would make methadone treatment more accessible for people who use drugs. One potential methadone delivery model under consideration is a take-away modality for clients who meet certain criteria. Though specific eligibility criteria have not been officially established, criteria proposed by the Ministry of Health and Social Welfare [Draft *Clinical Guidelines for Medically Assisted Treatment of Opioid Dependence for Health Facilities in Tanzania* October 2014] include:

- Mental health stability to assume responsibility to manage medication as prescribed;
- Stabilization in methadone treatment, indicated by enrollment in the MAT program for at least 3 months, demonstrated adherence to one's methadone treatment plan, refrainment from ongoing drug use for the last 3 months confirmed by urine toxicology and breathalyzer for alcohol;
- Social stability, indicated by stable social support and at least one methadone treatment adherence supporter, a stable living environment, and no proven engagement in criminal activities or other serious behavioral problems demonstrated at the clinic or in the community in the previous 3 months;
- Proof of access to a safe and secure place to store methadone and completion of an orientation on the safekeeping of medication; and
- A signed take-away dose agreement form that states that the client agrees to adhere to providers' instruction.

A take-away dose delivery method would help reduce methadone treatment interruptions and default due to transportation costs and travel, as clients would not have to present at the MAT clinic every day. Other models under consideration include expansion of MAT programs to health facilities in other regions, lower-level satellite sites that could dispense methadone with trained methadone prescribers and counselors, and the establishment of MAT programs within prison settings (Magimba 2015).

## 3.5 Responding to the Psychosocial and Environmental Vulnerabilities of People Who Inject Drugs Through the MAT Clinic

Though the cornerstone of the Muhimbili MAT clinic is its methadone maintenance treatment program, the clinic has adopted a holistic approach to addressing the psychosocial and environmental factors that impact the wellbeing of people who use drugs. As part of the enrollment process and prior to receiving methadone treatment, clients complete a comprehensive medical and psychosocial assessment through consultations with several providers, including a nurse, social worker, and psychiatrist. The assessment helps MAT clinic providers evaluate complications related to heroin and other substance use; medical and psychiatric disorders; high-risk behaviors; family, social, legal and employment situations; and any involvement with the judicial and/or criminal justice system. The information gathered from this comprehensive assessment allows providers to develop a treatment and referral plan for the client that addresses his or her unique circumstances. Clinicians refer clients to the relevant department at the national hospital for any medical conditions that cannot be managed at the MAT clinic.

In complement to the methadone maintenance treatment program, the MAT clinic offers a wide array of services that help to improve the physical, mental and social health of its clients, creating a 'one-stop shop' for comprehensive care. Costs can deter people from seeking treatment. To defray the economic costs to clients enrolled in the program who often lack income and employment opportunities, all services are offered free of charge.

Mental illnesses, including depression, are highly prevalent among people who inject drugs in Dar es Salaam (Nyandindi et al. 2014). Among a sample of 293 clients at the MAT clinic in 2012, when the total client population was 430, researchers found that about 10% of clients had suicidal thoughts at some point in their lives and 3% had ever attempted suicide (Ubuguyu et al. 2016). To address the burden of mental illness comorbidities among clients, psychiatrists based at the MAT clinic provide free treatment for mental disorders. Through the MAT clinic, which is strategically housed in the Department of Psychiatry and Mental Health at Muhimbili National Hospital, clients have access to a range of pharmacological, behavioral, and psychosocial treatment options for any mental disorders and other substance use disorders. Clients are also encouraged to attend mutual aid groups offered through their affiliated community-based organizations, including 12-step programs such as Alcoholics Anonymous, Narcotics Anonymous, and Methadone Anonymous. Methadone Anonymous grew out of a desire among MAT clients to have a group that focuses on the unique challenges of being enrolled in the methadone maintenance program. On-site Alcoholics Anonymous has also been established to allow easy access to such services for clients who may experience transportation or time barriers to attending meetings at community-based organizations.

To help mitigate the stigma that contributes to the social risk environment of clients enrolled in the methadone program, clients are provided access to social workers. Social workers play a key role in helping clients rebuild relationships with their families. The stigma and discrimination associated with drug addiction and HIV not only affects the emotional health and social support system of people who use drugs, but also their ability to access medical care. Internalized and anticipated HIV- and drug addiction-related stigma have been shown to negatively impact health service utilization for people who inject drugs (Burke et al. 2015; Calabrese et al. 2016; Saleem et al. 2016). Rebuilding the social support network of MAT clients helps to mitigate the effects of stigma and facilitate access to needed medical care, including HIV care and treatment (Saleem et al. 2016). According to MAT clients participating in a PEPFAR/US Centers for Disease Control and Prevention-sponsored study conducted on take-away methadone doses in Tanzania, family support, in the form of emotional and financial support to attend the clinic every day, was key to them remaining in treatment [unpublished data].

Social workers are also able to help clients navigate through legal matters. A history of involvement in the criminal justice system is common among MAT clients, with about half of clients enrolling in MAT reporting ever being arrested (Lambdin et al. 2014). MAT aims to provide relief from heroin cravings and the pains of heroin withdrawal, so MAT clients no longer need to resort to engaging in illicit activities to feed their addiction and stave off withdrawal. In establishing the MAT clinic, law enforcement officials were engaged and sensitized on methadone as a treatment option for those dependent on heroin. There has been movement in Tanzania to seeing opioid use as a health problem to be treated in the health care system rather than in the criminal justice system, with treatment as an alternative to incarceration for opioid dependent offenders (United Republic of Tanzania 2015). However, much remains to be accomplished in improving coordination between the MAT clinic and criminal justice systems (MoHSW and DCC 2015), since incarceration is one of the factors that can lead to interruption and/or default from methadone treatment.

Drug dependence affects the ability to perform daily activities as one's focus becomes getting the next fix to stave off withdrawal symptoms. Once in recovery, it is important to support clients in improving daily functioning. An occupational therapist is available to support MAT clients in building skills and independence in performing daily activities, including activities essential to reintegrating in one's family and community. Unemployment is high among MAT clients and a majority of clients have less than a primary-level education (Lambdin et al. 2014), which exacerbates their inability to generate income. Methadone maintenance treatment reduces dependency on heroin, which increases self-awareness among clients and helps them to regain trust and respect within their communities. The positive changes that result from being on methadone allow clients to resume previous employment or seek new employment opportunities within the community. To further facilitate economic relief, the MAT program, through support from TAPP, offers adult learning and job training for MAT clients to improve their prospects for employment. In addition, the MAT clinic has instituted a *Work as Treatment* program that provides selected MAT clients with jobs tending the gardens and areas in and surrounding the clinic. The *Work as Treatment* program serves as a form of contingency management as it rewards MAT clients for progressing well in treatment. Some clients have even been employed by TAPP as community outreach workers based at the clinic. These community outreach workers help clients navigate and remain in treatment. Their service not only allows them to earn money, but also supports them in their recovery from heroin addiction. The demand for occupational and vocational services, as well as income generating activities, is high particularly because clients relied on illegal activities for livelihoods and sustaining their addiction prior to methadone treatment. The low education among clients further poses barriers to job opportunities.

Through the concerted efforts of the team of providers at the MAT clinic, improvements in wellbeing among clients have been documented. A study was recently conducted using medical records of MAT clients to examine the effect of methadone maintenance treatment on both physical and mental health-related quality of life (Ubuguyu et al. 2016). The research team, which included members of the clinic's staff, found that enrollment in the program resulted in short-term improvements in health-related quality of life. However, overall, MAT clients had lower physical and mental health quality scores than other patient populations, including people living with HIV, hypertensive clients, and survivors of critical illness. This is not surprising given the high levels of multiple and complex vulnerabilities experienced by people who inject drugs.

## 3.6 Linking MAT Clients to Tuberculosis and HIV Care Through Integration

The MAT program has been successful in linking clients to important medical services. New clients are seven times more likely than people who inject drugs in the community who are not enrolled in the program to have been screened for HIV, other sexually transmitted infections, tuberculosis, and Hepatitis B and C (Mlunde et al. 2016). The recruitment model of the MAT program leverages the access that community-based organizations have to people in the community who inject drugs, which helps to facilitate linkages to care.

### *3.6.1 Integrating Tuberculosis Treatment Services*

Not long after the MAT clinic opened its doors in early 2011, the death of a patient due to tuberculosis incited fear among MAT clinic staff that other clients might be infected with the disease. Undiagnosed cases of tuberculosis could pose an increased risk of infection for both clients and providers. High rates of HIV coupled with a history of arrest and imprisonment among people who inject drugs further exacerbates their risk of contracting tuberculosis. WHO recommends systematic screening for active tuberculosis for people with a drug dependency (WHO 2013). Later that year in response to this concern, the MAT clinic implemented an active case findings program to assess the prevalence of tuberculosis among clients and link those found to be positive to treatment (Gupta et al. 2014). The piloted active case findings program demonstrated that the rate of tuberculosis was high. Four percent of MAT clients screened tested positive for active pulmonary tuberculosis (Gupta et al. 2014), which was nearly 23 times higher than the prevalence in the general population in Tanzania (WHO 2012).

As part of the MAT clinic's active case findings program, providers use a symptom-based questionnaire as an initial screening tool for clients. Clients who report one or more symptoms are referred for sputum diagnostic testing. Those who test positive for tuberculosis are started on directly observed treatment short course (DOTS), in accordance with national tuberculosis treatment guidelines[2] at the clinic through co-dispensing with methadone throughout the duration of the treatment plan.

The active case findings program at the MAT clinic has yielded positive results, demonstrating that integrating active screening for tuberculosis within a MAT facility can be achieved in low-resource settings. Dozens of clients have been successfully treated for tuberculosis with DOTS. Without actively screening for tuberculosis at the clinic, many of these clients would not have been diagnosed and treated until it was too late.

### *3.6.2 Integrating HIV Care and Treatment Services at the MAT Clinic*

The availability of HIV counseling and testing and treatment services offered at the MAT clinic has evolved since its launch in 2011. The MAT program was originally conceived as a harm reduction intervention – a way to reduce injection drug use, prevent HIV transmission, and help those who inject drugs and are living with HIV engage in HIV care and treatment. To that end, the MAT clinic began by offering opt-out provider-initiated HIV testing and counseling early on for clients at enrollment and every 6 months thereafter for people who screen HIV-negative. Clients who tested positive for HIV were assessed for antiretroviral therapy (ART) eligibility – samples of blood drawn at the MAT clinic were sent to the Muhimbili National Hospital central pathology laboratory for CD4 testing. MAT providers escorted eligible clients to the HIV care and treatment clinic for ART initiation. Escorts were also available for MAT clients to subsequent HIV clinic visits for routine monitoring and monthly ART dispensing. Despite daily encounters with the health care system and procedures in place at the MAT clinic to encourage HIV care-seeking behaviors, less than half of all ART-eligible MAT clients at Muhimbili had initiated ART within 3 months of being deemed eligible for treatment (Tran et al. 2015).

In an effort to reduce these delays and failures to initiate ART among MAT clients and to improve clinical outcomes, an integrated HIV and MAT service delivery model was piloted at the clinic (Lambdin et al. 2015). As part of these efforts, for-

[2] The first-line tuberculosis treatment regimen in Tanzania includes Isoniazid, Rifampicin, Pyrazinamide, Ethambutol, and Streptomycin formulated in fixed drug combinations (United Republic of Tanzania 2013). The recommended standardized multi-drug resistant tuberculosis treatment regimen includes Amikacin, Ofloxacin/Levofloxacin, Pyrazinamide, Ethionamide, Cycloserine, and Ethambutol (if no resistance to Ethambutol is documented) (United Republic of Tanzania 2012).

mative research was conducted with MAT clients and providers to elucidate factors that hinder and facilitate ART initiation and how an integrated service delivery model could be developed to create a clinic environment that enables timely ART initiation (Saleem et al. 2016). We identified several barriers to ART initiation: delays in CD4 testing and receiving CD4 test results; the inconvenience of MAT clients having to go off-site for ART initiation at the HIV care and treatment clinic; HIV- and addiction-related stigma and discrimination; and inadequate ART counseling and follow-up from MAT clinic providers as clients navigate the HIV care and treatment system. A series of community and partner engagement meetings were held with diverse stakeholders, including MAT clients, community outreach workers, HIV care providers, representatives from civic organizations, and the MoHSW. These engagement meetings provided an avenue to disseminate findings from the formative research. Key stakeholders were also provided a platform to weigh in and offer recommendations in light of the findings on how the MAT clinic could effectively integrate HIV services in order to improve treatment outcomes for clients. Using findings from the formative research and discussions from the community and partner engagement meetings, an integrated methadone and ART delivery model that seeks to address the challenges identified was developed and implemented at the Muhimbili MAT clinic.

The resulting integrated model includes four key components: (1) in-house HIV care and treatment specialists; (2) in-house CD4 testing; (3) ART delivery through the MAT clinic; and (4) an electronic information system to monitor clients.

Three MAT clinic clinicians and two nurses were cross-trained as HIV treatment specialists. Our clinicians are now able to initiate and prescribe ART to clients at the MAT clinic. Having qualified HIV treatment specialists based at the MAT clinic reduces the need to refer clients to the off-site HIV clinic for care and treatment, and thus lowers their exposure to stigma and discrimination due to their history of addiction.

Novel point-of-care CD4 testing technology at the clinic streamlines ART delivery by reducing the time for CD4 testing to 20 min. This dramatically reduced delays in ART initiation by decreasing the time it took for clients to receive CD4 test results previously encountered at the MAT clinic, which was reported by MAT clinic providers and clients as taking up to a month or longer in some cases (Saleem et al. 2016). Three MAT providers were trained in using the CD4 testing machine. MAT clients found to be eligible to receive ART by a trained clinician at the MAT clinic are given the option to receive their ART as: (1) directly observed therapy (DOT) by a clinician in a private setting, (2) DOT at the methadone dispensing window, or (3) monthly supplies of ART (standard of care in Tanzania). In the standard operating procedures developed for HIV treatment management for MAT clients, preference is given to first-line ART regimens that have once-daily dosing, which helps facilitate co-dispensing and improve adherence.

To address the challenge of inadequate patient monitoring and follow-up related to HIV care and treatment identified at the MAT clinic (Saleem et al. 2016), an electronic information system that includes patient laboratory test results, HIV treatment status, and other key information was developed for use by providers to reinforce ART initiation and monitor clients. The electronic information system allows providers at the MAT clinic to identify clients who are due for HIV testing and clients diagnosed with HIV who are due for CD4 screening or ART initiation.

Though implementation of the piloted integrated methadone and ART service delivery model is still in an early phase, initial outputs look promising. Within the first 3 months of implementation of the integrated model, MAT service providers conducted over 100 CD4 tests. Nearly 40 clients were seen by HIV care and treatment-trained clinicians for ART initiation at the MAT clinic. At the beginning of 2016, the team received communication from the MoHSW to adopt a 'test and treat' model for HIV among people who inject drugs at the MAT clinic, thereby eliminating the reliance on a specific CD4 threshold to determine ART eligibility. The implementation of the integrated model has effectively enabled providers at the MAT clinic to operationalize the first 'test and treat' model for HIV among people who inject drugs in sub-Saharan Africa.

## 3.7 Conclusion

In this chapter, we used a risk environment framework for drug harm proposed by Rhodes (2009) to examine physical, social, economic, and policy environments at the micro- and macro-levels in the Tanzanian context. This work contributes to our understanding of how relations between the environment and people who inject drugs impacts the production of HIV risks in East Africa, and how the MAT clinic at Muhimbili National Hospital in Dar es Salaam is creating an environment conducive to harm reduction by decreasing injecting practices through methadone maintenance treatment and linking HIV-positive clients to essential HIV care and treatment.

For example, structural shifts in the type of heroin marketed and used in Tanzania, influenced by changes in drug trafficking routes in the physical macro-environment, led to an increase in heroin injection. By offering methadone treatment, the Muhimbili MAT clinic has been able to reduce heroin cravings and heroin injecting practices that place people who use drugs at increased risk of HIV. Broad gender inequalities that operate at the macro-level in the social environment contribute to violence against women who inject drugs in Tanzania. In response to the risks of violence in male-dominated drug hangout spaces, women who inject drugs responded by adopting the practice of *flashblood*, which increases the risk of HIV transmission. The high rates of engagement in sex work among women who use drugs also contribute to higher HIV rates in women compared to men. The Muhimbili MAT clinic has sought to expand outreach and enrollment services to women to increase their access to important addiction therapy and HIV care and treatment. Additionally, by offering free methadone and HIV treatment and linking clients to in-house occupational therapy, job training, and opportunities to earn money through performing tasks around the clinic, the Muhimbili MAT clinic attempts to address the economic hardships experienced by its clients.

The Muhimbili MAT clinic has made great strides in creating an environment that facilitates HIV harm reduction by offering an array of services, including methadone maintenance treatment and integrated HIV care and treatment that impact the wellbeing of its clients. It has served as a model for scaling up MAT services to other communities in Tanzania. Since its launch in 2011, three additional MAT clinics have been established at Mwananyamala Regional Hospital, Temeke Regional Hospital, and on the island of Zanzibar.

The successes of the MAT clinic are rooted in the commitment of staff to support clients on their road to recovery and reduce their risks of HIV and other illnesses. However, the clinic is limited in its ability to address some of the broader environmental factors that have led so many to addiction and continue to influence the everyday lives of people dependent on heroin. It is only through partnerships with civil society organizations, such as community-based organizations serving communities of people who use drugs, and law enforcement agencies, that the micro- and macro-environmental vulnerabilities underlying the HIV risks of people who inject drugs can be more holistically addressed. Clinic leaders have been advocating and will continue to advocate with Parliament and the police to change law enforcement policies and practices that discriminate against and intimidate people who use drugs from seeking treatment. The evidence presented in this chapter suggests that a comprehensive package of physical, social, economic, and policy interventions at the micro- and macro-levels of the risk environment should be implemented in order to effectively reduce HIV harm among people who inject drugs.

The research that our consortium is conducting at the MAT clinic plays a key role in providing the evidence base needed to scale-up methadone treatment and inform policies that protect the right to health of those dependent on drugs in Tanzania.

## References

Anderson, J. F., & Warren, L. D. (2004). Client retention in the British Columbia Methadone Program, 1996–1999. *Canadian Journal of Public Health, 95*(2), 104–109.

Beckerleg, S., Telfer, M., & Hundt, G. L. (2005). The rise of injecting drug use in East Africa: A case study from Kenya. *Harm Reduction Journal, 2*, 12. doi:10.1186/1477-7517-2-12.

Blankenship, K. M., Bray, S. J., Merson, M. H., Reinhard, E., Sherman, S. G., & El-Bassel, N. (2000). Structural interventions in public health. *AIDS, 14*(Suppl 1), S11–S21. doi:10.1097/00002030-200006001-00003.

Blankenship, K. M., Reinhard, E., Sherman, S. G., & El-Bassel, N. (2015). Structural interventions for HIV prevention among women who use drugs: A global perspective. *JAIDS Journal of Acquired Immune Deficiency Syndromes, 69*(Suppl 2), S140–S145. doi:10.1097/qai.0000000000000638.

Booth, R. E., Corsi, K. F., & Mikulich-Gilbertson, S. K. (2004). Factors associated with methadone maintenance treatment retention among street-recruited injection drug users. *Drug & Alcohol Dependence, 74*(2), 177–185. doi:10.1016/j.drugalcdep.2003.12.009.

Bruce, R. D. (2010). Methadone as HIV prevention: High volume methadone sites to decrease HIV incidence rates in resource limited settings. *International Journal of Drug Policy, 21*(2), 122–124. doi:10.1016/j.drugpo.2009.10.004.

Burke, S. E., Calabrese, S. K., Dovidio, J. F., Levina, O. S., Uuskula, A., Niccolai, L. M., Abel-Ollo, K., & Heimer, R. (2015). A tale of two cities: Stigma and health outcomes among people with HIV who inject drugs in St. Petersburg, Russia and Kohtla-Jarve, Estonia. *Social Science & Medicine, 130*, 154–161. doi:10.1016/j.socscimed.2015.02.018.

Calabrese, S. K., Burke, S. E., Dovidio, J. F., Levina, O. S., Uuskula, A., Niccolai, L. M., & Heimer, R. (2016). Internalized HIV and drug stigmas: Interacting forces threatening health status and health service utilization among people with HIV who inject drugs in St. Petersburg, Russia. *AIDS and Behavior, 20*(1), 85–97. doi:10.1007/s10461-015-1100-4.

Ciccarone, D. (2009). Heroin in brown, black and white: Structural factors and medical consequences in the US heroin market. *International Journal of Drug Policy, 20*(3), 277–282. doi:10.1016/j.drugpo.2008.08.003.

Connock, M., Juarez-Garcia, A., Jowett, S., Frew, E., Liu, Z., Taylor, R. J., Fry-Smith, A., Day, E., Lintzeris, N., Roberts, T., & Burls, A. (2007). Methadone and buprenorphine for the management of opioid dependence: A systematic review and economic evaluation. *Health Technology Assessment, 11*(9), 1–171, iii–iv. doi:10.3310/hta11090.

Des Jarlais, D. C. (2000). Structural interventions to reduce HIV transmission among injecting drug users. *AIDS, 14*(Suppl 1), S41–S46. doi:10.1097/00002030-200006001-00006.

Fullerton, C. A., Kim, M., Thomas, C. P., Lyman, D. R., Montejano, L. B., Dougherty, R. H., Daniels, A. S., Ghose, S. S., & Delphin-Rittmon, M. E. (2014). Medication-assisted treatment with methadone: Assessing the evidence. *Psychiatric Services, 65*(2), 146–157. doi:10.1176/appi.ps.201300235.

Gossop, M., Marsden, J., Stewart, D., & Treacy, S. (2001). Outcomes after methadone maintenance and methadone reduction treatments: Two-year follow-up results from the National Treatment Outcome Research Study. *Drug and Alcohol Dependence, 62*(3), 255–264. doi:10.1016/s0376-8716(00)00211-8.

Gupta, A., Mbwambo, J., Mteza, I., Shenoi, S., Lambdin, B., Nyandindi, C., Doula, B. I., Mfaume, S., & Bruce, R. D. (2014). Active case finding for tuberculosis among people who inject drugs on methadone treatment in Dar es Salaam, Tanzania. *International Journal of Tuberculosis and Lung Disease, 18*(7), 793–798. doi:10.5588/ijtld.13.0208.

Lambdin, B. H., Bruce, R. D., Chang, O., Nyandindi, C., Sabuni, N., Zamudio-Haas, S., McCurdy, S., Masao, F., Ivo, Y., Msami, A., & Ubuguy, O. (2013). Identifying programmatic gaps: Inequities in harm reduction service utilization among male and female drug users in Dar es Salaam, Tanzania. *PloS One, 8*(6), e67062. doi:10.1371/journal.pone.0067062.

Lambdin, B. H., Masao, F., Chang, O., Kaduri, P., Mbwambo, J., Magimba, A., Sabuni, N., & Bruce, R. D. (2014). Methadone treatment for HIV prevention-feasibility, retention, and predictors of attrition in Dar es Salaam, Tanzania: A retrospective cohort study. *Clinical Infectious Diseases, 59*(5), 735–742. doi:10.1093/cid/ciu382.

Lambdin, B. H., Mbwambo, J. K., Josiah, R. M., & Bruce, R. D. (2015). Service integration: Opportunities to expand access to antiretroviral therapy for people who inject drugs in Tanzania. *Journal of the International AIDS Society, 18*(1), 19936. doi:10.7448/ias.18.1.19936.

Liu, E., Liang, T., Shen, L., Zhong, H., Wang, B., Wu, Z., & Detels, R. (2009). Correlates of methadone client retention: A prospective cohort study in Guizhou province, China. *International Journal of Drug Policy, 20*(4), 304–308. doi:10.1016/j.drugpo.2008.09.004.

Magimba, A. (2015). *National scale up lan for medically assisted treatment using methadone for people who use drugs in Tanzania*. Dar es Salaam: Ministry of Health and Social Welfare.

Magura, S., Casriel, C., Goldsmith, D. S., Strug, D. L., & Lipton, D. S. (1988). Contingency contracting with polydrug-abusing methadone patients. *Addictive Behaviors, 13*(1), 113–118. doi:10.1016/0306-4603(88)90035-4.

McCurdy, S., & Kaduri, P. (2016). The political economy of heroin and crack in Tanzania. *Review of African Political Economy, 43*(148), 312–319. doi:10.1080/03056244.2016.1170678.

McCurdy, S., & Maruyama, H. (2013). Heroin use, trafficking, and intervention approache in Sub-saharan Africa: Local and global contexts. In T. Giles-Vernick & J. L. A. Webb Jr. (Eds.), *Global health in Africa: Historical perspectives on disease control* (pp. 211–232). Athens: Ohio University Press.

McCurdy, S. A., Williams, M. L., Kilonzo, G. P., Ross, M. W., & Leshabari, M. T. (2005a). Heroin and HIV risk in Dar es Salaam, Tanzania: Youth hangouts, mageto and injecting practices. *AIDS Care, 17*(Suppl 1), S65–S76. doi:10.1080/09540120500120930.

McCurdy, S. A., Williams, M. L., Ross, M. W., Kilonzo, G. P., & Leshabari, M. T. (2005b). A theme issue by, for, and about Africa: New injecting practice increases HIV risk among drug users in Tanzania. *BMJ, 331*(7519), 778. doi:10.1136/bmj.331.7519.778-a.

McCurdy, S. A., Ross, M. W., Kilonzo, G. P., Leshabari, M. T., & Williams, M. L. (2006). HIV/AIDS and injection drug use in the neighborhoods of Dar es Salaam, Tanzania. *Drug and Alcohol Dependence, 82*(Suppl 1), S23–S27. doi:10.1016/s0376-8716(06)80004-9.

McCurdy, S., Kilonzo, G. P., Williams, M., & Kaaya, S. (2007). Harm reduction in Tanzania: An urgent need for multisectoral intervention. *International Journal of Drug Policy, 18*(3), 155–159. doi:10.1016/j.drugpo.2007.05.001.

McCurdy, S. A., Ross, M. W., Williams, M. L., Kilonzo, G. P., & Leshabari, M. T. (2010). Flashblood: Blood sharing among female injecting drug users in Tanzania. *Addiction, 105*(6), 1062–1070. doi:10.1111/j.1360-0443.2010.02908.x.

McNeil, D Jr. (2010). Desperate addicts inject others' blood. *New York Times*. New York City.

Metzger, D. S., Woody, G. E., McLellan, A. T., O'Brien, C. P., Druley, P., Navaline, H., DePhilippis, D., Stolley, P., & Abrutyn, E. (1993). Human immunodeficiency virus seroconversion among intravenous drug users in- and out-of-treatment: An 18-month prospective follow-up. *Journal of Acquired Immune Deficiency Syndromes, 6*(9), 1049–1056.

Mlunde, L. B., Sunguya, B. F., Mbwambo, J. K., Ubuguyu, O. S., Shibanuma, A., Yasuoka, J., & Jimba, M. (2016). A mismatch between high-risk behaviors and screening of infectious diseases among people who inject drugs in Dar es Salaam, Tanzania. *PloS One, 11*(2), e0148598. doi:10.1371/journal.pone.0148598.

MoHSW & DCC. (2014). *Guideline for medically-assisted treatment of opioid dependence in Tanzania*. Unpublished Draft.

MoHSW & DCC (2015). *Guideline for medically assisted treatment of opioid dependence in Tanzania* (2nd ed.). Dar es Salaam.

NACP (2014). Consensus estimates on key population size and HIV prevalence in Tanzania. Dar es Salaam: National AIDS Control Program.

Njenga, F., Kiima, D., Siminyu, M., Munyi, E., Abdool, R., Muthui, M., Lambdin, B., Mbwambo, J., Mwamburi, E., McCurdy, S., Pick, B., Anderson, G., Mital, S., & Needle, R. (2012). Heroin scarcity in coastal Kenya: Consequence for persons who inject drugs (PWID) and national and provincial response to the crisis. *XIX International AIDS Conference*. Washington, DC.

Nyandindi, C., Mbwambo, J., McCurdy, S., Lambdin, B., Copenhaver, M., & Bruce, R. (2014). Prevalence of HIV, hepatitis C and depression among people who inject drugs in the Kinondoni Municipality in Dar Es Salaam, Tanzania. *Drug & Alcohol Dependence, 140*, e164. doi:10.1016/j.drugalcdep.2014.02.461.

Office of National Drug Control Policy. (n.d.). *The international heroin market*. https://www.whitehouse.gov/ondcp/global-heroin-market. Accessed 14 Oct 2016.

Ratliff, E. A., Kaduri, P., Masao, F., Mbwambo, J. K., & McCurdy, S. A. (2016). Harm reduction as a complex adaptive system: A dynamic framework for analyzing Tanzanian policies concerning heroin use. *International Journal of Drug Policy, 30*, 7–16. doi:10.1016/j.drugpo.2015.12.008.

Rhodes, T. (2009). Risk environments and drug harms: A social science for harm reduction approach. *International Journal of Drug Policy, 20*(3), 193–201. doi:10.1016/j.drugpo.2008.10.003.

Rhodes, T., Singer, M., Bourgois, P., Friedman, S. R., & Strathdee, S. A. (2005). The social structural production of HIV risk among injecting drug users. *Social Science & Medicine, 61*, 1026–1044. doi:10.1016/j.socscimed.2004.12.024.

Saleem, H. T., Mushi, D., Hassan, S., Douglas Bruce, R., Cooke, A., Mbwambo, J., & Lambdin, B. H. (2016). 'Can't you initiate me here?': Challenges to timely initiation on antiretroviral therapy among methadone clients in Dar es Salaam, Tanzania. *International Journal of Drug Policy, 30*, 59–65. doi:10.1016/j.drugpo.2015.12.009.

Sarasvita, R., Tonkin, A., Utomo, B., & Ali, R. (2012). Predictive factors for treatment retention in methadone programs in Indonesia. *Journal of Substance Abuse Treatment, 42*(3), 239–246. doi:10.1016/j.jsat.2011.07.009.

Soyka, M., Zingg, C., Koller, G., & Kuefner, H. (2008). Retention rate and substance use in methadone and buprenorphine maintenance therapy and predictors of outcome: Results from a randomized study. *International Journal of Neuropsychopharmacology, 11*(5), 641–653. doi:10.1017/s146114570700836x.

The Economist. (2015). *The smack track: Drug smuggling in Africa.* 17 January 2015. http://www.economist.com/news/middle-east-and-africa/21639560-east-african-states-are-being-undermined-heroin-smuggling-smack-track. Accessed 29 Apr 2017.

Tran, O. C., Bruce, R. D., Masao, F., Ubuguyu, O., Sabuni, N., Mbwambo, J., & Lambdin, B. H. (2015). Implementation and operational research: Linkage to care among methadone clients living with HIV in Dar es Salaam, Tanzania. *Journal of Acquired Immune Deficiency Syndromes, 69*(2), e43–e48. doi:10.1097/qai.0000000000000582.

Ubuguyu, O., Tran, O. C., Bruce, R. D., Masao, F., Nyandindi, C., Sabuni, N., McCurdy, S., Mbwambo, J., & Lambdin, B. H. (2016). Improvements in health-related quality of life among methadone maintenance clients in Dar es Salaam, Tanzania. *International Journal of Drug Policy, 30*, 74–81. doi:10.1016/j.drugpo.2016.03.005.

United Republic of Tanzania. (1995). *The Drugs and Prevention of Illicit Traffic in Drugs Act, Act No. 9 of 1995.* United Republic of Tanzania. https://www.fiu.go.tz/PreventionOfIllicitTrafficInDrugsAct.pdf. Accessed 29 Apr 2017.

United Republic of Tanzania. (2012). *Operational guidelines for the management of drug resistant TB in Tanzania* (1st ed.). Dar es Salaam: National TB and Leprosy Programme, Ministry of Health and Social Welfare. https://drive.google.com/file/d/0By0MeTLkdAyFbmhORUtqa09hWUE/view. Accessed 29 Apr 2017.

United Republic of Tanzania. (2013). *Manual for the management of tuberculosis and leprosy* (6th ed.). Dar es Salaam: National TB and Leprosy Programme Ministry of Health and Social Welfare.

United Republic of Tanzania. (2014). *Global AIDS response country progress report.* Dar es Salaam: Ministry of Health and Social Welfare. http://www.unaids.org/sites/default/files/country/documents/TZA_narrative_report_2014.pdf. Accessed 29 Apr 2017.

United Republic of Tanzania. (2015). *The Drug Control and Enforcement Act, Act No. 5 of 2015.* United Republic of Tanzania. http://www.parliament.go.tz/uploads/documents/1476204842-GN%20173-DRUGS%20CONTROL%20AND%20ENFORCEMENT%20(GENERAL)%20REGULATIONS,%202016.pdf. Accessed 29 Apr 2017.

WHO. (2012). *Global tuberculosis report 2012.* Geneva: WHO.

WHO. (2013). *Systematic screening for active tuberculosis: Principles and recommendations.* Geneva: WHO.

WHO, UNODC, & UNAIDS. (2012). *WHO, UNODC, UNAIDS technical guide for countries to set targets for universal acces to HIV prevention, treatment and care for injecting drug users – 2012 revision.* Geneva: WHO.

Wolfe, D., Carrieri, M. P., & Shepard, D. (2010). Treatment and care for injecting drug users with HIV infection: A review of barriers and ways forward. *Lancet, 376*(9738), 355–366. doi:10.1016/s0140-6736(10)60832-x.

Zamudio-Haas, S. (2013). *Providing medication assisted treatment (MAT) as an HIV prevention intervention: Programmatic strategies to maximize service utilization in Dar es Salaam, Tanzania.* Doctoral dissertation, University of California-Berkeley.

Zamudio-Haas, S., Mahenge, B., Saleem, H., Mbwambo, J., & Lambdin, B. H. (2016). Generating trust: Programmatic strategies to reach women who inject drugs with harm reduction services in Dar es Salaam, Tanzania. *International Journal of Drug Policy, 30*, 43–51. doi:10.1016/j.drugpo.2016.01.012.

# Part II
# Resilience

# Chapter 4
# No-One-Size-Fits-All: Addressing the Social and Structural Dimensions of Sex Worker Vulnerability to HIV Through Community Mobilization in Avahan

**Nimesh Dhungana, Kim M. Blankenship, Monica R. Biradavolu, Nehanda Tankasala, and Annie George**

## 4.1 Introduction

In recent years, community mobilization (CM) has gained prominence as a type of intervention to address structural conditions that produce HIV risk (Blankenship et al. 2006; Campbell and Cornish 2010; Cornish et al. 2010; Evans et al. 2010). Specifically, though CM can refer to community participation in intervention planning and implementation, it is a structural intervention when it involves the collective organization of marginalized communities for the purposes of challenging unequal relations and structures of power that underlie their vulnerability, including their vulnerability to HIV (Blankenship et al. 2006; Cornish et al. 2014; Evans et al. 2010). While increasingly recognized as a structural intervention, analyses of the various ways in which CM is conceptualized and operationalized for HIV prevention remain relatively scant. Attempting to advance a theory-based model of CM for HIV prevention, a recent study reviewed the literatures on social movements and community empowerment and development to suggest six key domains of CM that can be used for the development of CM interventions for HIV prevention (Lippman et al. 2013). In their systematic review of the impact of CM in HIV prevention interventions, Cornish et al. (2014) found that CM has stronger impacts on behavioral and social outcomes related to HIV prevention than on biomedical outcomes, and has reasonably consistent impacts among sex workers but less clear impacts on other communities. In contrast, in a systematic review, Kerrigan et al. (2015) found that community empowerment interventions among female sex workers (FSW) are associated with reductions in HIV prevalence and sexually transmitted infections (STI), as well as with increases in condom use (with clients but not non-client

N. Dhungana (✉) • K.M. Blankenship • M.R. Biradavolu • N. Tankasala • A. George
Department of Methodology, London School of Economics and Political Science, London, UK
e-mail: n.dhungana@lse.ac.uk



D. Kerrigan, C. Barrington (eds.), *Structural Dynamics of HIV*, Social Aspects of HIV 4, DOI 10.1007/978-3-319-63522-4_4

partners). Both reviews highlight variation with regards to operationalization of CM and measurement of CM impacts (Cornish et al. 2014; Kerrigan et al. 2015). Indeed, they each define their tasks somewhat differently, with one using the language of CM (Cornish et al. 2014) and the other the language of community empowerment (Kerrigan et al. 2015), and these differences may partly explain their varied results. In this chapter, we contribute further to understandings of CM interventions in HIV prevention – their implementation and impact – by focusing on the Avahan India AIDS Initiative (Avahan).

In December of 2003, the Bill & Melinda Gates Foundation (BMGF) launched Avahan as a large-scale HIV prevention program to control the spread of HIV in six high-prevalence states of India. A multi-level, multi-component intervention, Avahan aimed to address both 'proximal' (e.g. HIV knowledge, condom use and other sexual behaviors, drug use and related behaviors, STI) and 'distal' (e.g. stigma, violence, economic inequality, gender inequality) determinants of HIV (Avahan India AIDS Initiative 2010). Accordingly, it involved a combination of behavior change communication activities; activities to increase the availability and accessibility of services and products, such as establishing static and mobile STI clinics, distributing free condoms (including through peer outreach and social marketing), and providing for syringe exchange (for injection drug users); and activities targeted to the social and economic environment that marginalizes FSW, such as media advocacy to encourage more positive depictions of FSW, creation of violence response teams, and promotion of greater access to social entitlement programs (Avahan India AIDS Initiative 2008). CM was a cross-cutting and integral part of the intervention, with mobilized FSW engaging in all of these activities. Additionally, the CM model worked to create community-based organizations of FSW that would take ownership of the intervention and become responsible for its implementation and maintenance (Avahan India AIDS Initiative 2008, 2010).

Over the course of its implementation, a growing body of literature has analyzed the processes and impacts of Avahan's CM. These studies have described variations in both uptake and outcomes of CM across various geographic locations (Wheeler et al. 2012) and highlighted the complexity of evaluating a multi-pronged CM intervention (Galavotti et al. 2012; Laga and Vuylsteke 2011). In this chapter, we present a synthetic review of the existing literature (through 2014) on Avahan's CM approach to identify major findings from analyses of the implementation and evaluation of CM among FSW, as well as gaps in knowledge that have bearing on the future research and practice of CM, and on structural interventions more generally.

## 4.2 Methods

We draw on the method of Critical Interpretive Synthesis (CIS) associated with an interdisciplinary group of scholars led by Mary Dixon-Woods (Dixon-Woods et al. 2006, 2007). The method originated from the growing concern that traditional forms of systematic review are primarily limited to collecting and aggregating quantitative evaluation findings, and thus have the tendency to exclude non-experimental and qualitative research. In so doing, Dixon-Woods and colleagues argue systematic reviews are best for testing theories about 'what works' (Dixon-Woods et al. 2006: 2). In contrast, the CIS method allows for critically interpreting diverse sets of evidence (quantitative, qualitative, programmatic) in an ongoing effort to generate understanding not only of '*what*' an intervention has achieved, but also '*how*' and in '*what context*' it is implemented and how this may, in turn, relate to what it has achieved. Using this approach, rather than starting with pre-defined terms or focusing only on the impact of CM on specific outcomes, we used a series of guiding questions including: How is CM conceptualized and operationalized under Avahan?; How is CM measured under Avahan?; What are the main outcomes of Avahan's CM?; What are the implications of the study of implementation and evaluation of Avahan for the future practice of and research on HIV prevention? We then sought materials discussing and analyzing Avahan, including peer-reviewed articles, commentaries, case studies, programmatic monographs, and project reports. In total, we identified 209 journal articles (research articles and commentaries), 2 case studies, 76 monographs/reports and 8 book chapters. Abstracts of all 209 journal articles and all other materials were screened to select only those related to FSW. We conducted full-text review of materials that explicitly used the term 'community mobilization' or related terms, with the latter, in keeping with the iterative nature of CIS, continuing to be refined as the papers were reviewed to include community empowerment, participatory development, and collectivization. Through this process, we selected for detailed review and analysis a final group of 38 journal articles (research articles, commentaries) and 15 monographs/reports, of which 7 were from a combination of State Lead Partners, Capacity Building Partners and Knowledge Building Partners of Avahan, and 8 were BMGF's own reports/ policy guidelines. The process chart (Fig. 4.1) further explains the review methods and classification of materials.

Data extraction was done by two independent reviewers (first and fourth author) using an Excel spreadsheet. Qualitative and quantitative data for journal articles were extracted and coded along the following broad criteria: study characteristics (study location, study participants, time of study, sampling techniques, data collection methods); concepts and theories discussed; intervention characteristics; and key results/outcomes. Since most of the programmatic literature was not research-based but instead was comprised of guidelines and project descriptions by funder and implementation agencies, we focused data extraction and coding on the following dimensions: program/project description; strategies/approaches to CM; and programmatic outcomes of CM.

We also kept detailed notes on specific challenges of CM discussed in each study. These notes were subsequently compiled and grouped as emergent data related to inconsistencies and key gaps in implementation and evaluation of CM.

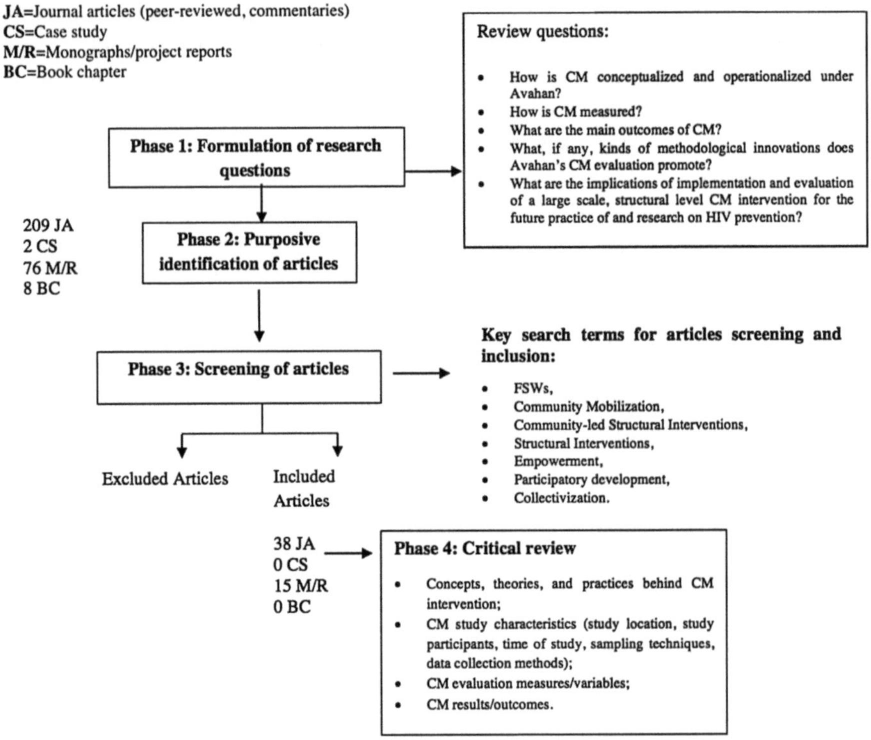


**Fig. 4.1** Review processs overview

## 4.3 Findings

We begin our discussion of the multiple ways that CM has been conceptualized, operationalized, and implemented in the context of Avahan, by highlighting key features of Avahan's overall implementation and rollout. From the outset, both organizationally and programmatically, Avahan was envisioned and implemented centrally as well as locally, reflecting a commitment to having a common multi-component intervention that would be adapted and reshaped in response to specific community needs and priorities, and diverse social and cultural contexts. Accordingly, Avahan was launched as a 10-year charter to change the course of the Indian HIV epidemic. The CM component was embedded as part of the overall initiative that followed three distinct phases of implementation: *start-up, scale-up* and *transition* (Wheeler et al. 2012). The *start-up* phase (2004–2005) involved conceptualization of the CM model alongside other components of the intervention. It was also marked by identification and selection of nine state-level implementing partners (State Lead Partners or SLPs) and capacity development partners (Avahan India AIDS Initiative 2008). SLPs, including a combination of national and international non-governmental organizations (NGOs), in turn, subcontracted major CM activities to local NGOs, to whom they provided technical and implementation support. The capacity development partners, on the other hand, assisted both the SLPs and local NGOs in the design and implementation of technical standards of community-led interventions and facilitated cross-sharing of findings from implementation. The second phase of *scale-up* (2006–2010) involved massive uptake of CM in conjunction with other intervention activities, including social marketing and distribution of free condoms, establishment of static and mobile STI diagnosis/treatment services and Drop-in-Centers (DICs), and dissemination of informational, educational, and communication (IEC) materials. In the final stage of *transition* (2010–2015) the financial and administrative responsibility for the intervention was handed over to the Government of India and community-based organizations (CBOs). Although our review included materials related to each of these different phases, we focus here primarily on findings related to the *start-up* and *scale-up* phases of the implementation, as these are the periods most covered by the extant literature.

### 4.3.1 Community Mobilization: Variation in Terminology, Definitions and Concepts

In our review of key programmatic documents, we identified multiple conceptualizations and operational definitions of CM beginning with the terminology itself. Originally, in defining its vision for CM, Avahan used the language of 'Community Led Structural Interventions (CLSI)', with FSW ownership and management of the intervention, empowerment of FSW, and capacity building as central programmatic goals (Avahan India AIDS Initiative 2005). This initial definition drew on inputs from individuals, such as Dr. Smarajit Jana, who were in the forefront of designing and implementing the Sonagachi project in Kolkata, India, a widely acclaimed FSW-led CM intervention. Indeed, at start-up, Dr. Jana was based at CARE India and the PI on a grant from BMGF to build capacity for implementing CM, defined as community led structural interventions (Ghose et al. 2008; Jana et al. 2004). Over the course of the start-up phase, however, Avahan adopted new terminology for CM, 'Peer Outreach, Community Mobilization, and Local Advocacy for Vulnerability Reduction' (Avahan India AIDS Initiative 2010), where community participation remained the central tenet, but the term *community mobilization* was made an explicit focus. The new conceptualization saw inclusion of 'collective efficacy', 'collective agency', 'social cohesion', and 'collective action' as elements of CM. In addition, creation of an enabling environment for HIV prevention received prominence as one of the central intervention outcomes. To a degree, these changes in the conceptualization and operational definition of CM resulted from intense critiques, contestations, and negotiations of the CLSI framing among a web of stakeholders, including Avahan leadership, SLPs, and capacity building partners, with each representing differing notions and visions of CM. Avahan leadership, who came from mostly business management and, to a lesser extent, public health backgrounds

(Laga and Vuylsteke 2011), had to realign the concepts and use of terms by engaging in a series of workshops, trainings, and consultations with implementing agencies and capacity building partners, who represented diverse fields of community activism, participatory development, organizational development, and health promotion. This process of sharing and critiquing was critical in stimulating programmatic adjustments. As one example, the 24-h Crisis Response System, which is managed and run by FSW volunteers, was not part of the original CM design. However, after the initial rounds of interactions with implementing agencies and FSW communities, it became clear that violence and discrimination were barriers to the adoption of safe sex practices. Consequently, the Crisis Response System, initially implemented by a few NGOs within Avahan, was incorporated and scaled up as a major CM component (Avahan India AIDS Initiative 2009a).

In Table 4.1, we present a sample inventory of the range of different approaches to CM within and across different intervention sites. The third column reflects the variation in terminology used to refer to CM, even within the Avahan program. It includes 'Community-led HIV/AIDS prevention project' (Argento et al. 2011), 'Multi-layered violence prevention program' (Beattie et al. 2010), 'Community-led structural intervention' (Blankenship et al. 2008), 'Rights-based approach' (Reza-Paul et al. 2008), 'Community collectivization strategy' (Gaikwad et al. 2012), and 'Community-to-CBO learning strategy' (Sadhu et al. 2014).

Beyond terminology, a range of strategies is used to accomplish CM (Table 4.1, Column 4). Many of these share a lineage with established and emergent practices of participatory development, community organizing, and organizational development, among others (Avahan India AIDS Initiative 2008, 2009a, b; Gaikwad et al. 2012; Reza-Paul et al. 2008; Sadhu et al. 2014; Wheeler et al. 2012). Peer outreach, for instance, draws on the concepts of participatory development to increase FSW involvement not only in utilization of prevention services, but also in planning, management, and monitoring of DICs and STI clinics. These DICs and STI clinics are, in turn, used as sites for collective action to challenge power imbalances that put FSW at risk of HIV. We also see CM taking a combined character of organizational development and community organizing through establishment of FSW-led CBOs. For instance, the Aastha Project in Maharashtra focuses on a FSW-led capacity building strategy that draws on a bottom-up approach to community organizing. This is achieved by establishing Aastha *gat*, a self-help group with a FSW-led structure at the grass-roots level, which would in turn affiliate with a regional-level federation of CBOs (Aastha Family) for policy advocacy (Aastha Monograph 2010 2010; Gaikwad et al. 2012). Likewise, some activities leveraged social capital practices by building and linking FSW networks with more powerful, yet like-minded, rights groups/organizations (Rau 2013b) to make government agencies accountable to FSW needs (Rau 2013a).

Specific CM activities are carried out to address distinct forms of risk environments facing specific intervention sites. For instance, by framing HIV as an occupational health issue, Ashodhaya collective in Mysore, Karnataka tailored their activities to address sex work-related stigma and violence (Argento et al. 2011). Likewise, Care Saksham, a local chapter of international NGO Care, based in the

**Table 4.1** Community mobilization intervention: multiple approaches and definitions

| Study | Site | Intervention referred to as | Key CM strategies |
|---|---|---|---|
| Argento et al. (2011) | Mysore City, Karnataka | Community-led HIV/AIDS Prevention Project | DICs |
| | | | Crisis response |
| | | | Police and public advocacy |
| | | | Community patrolling |
| Beattie et al. (2010) | Mysore City, Karnataka | Multi-layered Violence Prevention Program | Policy-level advocacy with government officials |
| | | | Sensitization/training with police, lawyers, and the media |
| | | | Psychological enhancement of sex workers through peer-mediated outreach |
| Beattie et al. (2014) | Four districts in Karnataka (Belgaum, Bellary, Shimoga, and Bangalore) | Community mobilization and Empowerment Strategy | Phased implementation of the CM intervention: |
| | | | Recruitment of peer educators and establishment of safe DICs with provision of clinical services |
| | | | Development of critical thinking skills of FSW; support collective action to work with policy makers, the police, government officials, human rights lawyers, and the media |
| | | | Formation of community based institutions like peer groups or collectives to sustain CM activities |
| Blankenship et al. (2010) | Rajahmundry, East Godavari District, Andhra Pradesh | Community-led Structural Intervention (*Saksham* Project) | Mobilizing through Social Change Agents |
| | | | Health literacy training |
| | | | DICs |
| | | | Public awareness, advocacy on behalf of FSW |
| | | | Sensitization programs targeted to police |
| | | | Establishment of CBOs |
| | | | Training community members for CBO participation |
| | | | Credit services and income generation activities for FSW |
| | | | Media events and rallies |
| | | | Community kitchens as part of income generating activities |
| | | | Exposure visits to other intervention sites |
| | | | Advocacy-related capacity building efforts |

(continued)

**Table 4.1** (continued)

| Study | Site | Intervention referred to as | Key CM strategies |
|---|---|---|---|
| Chakravarthy et al. (2012) | 9 Coastal Districts of Andhra Pradesh | Community mobilization intervention (*Swagati* Project) | Participatory site assessment with NGO involvement |
| | | | Identification of FSW 'hotspots' |
| | | | Recruiting and training community guides (peer educators) |
| | | | Formation of small groups (hotspot groups) and Community Mobilization Committees |
| Gaikwad et al. (2012) | Mumbai and Thane, Maharashtra | Community Collectivization Strategy (*Aastha* Project) | Legal literacy training |
| | | | Networking meetings with bar owners |
| | | | Peer-educator led meetings |
| | | | Training to develop negotiation skills to help others in times of crisis |
| | | | CBO building |
| Gurnani et al. (2011) | 18 districts of Karnataka | Rights-based approach | Trainings and sensitization programs |
| | | | Representation in District AIDS Committees (DACs) |
| | | | Peer-mediated outreach |
| | | | DICs |
| | | | Literacy classes |
| | | | Social entitlement workshops |
| Reza-Paul et al. (2008) | Mysore City, Karnataka | Rights-based approach to CM (*Asodhaya* Collective) | Participatory mapping and enumeration |
| | | | Peer-mediated outreach |
| | | | Advocacy with different stakeholders-government people, local shopkeepers, clients and partners, police; |
| | | | Provide DICs as safe space for collectivization, and promotion of sense of camaraderie and kinship |
| | | | Crisis Intervention Teams |
| | | | Advocacy to address occupational hazards such as violence |
| | | | Legal literacy, negotiation skills, and on-the-job training on how to handle crises |

(continued)

East Godavari district of Andhra Pradesh, recruited and trained Peer Educators (PEs) known as Social Change Agents, to support FSW in addressing both proximal causes, such as lack of HIV knowledge, and distal causes of HIV risk, such as unequal power relationships between sex workers and their male clients, and violence from clients and police (CARE 2009; George et al. 2015; Magar et al. 2009). CM activities are also adapted based on different typologies of sex work – brothel-,

**Table 4.1** (continued)

| Study | Site | Intervention referred to as | Key CM strategies |
|---|---|---|---|
| Sadhu et al. (2014) | Eight districts of Andhra Pradesh | The community-to-CBO learning strategy (under the SAKSHAM) | Phased implementation: |
| | | | Identifying learning or intervention sites that have successfully formed FSW CBOs |
| | | | Selection and capacity building of community faculty |
| | | | Organizing on-site capacity building workshops to demonstrate community mobilization learning elements (covered various aspects of community mobilization, such as understanding the community, self-esteem, attitudinal adjustment, and orientation on the National AIDS Control Program's (NACO) community mobilization strategy) |
| | | | Organizing skills-building workshops |
| | | | Community faculty to enhance their training skills |
| | | | Recruiting a mentoring team and providing on-site mentoring |
| | | | Reviewing progress through participatory sharing meetings |
| | | | Evaluating the impact of the community development strategy |

bar- home-, and street-based – and can take multiple forms when implemented in areas where sex work itself takes multiple forms (Gaikwad et al. 2012). There are also examples of context-specific approaches to CM where the governance of STI clinics is managed by FSW, leading to increased levels of service acceptance and utilization (Beattie et al. 2012). In some instances, community acceptance and ownership has been generated by providing FSW communities the authority to name the specific component of the CM interventions, such as Crisis Intervention Teams. Such efforts, although symbolic, are viewed as instrumental in generating community ownership of the process of collectivization (Avahan India AIDS Initiative 2009b).

The above highlights that definitions of, and approaches to, CM are variedly adapted to suit local needs and contexts. Nevertheless, our analysis shows considerable similarities in the use of terms and approaches to CM. In particular, *participation*, *empowerment* and *collectivization* of FSW are recurring terms. While in some instances they are used interchangeably, in others they represent distinct approaches and outcomes. Participation mostly entails a multi-pronged strategy for increasing

FSW involvement in the design and implementation of specific prevention activities (e.g. participatory needs assessment, micro-planning, community mapping, peer-outreach). Empowerment (e.g. psycho-social training, mentorship support, leadership development) and collectivization (e.g. FSW-led CBO formation, advocacy), on the other hand, serve as broader goals, aimed at influencing both the individual and structural conditions that increase FSW's exposure to HIV. By clustering these approaches to three recurring and broad themes, we do not intend to suggest a comprehensive, evidence-based model of CM. Consistent with findings from newly published research on systematic assessment of implementation of CM interventions (Cornish et al. 2014; Kerrigan et al. 2015; Lippman et al. 2013), we call for further research in constructing an evidence-based and theoretically-informed classification of definitions of and approaches to CM for HIV prevention that can be tailored and adapted to the needs of specific local settings.

### 4.3.2 *Community Mobilization: Shared Features and Recurring Strategies*

Despite a multitude of meanings, interpretations, and operational strategies, there are also important similarities in approaches to CM across different intervention sites. Each shares a common goal to address various forms of *power* inequalities that make FSW vulnerable to HIV. In particular, we found the following as recurring approaches to CM under Avahan:

- **Outreach through Peer Educators (PEs) often operating simultaneously as community organizers:** PEs are FSW who provide HIV prevention outreach to other members of the FSW community. Under Avahan's CM model, PEs are involved in mapping, outreach, and micro-planning[1] ('Micro-planning in peer led outreach programs' 2013). Besides providing FSW peers with a package of HIV services (e.g. condom distribution, IEC materials), Avahan's PEs also organize FSW to address issues such as access to health and educational services, stigma and discrimination, and violence. Additionally, PEs use various forms of community-based monitoring tools to capture vulnerabilities to HIV, including experiences of violence (reported violence from regular partners, pimps, police, and local thugs) and alcohol or substance abuse (reported by the individual or by colleagues) (Avahan India AIDS Initiative 2009b, d). In some instances, PEs explicitly act as community organizers, working to promote broad social change goals (George et al. 2015).
- **Crisis Intervention Teams (CITs)**: The crisis response is primarily created to address violence and harassment faced by FSW. The CITs are equipped with

[1] Micro-planning is a process that decentralizes outreach management and planning to grassroots-level workers – outreach workers and peer educators – and allows them to make decisions on how to best reach the maximum number of community members.

trained teams of FSW who respond rapidly and in person to incidents of violence against other FSW. CITs also include external members like lawyers, human rights activists, state human rights council members, youth leaders, doctors, political leaders, and representatives from underprivileged communities (Avahan India AIDS Initiative 2009c; Magar et al. 2009).

- **Advocacy**: Advocacy and sensitization activities targeted to police, media, policy makers, and lawmakers are found consistently across different sites. These activities are intended to address stigma and discrimination facing FSW and make government and police responsive to FSW needs.
- **Drop in Centers (DICs)**: DICs, which are often referred to as safe spaces, are used by FSW to rest and share HIV and other related information. DICs may be attached to STI clinics or housed separately to serve the distinct objective of increasing cohesion among FSW groups that may later develop into CBOs (Rau 2013a).
- **Social Entitlement:** A major source of FSW vulnerability to HIV is their lack of welfare and access to social entitlement programs such as ration cards and voter ID. CM involves collectivizing FSW to ensure access to these services. Similarly, CM has played a synergistic role in linking and referring FSW to other social/health services, as well as other like-minded institutions.
- **Capacity Building**: Trainings in FSW leadership development, legal literacy, self-esteem, and confidence enhancement are a standard component of the CM model. There is also a focus on organizational development involving establishment and support of self-help groups, increasing FSW membership in CBOs, and formation of committees and CBOs run by FSW. This two-pronged approach to individual and organization building is observed across multiple intervention sites.

### 4.3.3 *Community Mobilization Evaluation: Distinctions in Measurement and Outcomes*

Structural interventions are challenging to evaluate. In particular, structural interventions that lack specific control and treatment groups call for innovation in evaluation designs to understand the dynamic processes that shape HIV outcomes (Auerbach et al. 2011). Mixed-methods analysis, identification of long- and short-term measures, as well as consideration of contexts are critical in designing and evaluating them (Pronyk et al. 2013).

In the case of Avahan, the absence of a randomized controlled trial and the lack of comprehensive baseline data have posed challenges for attributing outcomes to the intervention in general and CM in particular (Bertozzi et al. 2010; Evans et al. 2010). Lack of adequate CM measures in the initial evaluation design, coupled with the overlapping nature of intervention components, have further contributed to the challenge (Chandrasekaran et al. 2008). This challenge, to a greater or lesser extent, has been addressed through internal and external impact evaluation components supported by Avahan. Internally, Avahan's CM is informed by a theory-of-change that guides its major outputs, activities, and measures of progress (Wheeler et al. 2012). Indicators of CM are integrated into the computerized system for continuous reporting, monitoring, and programmatic decision-making. As an external evaluation component, a varied group of researchers with different disciplinary backgrounds – anthropology, demography, economics, family health sciences, public health, and sociology – have sought to unravel the impacts of CM using a combination of data sources, including integrated biological and behavioral surveys, cross-sectional surveys, ethnographic research, case studies, and participatory research.

As discussed, we observed significant conceptual and definitional differences within and among these studies and in turn distinct methodological approaches utilized for CM evaluation. From a rights-based framework (Argento et al. 2011) to structural intervention (Blankenship et al. 2006; Reza-Paul et al. 2012), networked governance (Biradavolu et al. 2009) to collective empowerment (Blanchard et al. 2013), social cognitive theory (Gaikwad et al. 2012) to organizational development (Chakravarthy et al. 2012), researchers have used a wide range of theoretical constructs to inform their evaluation of CM as implemented under Avahan. The variables and measures used for impact assessment also represent a diversity of interests and evaluation agendas of researchers. While some have focused on understanding the causal relationship between program exposure (e.g. contact by PE) and service utilization (e.g. attendance at STI clinics, DICs) (Blankenship et al. 2010), others have sought to examine how specific components of CM, such as membership in and collective action through FSW-led CBOs are independently associated with program outcomes (Gaikwad et al. 2012). Still, others have sought to examine the interplay between FSW collective power and sources of HIV risk (e.g. violence, stigma) through both quantitative and qualitative techniques (Argento et al. 2011; Beattie et al. 2010; Biradavolu et al. 2012).

Major evaluation findings can be clustered into three categories: *service outcome*, *epidemic outcome* and *social outcome*. *Service outcome* entails availability and utilization of CM services, broadly measured in terms of outreach by PE, increased awareness about the intervention, and utilization of key services such as peer support, STI clinics, and DICs. *Epidemic outcome* involves measures that are critical in improving safe sexual risk practices that, in turn, reduce HIV acquisition and transmission. We cluster these in terms of consistent condom use with different clients, HIV testing, reduction in HIV prevalence and infections, and decline in STI infections. *Social outcome* represents changes in social and structural conditions that are vital not only in attaining HIV prevention goals, but in addressing HIV-related vulnerability confronting FSW communities more generally. These are broadly measured by reduction in level of violence, reduction in cases of stigma and discrimination, improvement in FSW's access to social entitlements, increased control over sex work (e.g. ability to decide type of sex, amount of money charged) and improvement in collectivization of FSW (e.g. membership in FSW-led CBOs).

As Table 4.2 demonstrates, various studies have found Avahan CM interventions to produce *service outcome,* in terms of increased availability and coverage of peer

**Table 4.2** Community mobilization: multiple types of intervention outcomes

| Citation | Study design | Service outcome | Epidemic outcome | Social outcome |
|---|---|---|---|---|
| Argento et al. (2011) | Ethnographic data | NA* | NA | Increased empowerment of FSW to recognize and speak out against violence and stigma |
| | | | | Decreased violence from police |
| | | | | Increased self esteem |
| | | | | Reduced level of stigma |
| Beattie et al. (2010) | Integrated Behavioral-Biological Assessments (IBBA) (n = 3852) + Polling Booth Survey (PBS) (n = 7638) | NA | NA | By the follow-up surveys, significant reductions in FSW reporting violence (IBBA 13.0 % vs. 9.0 %, aOR 0.7, 95 % CI 0.5–0.9, p < 0.01; PBS 27.3 % vs. 18.9 %, crude OR 0.5, 95 % CI 0.4–0.5, p < 0.001) |
| | Location: Karnataka | | | |
| Beattie et al. (2014) | IBBA Surveys I and II (In 2008, n = 1975; in 2011, n = 1934) | By the 2008 survey, 95.3 % of FSW reported having met a peer educator; 82.0 % reported having attended an NGO meeting; 73.5 % reported that they had visited a project drop-in center | FSW with high CM exposure were more likely to have been tested for HIV (aOR 25.13, CI 13.07 to 48.34) and less likely to be infected with gonorrhea and/or chlamydia (aOR 0.53, CI 0.31–0.87) | FSW who were highly exposed to CM were significantly more likely than those with low exposure to report all measures of collective and individual power such as: |
| | Location: Four districts in Karnataka (Belgaum, Bellary, Shimoga, and Bangalore) | | No significant associations between level of CM exposure and HIV or syphilis prevalence | I feel a strong sense of unity with FSW I do not know (78.5 % vs. 95.0 %, aOR 3.99, CI 2.34–6.80, p < 0.01) |
| | | | | In last 6 months attended rally or other public event where could be identified as FSW (1.2 % vs. 19.1 %, aOR 13.90, CI 3.26–59.22, p < 0.01) |

(continued)

**Table 4.2** (continued)

| Citation | Study design | Service outcome | Epidemic outcome | Social outcome |
|---|---|---|---|---|
| Bhattacharjee et al.(2013) | Behavioral Tracking Survey (BTS) (n = 1750), IBBA I (n = 2312) and II (n = 2387) | NA | Compared to non-members, peer group members (IBBA participants) had a lower prevalence of: gonorrhea and/or chlamydia (5.2 % vs. 9.6 %, $p < 0.001$), and of syphilis (8.2 % vs. 10.3 %, $p < 0.05$) | FSW with CBO membership (BTS participants), compared to non-members, reported: |
| | Location: Karnataka | | | Less physical violence in the past 6 months (19.7 % vs. 28.2 %, $p < 0.001$) |
| | | | | Having paid less bribes to police to avoid trouble (88.5 % vs. 82.3 %, $p < 0.001$) |
| | | | | Less instances of forced sex (15.8 % vs. 19.5 %, $p < 0.10$) |
| Biradavolu et al. (2009) | Ethnographic data | NA | NA | Increased feelings of individual and collective power against violence and stigma |
| | Location: Rajahmundry, Andhra Pradesh | | | Increased collectivization of FSW community following NGO and CBO-led CM intervention |
| | | | | Development of networked governance model of the CIT critical to effective FSW collectivization |
| Biradavolu et al. (2012) | Ethnographic data | NA | NA | CBOs were instrumental in addressing sex worker stigma among FSW |
| | Location: Rajahmun dry, AP | | | FSW members associated with CBOs more likely to consider sex work as legitimate work |

| | | | | |
|---|---|---|---|---|
| Blanchard et al. (2013) | BTS (n = 1750) | NA | NA | In Solapur and Dharwad (lower intensity CM programs), 62 % and 71 % of FSW respectively, reported membership in a CBO, compared to > than 80 % in the higher intensity CM districts ($p < 0.001$) |
| | Karnataka, 4 districts-Belgaum, Gulbarga, Gadag, and Dharwad; Maharashtra, 1 district-Solapur | | | The odds of having a high versus low autonomy level and never versus ever experiencing violence were 1.22 and 1.43 times higher respectively for every one unit increase in power within level in the high-intensity districts ($p < 0.01$) |
| Blankenship et al. (2008) | Parivartan Serial cross sectional survey (Apr-June 2006; n = 812) | NA | FSW reporting both program exposure and collective agency 2.5 times more likely than other FSW to report consistent condom use (CCU) ($p < 0.005$) | Active utilization of CM services associated with *collective power* (collective identity aOR 2.47, CI 1.56–3.92, $p < 0.001$; collective efficacy aOR 3.66, CI 2.52–5.3, $p < 0.001$; collective agency aOR 11.43, CI 7.63–17.14, $p < 0.001$) |
| | Location: East Godavari, Andhra Pradesh | | | |
| Blankenship et al. (2010) | Parivartan Serial cross sectional surveys I and II (Apr–June 2006, n = 812; Mar–May 2007, n = 673) | Increased awareness of the intervention between baseline and follow up (41.8 % vs. 69.6 %) | NA | NA |
| | Location: East Godavari, Andhra Pradesh | Active utilization of the intervention between baseline and follow up (49.2 % vs. 61.0 %) | | |

(continued)

**Table 4.2** (continued)

| Citation | Study design | Service outcome | Epidemic outcome | Social outcome |
|---|---|---|---|---|
| Chakaravarthy et al. (2012) | Community Ownership and Preparedness (COPI) Assessment (n = 11 CBOs) and BTS (Krishna district: n = 400; Vizianagaram district: n = 395) | NA | NA | Empowerment of FSW in terms of accessing services from government and nongovernment sources |
| | | | | CBOs instrumental in enhancing social cohesion among the sex workers and their capacity to address local barriers to safe sex practices |
| Dixon et al. (2012) | Ethnographic data | Increased utilization of STI services by FSW through promotion of sexual health as occupational health | NA | Decreased stigma around sex work and STIs |
| | | | | Increased feelings of sense of sex work as work |
| | | | | Increased self esteem |
| Erausquin et al. (2012) | Parivartan Serial cross sectional surveys I, II, III (Apr–June 2006, n = 812; March–May 2007, n = 673; and Nov 2009 – Feb 2010; n = 850) | NA | CCU with clients showed a trend of increasing over time (56.3 %, 72.0 % and 75.3 % in rounds I, II and III respectively; $p < 0.001$) | NA |
| | Location: East Godavari, Andhra Pradesh | | | |

| | | | | |
|---|---|---|---|---|
| Gaikwad et al. (2012) | Behavior Tracking Survey (n = 2106) | NA | FSW reporting higher collective efficacy are more likely than those reporting low collective efficacy to negotiate condom use with occasional clients (60.3 % vs. 19.7 %, aOR 6.3, 95 % CI 4.8–8.4) and with regular partners (62.8 % vs. 20.2 %, aOR 6.4, 95 % CI 4.9–8.4) | FSW (with high degree of collective efficacy) more likely to: |
| | Location: 411 intervention sites in Mumbai and Thane, Maharashtra | | | Stand up to police and madams/brokers to help fellow FSW (5.8 % vs. 3.3 %, aOR 2.7, 95 % CI 1.5–4.9); |
| | | | | More confident in supporting fellow FSW in a crisis (76.1 % vs. 49.6 %, aOR 2.9, 95 % CI 2.2–3.7) |
| Gurnani et al. (2011) | Routine program data (MIS), media reports | Across 83 project sites, an average of 50,000 FSW are contacted by peer educators each month | NA | Between 2006 and 2009, a total of 46,194 FSW were referred for social entitlement programs (voter identification, bank account, subsidized housing, and children for subsidized school or hostel admission food ration cards), with 27,355 (59 %) receiving these by the end of 2009 |
| | Location: 18 districts of Karnataka | | | Increase in the number of FSW becoming members of FSW organizations (CBOs, self-help groups and community committees) [8,000 in January 2007 to 37,000 by October 2009] |
| Kuhlmann et al. (2014) | BTS IV (n = 1986), Cluster-Level Community Participation Survey (CLCPS), Andhra Pradesh | NA | 61 % of the propensity weighted sample reported high CCU (i.e. using condoms at every sex act with both regular and occasional clients) | Strength of CM was positively associated with psychosocial mediators and collectivization at the cluster level, including: increased self-confidence for advice/opinion giving ($p < 0.05$), increased collective identity ($p < 0.05$), increased collective efficacy for working toward specific goals ($p < 0.01$), and increased social cohesion ($p < 0.01$) |

(continued)

**Table 4.2** (continued)

| Citation | Study design | Service outcome | Epidemic outcome | Social outcome |
|---|---|---|---|---|
| Parimi et al. (2012) | BTS (n = 1986)<br>Location: Five districts (Khammam, Warangal, Kurnool, Medak and Ananthapur) of Andhra Pradesh | NA | NA | Compared to FSW with low degree of overall collectivization, FSW with high degree of collectivization were significantly more likely to report: high self-efficacy to use government health facilities (75.0 % vs. 57.3 %, aOR 2.5, 95 % CI 2.0 to 3.1) and to use government health centers for STI treatment in past year (78.1 % vs. 63.2 %, aOR 2.1, 95 % CI 1.6 to 2.8) |
| Punyam et al. (2012) | BTS (n = 1986) and interview with outreach workers<br>Location: In five districts of Andhra Pradesh, namely Khammam, Warangal, Kurnool, Medak and Ananthapur | NA | NA | Sites with active community advisory groups (CAGs), compared to their counterparts, had a significantly higher mean number of FSW linked to: ration cards (12.8 vs. 6.8, $p < 0.01$), bank accounts (9.3 vs. 5.9, $p < 0.05$) and health insurance (13.1 vs. 7.0, $p < 0.02$); They also reported fairer treatment by police now compared to year prior (79.7 % vs. 70.3 %; $p < 0.05$) and that the police explained the reasons for arrest when arrested the last time (95.7 % vs. 87 %; $p < 0.05$) |

| | | | | |
|---|---|---|---|---|
| Ramesh et al. (2010) | IBBA I and II (n = 4712) | NA | By IBBA II, there were reductions in the prevalence of HIV (19.6 % vs. 16.4 %, aOR 0.81, 95 % CI 0.67 to 0.99, p = 0.04); high-titre syphilis (5.9 % vs. 3.4 %, aOR 0.53, 95 % CI 0.37–0.77, p = 0.001); and chlamydia and/or gonorrhea (8.9 % vs. 7.0 %, aOR 0.72, 95 % CI, 0.54–0.94, p = 0.02) | NA |
| | Location: Five districts of Karnataka (Mysore, Belagaum, Shimoga, Bellary, and Bangalore Urban) | | Reported condom use at last sex increased significantly for repeat clients (66.1 % vs. 0.84.1 %, aOR 1.98, 95 % CI 1.58–2.48, p < 0.001) and marginally for occasional clients (82.9 % vs. 88.0 %, aOR 1.22, 95 % CI 0.89–1.66, p = 0.2), but remained stable for regular partners (32 %) | |
| Reza-Paul et al. (2008) | IBBA and II (in 2004, n = 429; in 2006, n = 425) | Increased number of FSW visited by a peer educator from baseline to follow up (64.1 % vs. 95.1 %, aOR 13.77, CI 7.84–24.19, p < 0.001) | CCU increased between baseline and follow-up surveys with: occasional clients (65 % vs. 90 %, p < 0001); repeat clients (53 % vs, 66 %, p < 0.001); and regular partners (7 % vs. 30 %, p < 0.001) | NA |
| | Location: Mysore, Karnataka | Increased proportion of FSW visiting the DIC (56.5 % vs. 89.6 %, aOR 7.80, CI 5.04–12.07, p < 0.001) | STI prevalence declined from baseline to follow-up: syphilis (25 % vs. 12 %, p < 0.001); trichomonas infection (33 % vs. 14 %, p < 0.00); chlamydial infection (11 % vs. 5 %, p < 0.001); gonorrhea (5 % vs. 2 %, p < 0.03). HIV prevalence remained stable (26 % vs. 24 %) | |

(continued)

**Table 4.2** (continued)

| Citation | Study design | Service outcome | Epidemic outcome | Social outcome |
|---|---|---|---|---|
| Saggurti et al. (2013) | BTS (n = 3557) | NA | Compared to FSW who reported low collective efficacy, FSW with high collective efficacy were more likely to report CCU with occasional clients (76.7 % vs. 71.6 %, aOR 1.3, 95 % CI 1.1–1.7) and with regular clients (69.1 % vs. 61.9 %, aOR 1.4, 95 % CI 1.1–1.9) | FSW with high level of collective efficacy were more likely to report self-efficacy for: |
| | Location: AP, 9 program districts | | | Condom use (71.4 % vs. 63.5 %, aOR 1.5, 95 % CI: 1.1–2.0) |
| | | | | STI service utilization from government health facilities (60.5 % vs. 37.3 %, aOR 2.6, 95 % CI: 2.1–3.2) |
| Yadav et al. (2013) | IBBA 2009–2010 (n = 7806) | NA | Exposure to community groups associated with: | NA |
| | Location: 3 administrative districts of Andhra Pradesh, Maharashtra and Tamil Nadu. | | Lower STI presence by 4 % (95 % CI: –5.6 to – 3.4, $p < 0.001$), as compared to no exposure. However, this was not found in self-reporting of any STI symptoms | |
| | | | Increased self-reported STI symptom treatment-seeking behavior by 13.7 % (95 % CI: 12.0–17.1, $p < 0.001$), as compared to no exposure | |

NA* means data not applicable for particular outcome

outreach services and increased utilization of STI treatment services (Blankenship et al. 2010). Results also suggest significant outcomes in improving *epidemic outcome*, in terms of decreased HIV and STI prevalence (Bhattacharjee et al. 2013; Ramesh et al. 2010). Several studies have also found increased consistent condom use (based on client types) associated with exposure to community mobilization (Blankenship et al. 2008; Erausquin et al. 2012; Gaikwad et al. 2012; Saggurti et al. 2013). *Social outcomes* represent mutually reinforcing changes at the levels of individual, community, and society. At the individual-psychological level, CM has helped address self-stigmatization (Dixon et al. 2012) and increased levels of self-esteem and self-confidence (Argento et al. 2011; Dixon et al. 2012), as well as increased sense of individual empowerment to access prevention services (Chakravarthy et al. 2012). Similarly, community-level changes are reported through increased FSW group membership/organizational involvement, intended to safeguard one another against exploitative situations (Bhattacharjee et al. 2013; Chakravarthy et al. 2012; Gaikwad et al. 2012). Changes are observed at the broader/societal level in terms of reduction in physical and sexual violence facing the FSW community (Argento et al. 2011; Beattie et al. 2010; Reza-Paul et al. 2012), increased level of collective power among FSW (Blankenship et al. 2008; Blanchard et al. 2013), increased acceptance of sex work as a legitimate profession (Dixon et al. 2012), increased level of coalition between and among FSW and other social groups/NGOs (Biradavolu et al. 2009), reduced stigma affecting the FSW community (Biradavolu et al. 2012; Dixon et al. 2012), improvement in the enabling environment through provisions of entitlements (Gurnani et al. 2011; Punyam et al. 2012), and access to and use of government health facilities (Parimi et al. 2012).

## 4.4 Community Mobilization Implementation and Evaluation: Challenges and Gaps

While our review of the evidence points to promising results related to the use of CM to reduce FSW vulnerability to HIV, we also documented a number of challenges related to its implementation and evaluation. Some of these challenges likely reflect the ever-changing social and sex work environments within multiple locations in India, while others are related to the more universal nature and process of CM intervention and evaluation. Both types of challenges offer insights and directions for future research and practice related to structural interventions for HIV prevention among FSW and other key populations, in India and globally.

Though the previous section highlights various epidemic impacts, our review of analyses of CM under Avahan also indicates that the HIV epidemic continues to disproportionately affect the most vulnerable subpopulations of sex workers, especially survivors of violence, widows, divorcees, alcohol users, and young sex workers (Beattie et al. 2010; Bradley et al. 2010). This suggests an uneven distribution of CM benefits among different sub-populations. Such differential outcomes may reflect differences in intensity and duration of program implementation in different places (Blanchard et al. 2013; Kuhlmann et al. 2014). It may also be that, at the time of implementation, propensity for collectivization remained at a lower level among the most marginalized groups of FSW, leading to lower levels of service utilization post-intervention. Even after adjusting for treatment propensity, Kuhlmann et al. (2014) found the strength of CM, measured in terms of volunteer participation, to be varied across clusters within a single SLP-led intervention site. Gaikward et al. (2012), for instance, indicate that in brothel-based settings, increased level of control by madams and pimps allows limited time for FSW to mobilize outside of work. Meanwhile, Beattie et al. (2014) found that street-based sex workers represent a group that is most vulnerable and disempowered and therefore may have the greatest need for change or 'empowerment'. This suggests that differential outcomes may have resulted from characteristics associated with different sex worker groups and sex work settings. Together, these findings warrant further investigation of the link between program intensity and outcomes, and more generally, of how the characteristics of different forms of sex work may facilitate or impede CM efforts, or require tailoring of those efforts.

In addition to the implications of variation in the forms of sex work, each implementation context represents heterogeneity among FSW who may have competing interests and priorities. In Nagaland, for instance, polarization between native and non-native FSW, compounded by ethnic strife, posed a specific challenge to FSW collectivization (Devine et al. 2010). Likewise, the FSW community in Rajahmundry, Andhra Pradesh is diffused and fluid along geographic and socio-economic lines (Biradavolu et al. 2012). Mobilizing this heterogeneous group of FSW towards a common goal of HIV prevention and empowerment proved to be an ongoing struggle. The changing nature of sex work has posed further challenges to CM implementation. Our review shows that even in places with centers of fixed exchanges (i.e. brothel-based) like Mumbai, the conditions of sex work are becoming more fluid and, oftentimes, more hidden (i.e. home-based, contractual sex work) (Gaikwad et al. 2012). To further add to these complexities, modes of sex work solicitation that previously relied on networks of brokers/pimps are now shifting to solicitation by cell phones (Blanchard et al. 2013). This suggests that the environments for both CM and sex work may be influencing one another, and the existing forms of CM need to be adapted to suit the changing sex work environment.

Some have argued that the delivery, uptake, or effects of structural interventions are shaped by individuals, institutions, social norms, and values that may be broadly defined as contexts (Auerbach et al. 2011; Jana 2012). It has been argued, for example, that the unique history of West Bengal – with its traditions of trade unions, worker movements, and Marxist-left wing political parties – provided a context that has facilitated the collective organization of FSW (Campbell and Cornish 2010). Conversely, Guha et al. (2012) note that Mumbai is a challenging environment for sex worker mobilization due to its complex sex work typology, coupled with a limited history of HIV intervention involving CM. The nature of interventions and their outcomes also depends on the extent of broader alliances within and outside FSW networks (Chakravarthy et al. 2012). There are examples of organizational context – different types of organizations (from NGO to CBO) – affecting intervention outcomes (Sadhu et al. 2014; Yadav et al. 2013). Further research examining how social and institutional contexts shape the success or failures of interventions is warranted.

Some of the studies of Avahan suggest that implementation of CM involves, if not requires, making FSW publicly visible, as well as FSW speaking out and taking actions as a collective group (Blankenship et al. 2010). This poses a potential challenge for successful implementation, especially to home- or street-based sex workers who consider protection of FSW-identity from public scrutiny vital to their profession and well-being (Gaikwad et al. 2012). Limiting public visibility may be justifiable in a context where visibility makes FSW susceptible to a continuous cycle of stigma and discrimination, in addition to inviting opposition and backlash from powerful groups through newer forms of structural violence (retaliatory violence, abandonment by male partners, discrimination from service providers, economic extortion by pimps and police) (Avahan India AIDS Initiative 2009a). This represents a dilemma for CM as to how to mobilize FSW through public participation, while safeguarding their right to remain private.

Our review also points to several instances where the political and legal barriers facing FSW were confronted at the local level, primarily under the guises of Crisis Intervention Teams (CITs) and Advocacy Campaigns. In one instance, CITs in Andhra Pradesh played an instrumental role in informing local media and other parties (e.g. political organizations) of police excesses (Biradavolu et al. 2009). CITs also tackled cases of denial of educational services (school enrollment) to children of sex workers and other forms of discrimination and rights violations faced by FSW (Avahan India AIDS Initiative 2009a). Political and legal issues were also targeted through advocacy campaigns. Accordingly, FSW mass mobilized to influence existing sex work-related laws, primarily the 1986 Immoral Trafficking Prevention Act (ITPA), the Indian federal law governing sex work (Magar et al. 2009). Advocacy efforts were also organized to engage media in changing the perceptions of sex work and to make the national and state governments responsive to the FSW's needs for free public health care, Right To Information (RTI), and other social and welfare entitlements. Despite these notable examples (for further details, see Tables 4.1 and 4.2), it is unclear if influencing the political and legal discrimination facing FSW was initially part of the Avahan-wide, BMGF-induced CM strategy, or if it emerged more organically at the local levels, perhaps in part as a result of CM. It is possible that the political goals and indicators of CM may have been intentionally made less explicit by BMGF to avoid potential backlash from political actors who are supportive of FSW's participation in attaining HIV outcomes, but view CM's role in increasing FSW's political empowerment as either unrealistic or objectionable. Future research should examine to what extent an intervention such as Avahan, with primarily a health focus, can be further leveraged to advance the political empowerment of FSW.

Although the quantitative evidence establishes the contribution of CM to the overall intervention outcomes, it is lacking in its ability to isolate cause-effect relationships between specific components of CM and its outcomes. It must also be noted that all existing quantitative analyses on Avahan's CM have primarily relied on three sets of individual-level data: Integrated Behavioral and Biological Assessment (IBBA), Behavioral Tracking Survey (BTS), and Project Parivartan's Cross Sectional Survey in Andhra Pradesh (Project Parivartan 2007). Aside from the lattermost, the surveys are not designed to explicitly measure impacts of CM, which is a limitation. Qualitative research and rigorous forms of process evaluations may be instrumental in future research related to implementation and impact of CM, if not under Avahan, then in other locales. For example, process evaluations could be used to compare and contrast two or more distinct approaches of CM such as community-led peer-outreach and crisis response. Or even the same CM component, for example, peer outreach, could be compared and contrasted at two or multiple sites, or between two or more implementing agencies. As evident from our analysis of evaluation outcomes, qualitative studies may also continue to provide valuable data about the dynamic environment (e.g. sex work environment) that shapes intervention outcomes. It is our hope that some of the ongoing ex-post evaluation models of Avahan that examine community-level changes through a Community Ownership and Preparedness Index (COPI) (Thomas et al. 2012), consensus-based methods such as Delphi (Bennett et al. 2011), realist evaluation using cause-effect or pathway theory (Galavotti et al. 2012), and ethnographic study on intervention transition in Andhra Pradesh will further help address these research gaps. One noteworthy aspect of the COPI measure is its attempt to capture the changes in political environment facing FSW. Although the COPI is primarily designed to capture the readiness of FSW-led CBOs to sustain CM activities, these FSW-led CBOs are also assessed in their ability to engage with the Indian government and other socio-political actors. In another noteworthy study, Kuhlmann et al. (2014) sampled 104 geographic clusters in Andhra Pradesh to develop independent measures of CM strength, demonstrating a positive relationship between CM and HIV and psycho-social outcomes.

Auerbach et al. (2011) argue that a structural intervention for HIV prevention has to be based on social processes and interactions that are unique to each context. Our review suggests that Avahan's CM model was developed, negotiated, and renegotiated within the dynamic social and structural contexts in which it was implemented. Although implemented based on the standards prescribed by the funder, it was adapted based on findings of the partner NGOs, as well as multiple factors that are unique to each participating site (Wheeler et al. 2012). Further research is needed to understand the critical conditions and processes necessary for determining how to best standardize and/or adapt such a large-scale structural intervention program.

## 4.5 Limitations

Our synthetic review focused on articles with explicit reference to CM and/or related terms and its evaluation specific to the Avahan intervention among FSW in India. Additionally, given the purposive identification and selection of materials, certain studies did not meet the initial screening criteria and were subsequently excluded from the analysis. We note that the evidence that is synthesized in this paper may not be comprehensive, but rather suggestive of the varied characteristics, processes, and outcomes of CM. Although our review indicates Avahan's CM-encompassing elements of participatory development, community organizing, and organizational development, among others, we note that our analysis is limited to collection and synthesis of published data from one large-scale intervention. Further research involving interviews with key individuals from Avahan and others who have been instrumental in shaping the CM intervention and evaluation may supplement this analysis to develop a more robust understanding of the theoretical underpinnings of Avahan's CM model. Such analysis may also help identify elements that make CM interventions distinct from other established theories and practices of community-centered HIV prevention (Jana 2012). Finally, we have indicated in the discussion section above that the heterogeneity in both approaches and outcomes of CM are shaped by specific contexts. Caution should therefore be exercised in transferring these findings to other contexts.

## 4.6 Conclusion

Avahan's FSW-focused CM intervention represents a multicomponent, multidimensional HIV prevention model that is designed to address structural conditions that produce HIV risk. Even within one large-scale intervention, our review indicates no 'one-size-fits-all' strategy to CM conceptualization and implementation. It shows that CM has been adapted based on local resources, conditions, and risk environment. Despite variations in conceptualization and operationalization of CM, we suggest some standard approaches of CM that were vital for the rapid scale up of the Avahan intervention across 83 districts in 6 Indian states, including outreach/community organizing via peer educators, crisis intervention teams, advocacy, drop-in-centers, capacity building, and emphasis on social entitlements.

Our review also provides an inventory of evaluation designs, measures, and variables of CM that are indicative of the varied ways a multi-component, large scale CM intervention for HIV prevention may be evaluated. It suggests non-linear but mutually reinforcing outcomes of CM at the levels of service outcome (e.g. increased peer outreach, increased STI service utilization), epidemic outcome (e.g. decreased STI and HIV prevalence, increased condom use), and societal outcome (e.g. reduced violence, stigma and discrimination facing FSW, increased group membership). This underpins the transformative potential of CM in not only addressing HIV outcomes, but in altering societal conditions that put FSW at risk of HIV. Our review, in particular, shows that attempts to situate HIV as a shared community concern would enhance ownership and engagement of groups at higher risk in any form of HIV prevention tools and strategies. We hope that lessons from this review bear relevance in advancing the integration of community-led structural interventions and implementation of behavioral and biomedical HIV prevention tools.

## References


Aastha Monograph 2010. (2010). *Family health international*. https://www.indiahiv.org/Pages/Aastha-Monograph.aspx. Accessed 9 Dec 2014.

Argento, E., Reza-Paul, S., Lorway, R., Nain, J., Bhagya, M., Fathima, M., Sreeram, S. V., Hafeezur, R. S., & O'Neil, J. (2011). Confronting structural violence in sex work: Lessons from a community-led HIV prevention project in Mysore, India. *AIDS Care, 23*(1), 69–74. doi:0.1080/09540121.2010.498868.

Auerbach, J. D., Parkhurst, J. O., & Cáceres, C. F. (2011). Addressing social drivers of HIV/AIDS for the long-term response: Conceptual and methodological considerations. *Global Public Health, 6*(Suppl. 3), S293–S309. doi:10.1080/17441692.2011.594451.

Avahan India AIDS Initiative. (2005). *Avahan common minimum programme for sex worker interventions*. Unpublished report. The Bill & Melinda Gates Foundation.

Avahan India AIDS Initiative. (2008). *Avahan – The India AIDS Initiative: The business of HIV prevention at scale*. New Delhi: The Bill & Melinda Gates Foundation. https://docs.gatesfoundation.org/Documents/Avahan_HIVPrevention.pdf. Accessed 3 June 2016.

Avahan India AIDS Initiative. (2009a). *The power to tackle violence: Avahan's experience with community led crisis response in India*. New Delhi: Bill & Melinda Gates Foundation. https://docs.gatesfoundation.org/documents/avahan_powertotackleviolence.pdf. Accessed 6 May 2017.

Avahan India AIDS Initiative. (2009b). *Managing HIV prevention from the ground up: Peer led outreach at scale in India*. New Delhi: The experience of Avahan. The Bill & Melinda Gates Foundation. http://www.ghdonline.org/uploads/Avahan_Managing_HIV_Prevention_from_the_Ground_up_Peer_Outreach_2009.pdf. Accessed 6 May 2017.

Avahan India AIDS Initiative. (2009c). *Community led crisis response systems: A guide to implementation*. New Delhi: The Bill & Melinda Gates Foundation. https://docs.gatesfoundation.org/documents/community-led-crisis-response-systems.pdf. Accessed 6 May 2017.

Avahan India AIDS Initiative. (2009d). *Peer led outreach at scale: A guide to implementation*. New Delhi: The Bill & Melinda Gates Foundation. https://docs.gatesfoundation.org/Documents/Avahan_PeerLedOutreach.pdf. Accessed 6 May 2017.

Avahan India AIDS Initiative. (2010). *Common minimum program for HIV prevention in India*. New Delhi: The Bill & Melinda Gates Foundation. https://docs.gatesfoundation.org/Documents/cmp-monograph.pdf. Accessed 3 June 2016.

Beattie, T., Bhattacharjee, P., Ramesh, B. M., Gurnani, V., Anthony, J., Isac, S., Mohan, H. L., Ramakrishnan, A., Wheeler, T., Bradley, J., & Blanchard, J. F. (2010). Violence against female sex workers in Karnataka state, south India: Impact on health, and reductions in violence following an intervention program. *BMC Public Health, 10*(1), 476. doi:10.1186/1471-2458-10-476.

Beattie, T. S. H., Bhattacharjee, P., Suresh, M., Isac, S., Ramesh, B. M., & Moses, S. (2012). Personal, interpersonal and structural challenges to accessing HIV testing, treatment and care services among female sex workers, men who have sex with men and transgenders in Karnataka state, South India. *Journal of Epidemiology and Community Health, 66*(Suppl 2), ii42–ii48. doi:10.1136/jech-2011-200475.

Beattie, T. S. H., Mohan, H. L., Bhattacharjee, P., Chandrashekar, S., Isac, S., Wheeler, T., Prakash, R., Ramesh, B. M., Blanchard, J. F., Heise, L., & Vickerman, P. (2014). Community mobilization and empowerment of female sex workers in Karnataka state, south India: Associations with HIV and sexually transmitted infection risk. *American Journal of Public Health, 104*(8), 1516–1525. doi:10.2105/ajph.2014.301911.

Bennett, S., Singh, S., Ozawa, S., Tran, N., & Kang, J. S. (2011). Sustainability of donor programs: Evaluating and informing the transition of a large HIV prevention program in India to local ownership. *Global Health Action, 4*, 7360. doi:10.3402/gha.v4i0.7360.

Bertozzi, S., Padian, N., & Martz, T. (2010). Evaluation of HIV prevention programmes: The case of Avahan. *Sexually Transmitted Infections, 86*(Suppl 1), i4–i5. doi:10.1136/sti.2009.039263.

Bhattacharjee, P., Prakash, R., Pillai, P., Isac, S., Haranahalli, M., Blanchard, A., Shahmanesh, M., Blanchard, J., & Moses, S. (2013). Understanding the role of peer group membership in reducing HIV-related risk and vulnerability among female sex workers in Karnataka, India. *AIDS Care, 25*(Suppl 1), S46–S54. doi:10.1080/09540121.2012.736607.

Biradavolu, M. R., Burris, S., George, A., Jena, A., & Blankenship, K. M. (2009). Can sex workers regulate police?: Learning from an HIV prevention project for sex workers in southern India. *Social Science & Medicine, 68*(8), 1541–1547. doi:10.1016/j.socscimed.2009.01.040.

Biradavolu, M. R., Blankenship, K. M., Jena, A., & Dhungana, N. (2012). Structural stigma, sex work and HIV: Contradictions and lessons learnt from a community-led structural intervention in southern India. *Journal of Epidemiology and Community Health, 66*(Suppl 2), ii95–ii99. doi:10.1136/jech-2011-200508.

Blanchard, A. K., Mohan, H. L., Shahmanesh, M., Prakash, R., Isac, S., Ramesh, B. M., Bhattacharjee, P., Gurnani, V., Moses, S., & Blanchard, J. F. (2013). Community mobilization, empowerment and HIV prevention among female sex workers in south India. *BMC Public Health, 13*(1), 234. doi:10.1186/1471-2458-13-234.

Blankenship, K. M., Friedman, S. R., Dworkin, S., & Mantell, J. E. (2006). Structural interventions: Concepts, challenges and opportunities for research. *Journal of Urban Health, 83*(1), 59–72. doi:10.1007/s11524-005-9007-4.

Blankenship, K. M., West, B. S., Kershaw, T. S., & Biradavolu, M. R. (2008). Power, community mobilization, and condom use practices among female sex workers in Andhra Pradesh, India. *AIDS, 22*(Suppl 5), S109–S116. doi:10.1097/01.aids.0000343769.92949.dd.

Blankenship, K. M., Burroway, R., & Reed, E. (2010). Factors associated with awareness and utilisation of a community mobilisation intervention for female sex workers in Andhra Pradesh, India. *Sexually Transmitted Infections, 86*(Suppl 1), i69–i75. doi:10.1136/sti.2009.038653.

Bradley, J., Moses, S., Blanchard, J. F., Rajaram, S., Ramesh, B. M., Verma, S., & Alary, M. (2010). Assessing reported condom use among female sex workers in southern India through examination of condom availability. *Sexually Transmitted Infections, 86*(Suppl 1), i44–i48. doi:10.1136/sti.2009.038398.

Campbell, C., & Cornish, F. (2010). Towards a ' fourth generation' of approaches to HIV/AIDS management: Creating contexts for effective community mobilisation. *AIDS Care, 22*(Suppl 2), 1569–1579. doi:10.1080/09540121.2010.525812.

CARE. (2009). *Standing together, reducing risk: The power of groups*. Atlanta: CARE. http://www.care.org/sites/default/files/documents/HIV-2009-STRR_Report.pdf. Accessed 6 May 2017.

Chakravarthy, J., Joseph, S. V., Pelto, P., & Kovvali, D. (2012). Community mobilisation programme for female sex workers in coastal Andhra Pradesh, India: Processes and their effects. *Journal of Epidemiology and Community Health, 66*(Suppl 2), ii78–ii86. doi:10.1136/jech-2011-200487.

Chandrasekaran, P., Dallabetta, G., Loo, V., Mills, S., Saidel, T., Adhikary, R., Alary, M., Lowndes, C. M., Boily, M. C., & Moore, J. (2008). Evaluation design for large-scale HIV prevention programmes: The case of Avahan, the India AIDS initiative. *AIDS, 22*(Suppl 5), S1–S15. doi:10.1097/01.aids.0000343760.70078.89.

Cornish, F., Shukla, A., & Banerji, R. (2010). Persuading, protesting and exchanging favours: Strategies used by Indian sex workers to win local support for their HIV prevention programmes. *AIDS Care, 22*(Suppl 2), 1670–1678. doi:10.1080/09540121.2010.521545.

Cornish, F., Priego-Hernandez, J., Campbell, C., Mburu, G., & McLean, S. (2014). The impact of community mobilisation on HIV prevention in middle and low income countries: A systematic review and critique. *AIDS and Behavior, 18*(11), 2110–2134. doi:10.1007/s10461-014-0748-5.

Devine, A., Bowen, K., Dzuvichu, B., Rungsung, R., & Kermode, M. (2010). Pathways to sex-work in Nagaland, India: Implications for HIV prevention and community mobilisation. *AIDS Care, 22*(2), 228–237. doi:10.1080/09540120903039869.

Dixon, V., Reza-Paul, S., D'Souza, M. F., O'Neil, J., O'Brien, N., & Lorway, R. (2012). Increasing access and ownership of clinical services at an HIV prevention project for sex workers in Mysore, India. *Global Public Health, 7*(7), 779–791. doi:10.1080/17441692.2012.668918.

Dixon-Woods, M., Cavers, D., Agarwal, S., Annandale, E., Arthur, A., Harvey, J., Hsu, R., Katbamna, S., Olsen, R., Smith, L., & Riley, R. (2006). Conducting a critical interpretive synthesis of the literature on access to healthcare by vulnerable groups. *BMC Medical Research Methodology, 6*(1), 35. doi:10.1186/1471-2288-6-35.

Dixon-Woods, M., Booth, A., & Sutton, A. J. (2007). Synthesizing qualitative research: A review of published reports. *Qualitative Research, 7*(3), 375–422. doi:10.1177/1468794107078517.

Erausquin, J. T., Biradavolu, M., Reed, E., Burroway, R., & Blankenship, K. M. (2012). Trends in condom use among female sex workers in Andhra Pradesh, India: The impact of a community mobilisation intervention. *Journal of Epidemiology and Community Health, 66*(Suppl 2), ii49–ii54. doi:10.1136/jech-2011-200511.

Evans, C., Jana, S., & Lambert, H. (2010). What makes a structural intervention?: Reducing vulnerability to HIV in community settings, with particular reference to sex work. *Global Public Health, 5*(5), 449–461. doi:10.1080/17441690902942472.

Family Health International. (n.d.). Guidelines and standards for counseling high-risk groups in clinic settings. http://www.fhi360.org/sites/default/files/media/documents/Guidelines%20and%20Standards%20for%20Counseling%20High-risk%20Groups%20in%20Clinic%20Settings.pdf. Accessed 9 June 2016.

Gaikwad, S. S., Bhende, A., Nidhi, G., Saggurti, N., & Ranebennur, V. (2012). How effective is community mobilisation in HIV prevention among highly diverse sex workers in urban settings?: The Aastha intervention experience in Mumbai and Thane districts, India. *Journal of Epidemiology and Community Health, 66*(Suppl 2), ii69–ii77. doi:10.1136/jech-2011-200514.

Galavotti, C., Wheeler, T., Sebert Kuhlmann, A., Saggurti, N., Narayanan, P., Kiran, U., & Dallabetta, G. (2012). Navigating the swampy lowland: A framework for evaluating the effect of community mobilisation in female sex workers in Avahan, the India AIDS Initiative. *Journal of Epidemiology and Community Health, 66*(Suppl. 2), ii9–ii15. doi:10.1136/jech-2011-200465.

George, A., Blankenship, K. M., Biradavolu, M. R., Dhungana, N., & Tankasala, N. (2015). Sex workers in HIV prevention: From social change agents to peer educators. *Global Public Health, 10*(1), 28–40. doi:10.1080/17441692.2014.966251.

Ghose, T., Swendeman, D., George, S., & Chowdhury, D. (2008). Mobilizing collective identity to reduce HIV risk among sex workers in Sonagachi, India: The boundaries, consciousness, negotiation framework. *Social Science & Medicine, 67*(2), 311–320. doi:10.1016/j.socscimed.2008.03.045.

Guha, M., Baschieri, A., Hharat, S., Bhatnagar, T., Sane, S. S., Godbole, S. V., Saravanamurthy, P. S., Mainkar, M. K., Williams, J., & Collumbien, M. (2012). Risk reduction and perceived collective efficacy and community support among female sex workers in Tamil Nadu and Maharashtra, India: The importance of context. *Journal of Epidemiology and Community Health, 66*(Suppl 2), ii55–ii61. doi:10.1136/jech-2011-200562.

Gurnani, V., Beattie, T. S., Bhattacharjee, P., CFAR Team, Mohan, H. L., Maddur, S., Washington, R., Isac, S., Ramesh, B. M., Moses, S., & Blanchard, J. F. (2011). An integrated structural intervention to reduce vulnerability to HIV and sexually transmitted infections among female sex workers in Karnataka state, south India. *BMC Public Health, 11*(1), 755. doi:10.1186/1471-2458-11-755.

Jana, S. (2012). Community mobilisation: Myths and challenges. *Journal of Epidemiology and Community Health, 66*(Suppl 2), ii5–ii6. doi:0.1136/jech-2012-201573.

Jana, S., Basu, I., Rotheram-Borus, M. J., & Newman, P. A. (2004). The Sonagachi Project: A sustainable community intervention program. *AIDS Education and Prevention, 16*(5), 405–414. doi:10.1521/aeap.16.5.405.48734.

Kerrigan, D. L., Kennedy, C. E., Morgan-Thomas, R., Reza-Paul, S., Mwangi, P., Win, K. T., Win, K. T., McFall, A., Fonner, V. A., & Butler, J. (2015). A community empowerment approach to the HIV response among sex workers: Effectiveness, challenges, and considerations for implementation and scale-up. *The Lancet, 385*, 172–185. doi:10.1016/s0140-6736(14)60973-9.

Kuhlmann, A. S., Galavotti, C., Hastings, P., Narayanan, P., & Saggurti, N. (2014). Investing in communities: Evaluating the added value of community mobilization on HIV prevention outcomes among FSWs in India. *AIDS and Behavior, 18*(4), 752–766. doi:10.1007/s10461-013-0626-6.

Laga, M., & Vuylsteke, B. (2011). Evaluating AVAHAN's design, implementation and impact: Lessons learned for the HIV prevention community. *BMC Public Health, 11*(Suppl. 6), S16. http://www.biomedcentral.com/1471-2458/11/S6/S16.

Lippman, S. A., Maman, S., MacPhail, C., Twine, R., Peacock, D., Kahn, K., & Pettifor, A. (2013). Conceptualizing community mobilization for HIV prevention: Implications for HIV prevention programming in the African context. *PloS One, 8*(10), e78208. http://dx.doi.org/10.1371/journal.pone.0078208. doi: 10.1371/journal.pone.0078208.

Magar, V., Bandari, V., Rao, N., & Roy, D. (2009). *Final evaluation SAKSHAM Project: Report to CARE India*. https://researchaction4change.files.wordpress.com/2009/10/final-evaluation-saksham.pdf. Accessed 6 May 2017.

Micro-planning in peer led outreach programs-a handbook. (2013). *The Bill & Melinda Gates Foundation: New Delhi*. https://docs.gatesfoundation.org/documents/Microplanning%20Handbook%20(Web).pdf. Accessed 6 May 2017.

Parimi, P., Mishra, R. M., Tucker, S., & Saggurti, N. (2012). Mobilising community collectivisation among female sex workers to promote STI service utilisation from the government healthcare system in Andhra Pradesh, India. *Journal of Epidemiology and Community Health, 66*(Suppl 2), ii62–ii68. doi:10.1136/jech-2011-200832.

Project Parivartan. (2007). *Results of a cross-sectional survey of female sex workers in Rajahmundry, Andhra Pradesh: A summary report*. New Haven.

Pronyk, P., Schaefer, J., Somers, M., & Heise, L. (2013). Evaluating structural interventions in public health: Challenges, options and global practice. In M. Sommer & R. Parker (Eds.), *Structural approaches in public health* (pp. 187–205). New York: Routledge.

Punyam, S., Pullikalu, R. S., Mishra, R. M., Sandri, P., Mutupuru, B. P., Kokku, S. B., & Parimi, P. (2012). Community advocacy groups as a means to address the social environment of female sex workers: A case study in Andhra Pradesh, India. *Journal of Epidemiology and Community Health, 66*(Suppl. 2), ii87–ii94. doi:10.1136/jech-2011-200478.

Ramesh, B., Beattie, T. S. H., Shajy, I., Washington, R., Jagannathan, L., Reza-Paul, S., Blanchard, J. F., & Moses, S. (2010). Changes in risk behaviours and STI prevalence following HIV preventive interventions among female sex workers in five districts in Karnataka state, south India. *Sexually Transmitted Infections, 86*(Suppl 1), i17–i24. doi:10.1136/sti.2009.038513.

Rau, B. (2013a). *From isolation to solidarity: How community mobilization underpins HIV prevention in the Avahan India AIDS Initiative*. Washington, DC: Futures Group. http://futuresgroup.com/files/publications/Case_Study_Networks_1-30-13_Single.pdf.

Rau, B. (2013b). *Forming networks of community-based organizations: Early experiences from the Avahan India AIDS Initiative*. Washington, DC: Futures Group. http://futuresgroup.com/files/publications/Case_Study_CBO_(Web).pdf. Accessed 9 Dec 2014.

Reza-Paul, S., Beattie, T., Syed, H. U. R., Venukumar, K. T., Venugopal, M. S., Fathima, M. P., Raghavendra, H. R., Akram, P., Manjula, R., Lakshmi, M., & Isac, S. (2008). Declines in risk behaviour and sexually transmitted infection prevalence following a community-led HIV preventive intervention among female sex workers in Mysore, India. *AIDS, 22*(Suppl 5), S91–S100. doi:10.1097/01.aids.0000343767.08197.18.

Reza-Paul, S., Lorway, R., O'Brien, N., Lazarus, L., Jain, J., Bhagya, M., Fathima, M. P., Venukumar, K. T., Raviprakash, K. N., Baer, J., & Steen, R. (2012). Sex worker-led structural interventions in India: A case study on addressing violence in HIV prevention through the Ashodaya Samithi collective in Mysore. *The Indian Journal of Medical Research, 135*(1), 98–106. doi:10.4103/0971-5916.93431.

Sadhu, S., Manukonda, A. R., Yeruva, A. R., Patel, S. K., & Saggurti, N. (2014). Role of a community-to-community learning strategy in the institutionalization of community mobilization among female sex workers in India. *PloS One, 9*(3), e90592. doi:10.1371/journal.pone.0090592.

Saggurti, N., Mishra, R. M., Proddutoor, L., Tucker, S., Kovvall, D., Parimi, P., & Wheeler, T. (2013). Community collectivization and its association with selected outcomes among female sex workers and high-risk men who have sex with men/transgenders in Andhra Pradesh, India. *AIDS Care, 25*(Suppl 1), S55–S66. doi:10.1080/09540121.2012.749334.

Thomas, T., Narayanan, P., Wheeler, T., Kiran, U., Joseph, M. J., & Ramanathan, T. V. (2012). Design of a community ownership and preparedness index: Using data to inform the capacity development of community-based groups. *Journal of Epidemiology and Community Health, 66*(Suppl 2), ii26–ii33. doi:10.1136/jech-2011-200590.

Wheeler, T., Kiran, U., Dallabetta, G., Jayaram, M., Chandrasekaran, P., Tangri, A., Menon, H., Kumta, S., Sgaier, S., Ramakrishnan, A., & Moore, J. (2012). Learning about scale, measurement and community mobilisation: Reflections on the implementation of the Avahan HIV/AIDS Initiative in India. *Journal of Epidemiology and Community Health, 66*(Suppl 2), ii16–ii25. doi:10.1136/jech-2012-201081.

Yadav, D., Ramanathan, S., Goswami, P., Ramadrishnan, L., Saggurti, N., Sen, S., George, B., & Paranjape, R. (2013). Role of community group exposure in reducing sexually transmitted infection-related risk among female sex workers in India. *PloS One, 8*(10), e78361. doi:10.1371/journal.pone.0078361.

# Chapter 5
# *Abriendo Puertas*: A Multi-level Intervention to Improve HIV Outcomes by Addressing Stigma and Discrimination Among Female Sex Workers in the Dominican Republic

**Deanna Kerrigan, Clare Barrington, Maria Carrasco, Andrea Mantsios, Martha Perez, Hoisex Gomez, and Yeycy Donastorg**

## 5.1 Introduction

While the Dominican Republic (DR) has been previously recognized for community-led, structural interventions focused on HIV prevention among female sex workers (FSW), these prior efforts did not explicitly address the needs and realities of FSW living with HIV. In 2013, based on findings from formative research, we developed and implemented the *Abriendo Puertas* (Opening Doors) intervention in Santo Domingo, initially among 250 FSW living with HIV (Donastorg et al. 2014). The multi-level model has four core components: (1) individual counseling and health education; (2) peer-led HIV service navigation; (3) sensitivity trainings for clinical care providers; and (4) community solidarity and mobilization. Additionally, we piloted efforts to create access to HIV services for the regular male partners of FSW living with HIV. The model was found to be feasible and acceptable to the

D. Kerrigan (✉) • A. Mantsios
Johns Hopkins Bloomberg School of Public Health, Baltimore, MD 21205, USA
e-mail: dkerrig1@jhu.edu

C. Barrington
University of North Carolina (UNC) Gillings School of Global Public Health,
Chapel Hill, NC 27599, USA
e-mail: cbarring@email.unc.edu

M. Carrasco
Johns Hopkins Bloomberg School of Public Health, Baltimore, MD 21205, USA

United States Agency for International Development, Washington, DC, USA

M. Perez • H. Gomez • Y. Donastorg
Instituto Dermatológico y Cirugía de Piel Dr. Huberto Bogaert Díaz, HIV Vaccince Research Unit, Santo Domingo, Dominican Republic



D. Kerrigan, C. Barrington (eds.), *Structural Dynamics of HIV*, Social Aspects of HIV 4, DOI 10.1007/978-3-319-63522-4_5

community and other stakeholders and showed initial effectiveness in improving behavioral outcomes such as protected sex, engagement in HIV treatment and care services, and adherence to antiretroviral therapy (ART).

In this chapter, we describe the development, implementation and evaluation of the *Abriendo Puertas* model, with particular attention to how the intervention challenged both HIV and sex work-related stigma and discrimination. We examine how the intervention began to enable participants to resist and redefine stigmatized identities surrounding their HIV status and occupation by creating individual- and group-level safe spaces, which facilitated development of self-acceptance and social solidarity. Findings suggest the importance of both psychosocial support and collective action, as part of a community empowerment approach to improve the health and human rights of FSW living with HIV. We also examine challenges with the model's implementation, and ongoing gaps in HIV outcomes, highlighting the need for further research and implementation science.

## 5.2 Background

### *5.2.1 Structural Factors and HIV Vulnerability Among Female Sex Workers*

Female sex workers (FSW) have a 13.5-fold higher odds of being HIV-infected compared to women overall globally (Kerrigan et al. 2013; Baral et al. 2012). Structural factors including criminalization and legal constraints surrounding sex work, stigma and discrimination, violence, substance use and financial insecurity have been linked to the heightened vulnerability of FSW to HIV acquisition (Kerrigan et al. 2015). These structural factors have been found to affect the HIV risk of FSW through their negative impact on access to primary prevention services and clinical care for sexually transmitted infections, as well as inhibiting related protective behaviors such as consistent condom use with clients and other sexual partners (Shannon et al. 2015).

Despite the fact that FSW have been known to have significantly higher risk for HIV infection since the early days of the global HIV epidemic, relatively limited attention has been paid to the specific needs of FSW living with HIV. In fact, FSW living with HIV have been largely invisible in the literature and in programming. In the last 5 years, however, with the growth of Treatment as Prevention (TasP) programs for key populations, attention to FSW living with HIV has slowly increased (Mountain et al. 2014a). Similar structural factors to those described above have now been found to be associated with negative HIV care and treatment outcomes across the care continuum among FSW living with HIV. Specifically, stigma, discrimination and violence against FSW living with HIV have been linked to reduced access to HIV care and treatment services, as well as lower rates of adherence to antiretroviral therapy (ART), and sub-optimal rates of viral suppression (Mountain et al. 2014b).

### *5.2.2 Understanding and Addressing Intersecting Forms of Stigma and Discrimination*

In his seminal work, *The History of Sexuality,* Foucault analyzes the cultural production of differences, providing a nuanced understanding of culturally constituted stigmatization as key to the establishment and maintenance of the social order (Foucault 1978). From a Foucauldian perspective, HIV and sex work-related stigma and discrimination can be understood as strategies to enforce oppressive social norms around gender and sexuality and to discipline those who engage in behaviors that are deemed to violate established norms and threaten the status quo of existing hierarchical social and economic power relations and inequalities within a given setting.

In addition to drawing on Foucault's work to understand the nature and role of various forms of intersecting social stigmas, we consider social cohesion and community empowerment as a strategy of collective resistance to and subversion against such oppressive social norms and existing power structures (Link and Phelan 2014; Parker and Aggleton 2003). We explore how social cohesion, or the level and type of trust, solidarity and mutual aid in a given group, may create a platform for resistance against multiple forms of stigma experienced by FSW (Carrasco and Bilal 2016). Social cohesion has been shown to be an integral component of community empowerment approaches among FSW in various contexts that bring them together to analyze, articulate, and demand their human rights, including access to quality HIV services (Kerrigan et al. 2015). Social cohesion has surfaced as a necessary first step for community mobilization and subsequent alteration of the existing power structures that constrain the right to health (Kerrigan et al. 2015; Peterson and Hughey 2004). Thus, we take a structural perspective to examine how a marginalized group may challenge stigma collectively, while recognizing the multi-level nature of the empowerment process which may involve: individual conscientization (power within), working collectively (power with others), and using these collective resources to bring about change (power to), including improvements in overall health and HIV outcomes (Rowlands 1997).

### *5.2.3 Sex Work and HIV Prevention in the Dominican Republic*

The Dominican Republic (DR) is a relatively small country of approximately ten million people (UNdata 2016) with an estimated 80,000 FSW (Kerrigan et al. 2013). Since the late 1980s, the partnerships between non-governmental organizations (NGOs), government agencies and community groups have characterized the national response to HIV among key populations including FSW. The focus on key populations reflects the historically and currently concentrated nature of the epidemic in the DR

(COPRESIDA 2008; Halperin et al. 2009), with less than 1% of the general population currently estimated to be infected with HIV (UNAIDS 2013). However, among groups such as FSW, the median national HIV prevalence stands at 4.4%, approximately six times higher than the overall HIV prevalence (CONAVIHSIDA 2012).

Sex work is not illegal in the DR, however stigma and discrimination against sex workers still exists in the media, in families and communities, and in clinical care environments (Donastorg et al. 2014; Kennedy et al. 2013; Kerrigan et al. 2016). The relatively non-restrictive legal status of sex work in the DR has facilitated community-led interventions among FSW for almost three decades (Moreno and Kerrigan 2000; Kerrigan et al. 2001). Both NGOs and community groups working on HIV prevention among FSW exist in various regions of the country, implementing peer education, condom distribution and screening and treatment services for sexually transmitted infections (STI) (Kerrigan et al. 2006). Significant variation in the type and frequency of HIV prevention interventions is known to exist among FSW across different areas of the DR, particularly outside larger cities and towns. Yet, overall, the DR has been recognized regionally and internationally for its grassroots response to HIV among FSW, which has emphasized the promotion and protection of the human rights of sex workers, including the rights to both health and work (Kerrigan et al. 2013).

HIV prevention programs such as *Avancemos* (We Shall Overcome) and *Compromiso Colectivo* (Collective Commitment) were implemented in various cities in the DR to address the multi-level factors influencing the increased risk of FSW to HIV/STI including environmental-structural factors (Kerrigan et al. 2013). Both initiatives were grounded in a rights-based approach that recognizes sex work as work and promoted FSW's ability to advocate for their labor rights, including safe working conditions. In this process, the FSW community and its partners engaged with sex establishment owners, managers and staff to create an enabling environment for HIV prevention based on the principles and practices of solidarity and collective action (Kerrigan et al. 2013). Similar to global trends, these actions and programs in the DR were largely focused on primary prevention efforts with FSW, working to reduce and limit incident HIV infections and other STIs.

### *5.2.4 Developing a Multi-level Intervention with FSW Living with HIV*

In response to the dearth of research and programming addressing health outcomes for FSW living with HIV, in 2011 we conducted formative research in the DR including 40 in-depth interviews with FSW living with HIV and their regular male partners, four focus group discussions (FGD) among FSW, and 21 key informant interviews with policy makers and service providers working with this group. From this initial exploration, we identified challenges faced by FSW living with HIV in the DR including: stigma and discrimination associated with HIV and sex work; lack of social support and inclusion in existing interventions and services;

financial burden of transportation and medicines, beyond ART, related to HIV care and treatment; and mental health concerns such as anxiety and depression (Kennedy et al. 2013).

These challenges spoke to the structural dynamics surrounding sex work in the DR, and many other settings, where multiple forms of marginalization and exclusion produce both psychosocial and material constraints on FSW's access to care, health and human rights. In turn, these findings highlighted the need to extend prior rights-based frameworks and models of community empowerment and mobilization to FSW living with HIV. Drawing on the principles of community empowerment models among FSW (WHO et al. 2013), and findings from the formative work, in 2012 we developed a community-driven, multi-level intervention model to improve the overall health and well-being and HIV outcomes of FSW living with HIV in the DR (Donastorg et al. 2014). Our conceptual framing of this work is rooted in an understanding of the intersecting forms of stigma, discrimination and inequality experienced by FSW living with HIV related to their HIV status, occupation, socioeconomic position, and gender (Kerrigan et al. 2013). The *Abriendo Puertas* model sought to stimulate support systems to address both the psychosocial and structural dynamics of these intersecting forms of stigma, which have been documented as barriers to care and treatment among FSW in a variety of settings (Beattie et al. 2012; Beyrer et al. 2011; Ghimire and Van Teijlingen 2009; McClelland et al. 2011; Scambler and Paoli 2008).

The *Abriendo Puertas* (Opening Doors) model and related intervention research project was formulated and implemented through a partnership between multiple sectors and actors, including: researchers and clinicians at the *Instituto Dermatológico y Cirugía de la Piel* (IDCP) in Santo Domingo; researchers from the Johns Hopkins University (JHU) and the University of North Carolina (UNC) in the United States; the Dominican sex worker rights organization, *Movimiento de Mujeres Unidas* (MODEMU); and a local NGO, *Centro de Orientación e Investigación Integral* (COIN). Strong ties and coordination with the Dominican government through its National AIDS Programs (known as DIGECITSS and COPRESIDA) and network of public HIV treatment centers was also cultivated throughout the project. The formative and intervention research were funded by the United States Agency for International Development (USAID) through the Research to Prevention (R2P) project led by the Johns Hopkins University.

To respond to the multi-level factors found to influence care and treatment outcomes among FSW living with HIV in the formative work, the following core intervention elements were included at the individual, interpersonal, institutional and community levels (Table 5.1).

Systematic efforts were also made to refer and engage the regular male partners of FSW participating in the intervention, by offering them HIV counseling and testing (via referral from their FSW partner if, and only if, she saw fit), and linkages to HIV treatment and care when appropriate. Support services for disclosure and partner communication were also provided.

**Table 5.1** Multi-level intervention components of the *Abriendo Puertas (Opening Doors)* model

| Level | Component | Description | Key Elements |
|---|---|---|---|
| Individual | Individual counseling and education | Six sessions of counseling, reflective exercises, and health education. Session content was developed based on formative research and three existing curricula adapted for the study population: (1) a globally-established model of peer support networks for women living with HIV in Europe and the UK (the SHE Programme); (2) a locally developed model, *Podemos* (we can), developed for people living with HIV in the DR; and (3) the HIV vaccine trials HIV testing and counseling protocol for risk reduction | Counselors follow a predetermined but flexible curriculum that includes the following topics: |
| | | | Acceptance of diagnosis and stigma |
| | | | Adherence to care and ART |
| | | | Practicing safer sex |
| | | | Reproductive and sexual health |
| | | | Disclosure of HIV status |
| | | | Other topics such as substance use, family planning and partner violence are covered when relevant |
| Interpersonal | Peer navigation and support | Trained FSW peer navigators accompany women as they enroll, re-engage with and/or attend HIV-related care and treatment services. Navigators maintain regular contact with study participants, which is critical to sustained retention over time. While focused on HIV services, navigators at times also offer social support and logistical assistance to make connections with other health-related services, labor and human rights services, and social services | Examples of peer navigator activities include: |
| | | | Accompanying a participant to an appointment |
| | | | Serving as a patient advocate |
| | | | Visiting study participants' homes |
| | | | Helping women with disclosure of their HIV status to friends, family members or partners |
| Institutional | Healthcare provider training | Sensitivity trainings were conducted with providers at government and NGO HIV clinics where women from the cohort received their clinical care to raise awareness about the experiences and needs of FSW living with HIV. The trainings responded to formative research findings that FSW often felt stigmatized or discriminated against in HIV clinics. Trainings are conducted with groups of providers including physicians, nurses, and psychologists to facilitate exchange between the clinics | Sensitivity trainings are meant to: |
| | | | Raise awareness about FSW living with HIV |
| | | | Identify and improve current clinic attitudes and practices that may be stigmatizing or discriminatory |
| | | | Improve provider communication skills on topics such as sexual behavior, violence, substance use, and barriers and strategies to treatment adherence |

| | | | |
|---|---|---|---|
| Community | Social solidarity and community mobilization | MODEMU facilitated a series of '*casas abiertas*'—or open houses—where women from the cohort came together throughout the intervention. These gatherings were instituted in response to formative research findings that FSW living with HIV felt socially isolated. At the open houses, women joined together as a group and talked about topics of interest and learned practical skills to create income-generating opportunities, such as making cleaning products and decorative sandals that they can sell | *Casas abiertas* aim to:<br>Strengthen the social cohesion and solidarity among sex workers living with HIV and the larger sex worker community<br>Address stigma within and beyond the sex worker community<br>Help to address financial barriers to engagement in HIV care and adherence to treatment |

### *5.2.5 Evaluating the Feasibility and Initial Effects of Abriendo Puertas*

To evaluate the feasibility and initial effects of the *Abriendo Puertas* model, we established a cohort of 268 women between November 2012 and February 2013. The cohort was recruited using a hybrid sampling approach that relied primarily on peer navigators reaching out to the FSW community, combined with peer and key informant referrals. Of these women, 250 participated in the *Abriendo Puertas* intervention during its original implementation. Each woman participated in a pre- and post-intervention survey examining HIV-related behaviors and socio-structural factors surrounding care and treatment outcomes. Participants also provided biological samples for viral load (blood) and STI testing (urine). A subset of 24 women and 16 men participated in semi-structured in-depth interviews to explore their perceptions of and experiences with the intervention model and contextual factors that may have influenced its impact. Additionally, two focus group discussions were held, one with women who participated in community mobilization activities and one with women who did not. All participants provided informed consent and were compensated for each study visit (~$US5). The study was approved by the Institutional Review Boards of the JHU, UNC, IDCP and CONABIOS, which is the national biomedical ethical review board in the DR.

At baseline, the full cohort sample (n = 268) had a median age of 36 years. Most women (65%) had only a primary school education (range 0–8 years). The vast majority of women had at least one child (93%) and almost all women had a current regular non-paying partner (81%). Most had been sex workers for many years (median 15 years). The median number of years living with HIV was 5. On average, they charged approximately US$18 per date with clients. Alcohol use was common in the sample with 54% reporting drinking in the last week. Approximately one quarter (24%) reported having ever used illicit drugs. A minority perceived themselves to be in excellent health, while 38% reported being in fair or poor health at baseline. Almost a quarter (23%) had another STI beyond HIV at baseline. As shown in Fig. 5.1, the vast majority (92 %) of cohort participants were previously linked to HIV care and treatment services, and the majority were engaged in care in the last 6 months (85%) and currently on ART (72%) at baseline. However, only about half of the women in the cohort were virally suppressed (<50 copies/mL) (49%), indicating significant gaps in optimal engagement in the HIV care continuum at the time the *Abriendo Puertas* intervention began in 2012 among the initial 250 FSW participants.

During 10 months of follow-up with the cohort of 250 women who initiated the intervention, we achieved 91% retention (228/250). Engagement with the intervention was generally strong but varied across the different program elements. At 10 months follow-up, 86.4% of women had completed all six individual counseling sessions, 61.7 % reported having had contact with a peer navigator, and 50.4% reported having participated in at least one community mobilization activity, such as the *casas abiertas* (open houses). Only ten women (4.4%) reported having no exposure to any intervention component, while over one third (34.2%) reported

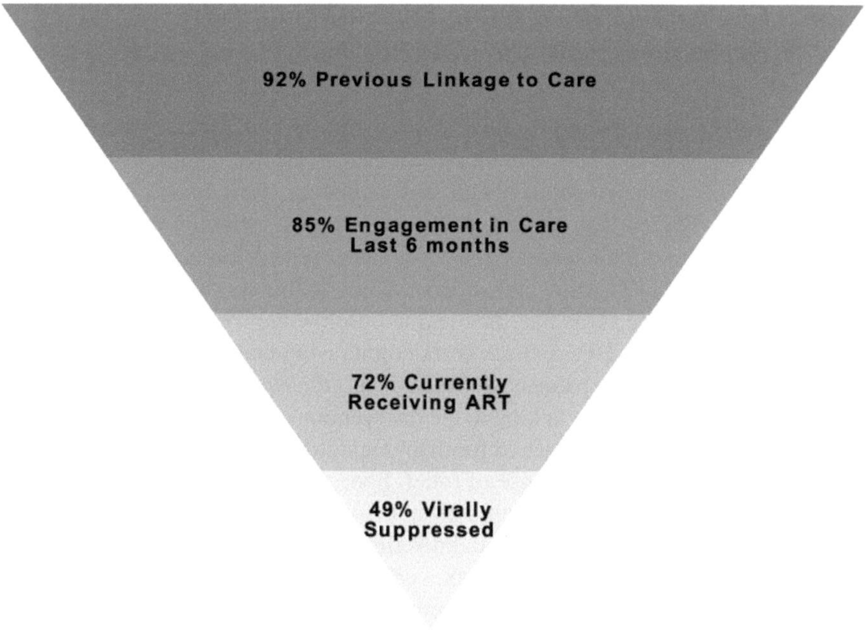


**Fig. 5.1** HIV care continuum among female sex workers living with HIV in the DR (n = 268)

exposure to all three components. Over half of the women in the cohort (68.4%) were categorized as having high/moderate exposure, defined as having participated in two or three intervention components.

Important changes were observed in terms of key HIV-related behaviors among the cohort during this 10-month period, including significant improvements in: protected sex, engagement in care, and adherence to ART. With regards to prevention outcomes, there were significantly increased odds of reporting protected sex across all partner types (aOR 2.35, 95% CI 1.30–4.43) from baseline to follow-up. Protected sex was initially defined for each type of sexual partner (new client, regular client, steady partner) and defined as 1 if the participant reported either no sex or always using condoms with that specific partner in the last 30 days, and 0 if otherwise. While reports of drug and alcohol use overall showed a non-significant declining trend, the rates of drug or alcohol use before sex dropped significantly at follow-up, with drug use before sex decreasing from 7.5 to 3.5 % ($p < 0.013$) and alcohol before sex from 47 to 40 % ($p < 0.034$). Engagement in care increased significantly from 86 to 95% ($p < 0.001$), although positive changes in retention in care were non-significant (64–69%). The percent of women on ART increased significantly from 70 to 78% ($p < 0.005$) over 10-month follow-up, as did adherence to ART in the last 4 days from 72 to 89% ($p < 0.001$). Higher intervention exposure was found to be significantly associated with changes in both ART adherence (aOR 2.42, 95% CI 1.23–4.51) and protected sex (aOR 1.76, 95% CI 1.09–2.84).

### 5.2.6 Challenging Intersecting Stigmas: Qualitative Experiences with Abriendo Puertas

Overall, women participating in the in-depth interviews and focus groups relayed that the intervention had a positive impact on their lives, their ability to manage living with HIV, and their overall health and wellbeing. Participants described the importance of different components of the intervention including the role of individual counseling on their sense of self-worth, peer service navigation in providing them with social and instrumental support, and community mobilization through both solidarity and the skills that they learned. Below we specifically explore how various aspects of both HIV and sex work stigma were understood and challenged by participants during the process of the *Abriendo Puertas* intervention.

Participants reported that talking to the intervention counselors and knowing that other people valued them and cared for them regardless of their HIV status or occupation provided them with a sense of relief, hope, and support. Many participants indicated that they had very low self-esteem before participating in the intervention and that this was due to the shame and discrimination that they experienced being both a person living with HIV and a sex worker. For example, when invited to participate in the *Abriendo Puertas* intervention, one participant indicated she was reluctant at first because she wondered: 'Why would they be interested in a prostitute living with HIV? I used to feel that I was insignificant.'

The women interviewed indicated that they learned coping strategies from their counselors to help them avoid internalizing stigma and discrimination related to both their HIV status and their occupation as sex workers. They also reported that they garnered strength and inspiration from the respect and kindness that they received from *Abriendo Puertas* intervention staff, which many women reported that they did not otherwise have in their lives.

Many participants highlighted that the intervention specifically helped them to change or shift their perspectives about the experience of living with HIV, which had been an ongoing struggle. They reported developing a sense that HIV was not insurmountable and was not in control of their fate. For example, one participant reported, that: 'I will die when God wants it, not when the disease decides it.' Another stated: 'This is a disease like any other disease; the main thing is that one has to take care of oneself.' A few participants indicated that before participating in the intervention they felt that HIV was a 'monster' that besieged them. Through *Abriendo Puertas*, many participants realized that a person living with HIV could lead a healthy life if she intentionally takes care of her health and adheres to treatment. The intervention helped many participants to more fully accept their HIV diagnosis, learn from their experiences and find a purpose again, and to personally and collectively empower themselves to not feel like victims, as the quote below relays.

> For me, [the intervention] was very good because I was very depressed and I thank God for coming here to Abriendo Puertas. Now, I feel great. I feel I can move forward; I have more faith in myself. All the staff members have helped me a lot. I thought that I was going to die;

> that my time was over. [At Abriendo Puertas] I got a very good psychologist. Whenever I came to see her she gave me support, she energized me, she always told me that I looked pretty. And here [at MODEMU] I participated in [casas abiertas] to learn to decorate sandals, and make hair products and candles. I thought to myself, 'But if I'm doing all of this, why can't I move forward?' I came here and they changed my life because I was so depressed, I felt dirty, I felt isolated.

In coming together to redefine stigmatizing narratives, participants were also able to describe positive aspects of their work and recognize the value of their occupation. Several women relayed how sex work gave them financial independence and the ability to provide for their children and fulfill their role as mothers, which was a source of pride rather than shame.

> I have worked, built my house, supported my children. In my household, I am man and woman... [and] we do what I say because I am the one who supports the house and provides.

Some women also indicated that the income earned from sex work helped them to avoid living in situations of domestic violence or being dependent on violent partners who threatened withdrawing financial support. A few women who reported facing ongoing violence, shared that through the intervention they learned the importance of respecting themselves and not letting other people abuse or mistreat them, and, in turn, separating from partners who abused them emotionally or verbally, while others separated from partners who refused to use condoms. Furthermore, several participants indicated that they were not using condoms consistently before participating in the intervention but that intervention counselors helped them to fully understand the importance of consistent condom use with their clients and regular partners. In the women's narratives, the importance of partner selection and consistent condom use was closely tied to and enhanced by challenging internalized stigma through the creation of solidarity with others.

While often participants' sense of personal empowerment was strengthened over the course of the intervention, many also indicated that they face a harsh socioeconomic reality in a country devoid of strong safety nets for the poor and with an HIV anti-discrimination law that is often not enforced. Many women could not follow recommended health practices due to lack of resources to attend clinic visits or not having the economic means to take medication with food as prescribed. Financial insecurity created stress related to responsibilities such as paying for rent and school fees for their children. A number of participants indicated that they were planning to or had already started making and selling some of the products that they learned to make at the *casas abiertas* implemented by MODEMU including decorative sandals, hair products, and candles. Most of the women interviewed said that one of their major hopes and dreams was to improve their financial security by starting their own business. Some were able to operationalize these dreams by continuing to produce and sell their products, or going back to school. There were examples of women who became hairdressers and one who became a nurse, each citing *Abriendo Puertas* as helping them find the motivation and strength to pursue these paths.

Through the *casas abiertas*, participants met other FSW living with HIV, some of whom were leading healthy lives and some who were struggling, which provided a rich space for exchanging experiences and support. These gatherings improved the women's sense of belonging and solidarity by creating a safe space where they could freely express themselves and connect with other women. Women who participated in the *casas abiertas* revealed in the FGD that they had developed friendships and networks with other program participants and kept in touch with them via phone or meetings after the intervention ended. These newly-formed connections enabled women to access broader networks to help themselves and other FSW and people living with HIV. The ability to help others also imbued a sense of meaning to the experience of living with HIV, coming from a sense of reciprocity and connection among FSW living with HIV, as seen in the quote from one *Abriendo Puertas* participant below.

> [Here] I met many women who are just like me. When they sent me to the casas abiertas, I did not want to go inside the room. When I sat down I wanted to run away but a lady said to me 'no [don't leave], you're just like me and if I have not left why would you leave?' I appreciated that; I stayed there. I used to think that I was the only one in this world who is living like this. At the casas abiertas I met all those women who live full of joy, that smile to life. I can smile to life too!

This sense of community, however, was not fully shared by all study participants. Women who did not participate in the *casas abiertas* revealed in the FGD that they felt it was impossible to create solidarity among FSW, many of them recounting stories of intense competition and fights among FSW at sex work establishments where they had worked. The comparison of both groups of women reveals that having the opportunity to openly interact with other FSW who were living with HIV in a safe environment helped to strengthen trust, solidarity, and reciprocity among participants. Several participants indicated the need to further strengthen the community mobilization component of the intervention by offering more opportunities for a greater number of FSW to come together in a safe space on a regular basis and to build practical financial and income-generating skills.

### 5.2.7 Engaging Male Partners of FSW Living with HIV

Approximately one-quarter of the women participating in the intervention referred their male regular partner for HIV counseling and testing, and participation in a brief socio-behavioral survey (n = 64 men). The majority of these men were living with the FSW partner who referred them to these services. We found that 35 of these 64 men were living with HIV; 27 were previously diagnosed and 8 were newly diagnosed during our study (Fleming et al. 2016). As a result, 45% of men were members of sero-discordant sexual partnerships. Of men with no previous HIV diagnosis (n = 37), 15 had never been tested for HIV and nine had not been tested in the past 2 years (Fleming et al. 2016). Low HIV testing was partly due to men not feeling at risk for HIV, despite having a partner who was living with HIV.

Among the 27 men who already knew that they were living with HIV, 93% had received HIV care in the past 6 months. The large majority (78%) was currently on ART. Of those currently on ART, almost all (90%) said they followed their prescribed doses 'perfectly'. A lack of tailored care inhibited engagement in anti-retroviral treatment for those infected. The time burden for clinic appointments and acquisition of medication was also a challenge.

> Well, actually I find it to be really difficult [to get my medication] because I think that if I'm just coming to get my medication, I shouldn't have to wait a long time...I don't think they should let someone who isn't there to see a doctor but rather is just looking for his medications to wait for 4 or 5 hours, I don't think that's right...We're just poor workers and I can't be paralyzed there.

This quote highlights the challenge of navigating HIV care around work schedules, which are a critical component of men's adherence to gender norms and expectations in this setting and others.

Like the women, the male partners of FSW interviewed also reported that they had a positive experience with the intervention, interacting with study staff and the services received. They reported feeling respected and validated by the *Abriendo Puertas* study team, which differed from their experiences in other clinical care environments, as described in the following quote by a male regular partner:

> When I climbed those 4 flights of stairs, I felt good, because I felt above all like an important person...I did an interview here, I liked it a lot, they treated me not like a person, but they treated me like an important executive.

Through this pilot effort to offer HIV testing and linkage to care to men through their steady FSW partner, we found that such referrals were acceptable within the context of a substantial number of partnerships in the cohort. We also identified that structural factors, in particular gender norms and lack of accessible and tailored services for men, were important determinants of testing, engagement and retention in care among male steady partners of FSW.

## 5.3 Discussion

Through our mixed methods evaluation of *Abriendo Puertas,* we found that the intervention is feasible and effective in improving key behavioral outcomes related to HIV prevention, treatment and care among FSW living with HIV, including protected sex and ART adherence. Additionally, qualitative data sheds light on the process of dismantling the negative impact of both HIV and sex work-related stigma and discrimination in the lives of FSW living with HIV, including how these forces shape their health behaviors and access to HIV treatment and care.

Our findings depict the importance of both internalized and enacted stigma related to HIV and sex work in the lives of FSW living with HIV and show that through their participation in the *Abriendo Puertas* intervention, the women were able to come together to develop and put into practice new de-stigmatizing narratives, opening up possibilities for both health behaviors and collective action and social change. Such a process has been documented among sex workers in other settings, including participants in the *Encontros* intervention in Brazil, which also documented the importance of having a safe shared space, enabling participants to gather and construct a positive social identity, which could be then leveraged to influence both individual behavior and broader access to resources and services (Murray et al. 2010).

The importance of employing a Foucauldian perspective to understanding stigma and discrimination in this work lies in the possibility of uncovering underlying power dynamics that fuel stigma and in identifying both psychosocial and collective strategies to address it. If stigma is indeed a tactic through which power is deployed, methods to effectively address it must subvert the norms through which stigmatizing differences are created. Such subversion entails resistance against the ways in which we are defined, categorized and classified (Rajchman 1983). The women in the *Abriendo Puertas* intervention learned to jointly challenge the negative, devaluing, constraining labels imposed on them by society. We found that this process was made possible by both the individual counseling provided and the social cohesion generated in a safe physical and social space. The solidarity created in that space through the process of the women coming together and realizing that they were not alone in facing these issues and challenges, is a critical first step to overcoming the structural stigma and marginalization they face as a group.

### 5.3.1 Challenges Shaping Future Research and Program Directions

Despite the positive social and behavioral changes found in our initial evaluation of the *Abriendo Puertas* intervention, there were and are ongoing challenges and gaps in HIV outcomes. For example, the rates of women with a detectable viral load remained virtually the same between baseline and follow-up (50–51%; $p = 0.715$). While there could be issues with the appropriateness of HIV treatment regimens being prescribed and possible resistance, further analysis also indicates that there may be gaps in the quality of clinical care being provided to FSW living with HIV, including sex work stigma and discrimination by HIV providers (Zulliger et al. 2015a, b). Additionally, we found that one of the most powerful predictors of a detectable viral load over time, was substance use, highlighting the importance of further research and programming for FSW living with HIV who also use drugs or alcohol (Kerrigan et al. 2016). Based on our findings to date, including both achievements and challenges, we developed (Fig. 5.2) a conceptual and operational model mapping the pathways from intervention elements through socio-structural pathways to key behavioral changes which can lead to improved viral suppression among FSW living with HIV.

Moving forward, further implementation science research is needed to examine how the principles, pathways and intervention elements of community empower-

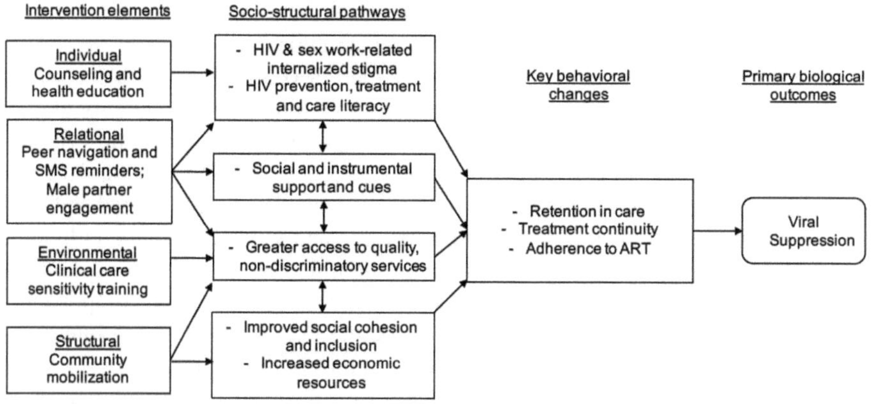


**Fig. 5.2** *Abriendo Puertas* model and socio-structural pathways to improving HIV outcomes among female sex workers living with HIV

ment, including specific attention to structural factors such as intersecting stigma and discrimination, can be utilized to optimize HIV outcomes and the health and human rights of FSW living with HIV. Our findings to date highlight the importance of ensuring that interventions provide FSW living with HIV opportunities to challenge intersecting stigmas that inhibit their health, well-being and HIV outcomes through solidarity and collective action.

However, in light of the aforementioned gaps in improved biological outcomes, we continue to consider how to further strengthen the *Abriendo Puertas* intervention. Future implementation efforts may in turn consider using a screening and triaging model, which has been utilized in other settings including with people living with HIV (Broaddus et al. 2015; Reay et al. 2016), to assess the specific needs of FSW who are not virally suppressed over time in terms of counseling, navigation, social support and mobilization to tailor the intervention and increase its impact.

Since the promising findings from the initial implementation of *Abriendo Puertas* in 2014, the project received additional funding from the Advancing Partners and Communities (APC) project of John Snow International, with support from USAID, to expand the model and integrate it into three government-sponsored HIV clinics in Santo Domingo. In this second phase of the project, an additional 90 women were added to the cohort and offered the multi-level intervention package. These women were recruited directly from public clinics serving people living with HIV and the staff (social workers and psychologists) of these clinics were trained to offer the individual health education and counseling sessions in the clinic. Additionally, starting in 2015, we adapted the model for transgender women sex workers living with HIV. We piloted this adapted intervention with 30 transgender women sex workers living with HIV and conducted a mixed methods evaluation of their experiences. Evaluations of these adaptations and scale-up are still underway, but initial findings underscore the positive potential of utilizing the principles and elements of the *Abriendo Puertas* model in other populations and contexts. They have also highlighted the challenges of integrating a model like *Abriendo Puertas* into public health clinics with limited staff, space, and resources for such activities.

In a third phase of scale up, sponsored by the USAID Linkages Project, led by FHI 360, *Abriendo Puertas* is being viewed as a tool to improve the quality of HIV care services for sex workers living with HIV by providing more holistic, comprehensive services that directly address the key psychosocial and structural factors that shape HIV care and treatment outcomes. We have developed, piloted and integrated two new sessions focused on substance use and violence into the individual counseling component as these factors were identified as critical determinants of HIV outcomes. We are also developing manuals for each intervention component to facilitate broader scale up and training. Within the DR, we are training interdisciplinary clinic teams from 11 public and NGO clinics in three cities in the *Abriendo Puertas* model. To date, the model has been well received with psychologists in particular praising the framework and tools provided by the individual counseling sessions, which allow them to do the work they were trained to do. A challenge that will be critical in this third phase of scale up is how to support community mobilization activities in smaller cities where there is not a large or strong FSW rights group. While recognizing the need for continued refinement, as one of the first models specifically developed for FSW living with HIV, *Abriendo Puertas* serves as a guide for critical future work among FSW in the DR and globally to improve their health, well-being and human rights.

## References

Baral, S., Beyrer, C., Muessig, K., Poteat, T., Wirtz, A. L., Decker, M. R., Sherman, S. G., & Kerrigan, D. (2012). Burden of HIV among female sex workers in low-income and middle-income countries: A systematic review and meta-analysis. *Lancet Infectious Diseases, 12*(7), 538–549. doi:10.1016/s1473-3099(12)70066-x.

Beattie, T. S., Bhattacharjee, P., Suresh, M., Isac, S., Ramesh, B. M., & Moses, S. (2012). Personal, interpersonal and structural challenges to accessing HIV testing, treatment and care services among female sex workers, men who have sex with men and transgenders in Karnataka state, South India. *Journal of Epidemiology and Community Health, 66*(Suppl 2), ii42–ii48. doi:10.1136/jech-2011-200475.

Beyrer, C., Baral, S., Kerrigan, D., El-Bassel, N., Bekker, L. G., & Celentano, D. D. (2011). Expanding the space: Inclusion of most-at-risk populations in HIV prevention, treatment, and care services. *Journal of Acquired Immune Deficiency Syndromes, 57*(Suppl 2), S96–S99. doi:10.1097/QAI.0b013e31821db944.

Broaddus, M. R., Hanna, C. R., Schumann, C., & Meier, A. (2015). "She makes me feel that I'm not alone": Linkage to care specialists provide social support to people living with HIV. *AIDS Care, 27*(9), 1104–1107. doi:10.1080/09540121.2015.1028882.

Carrasco, M. A., & Bilal, U. (2016). A sign of the times: To have or to be? Social capital or social cohesion? *Social Science & Medicine, 159*, 127–131. doi:10.1016/j.socscimed.2016.05.012.

CONAVIHSIDA. (2012). *Segunda encuesta de vigilancia de comportamiento con vinculación serológica en poblaciones claves: Gais, trans y hombres que tienen sexo con hombres (GTH), trabajadoras sexuales (TRSX), usuarios de drogas (UD).* http://www.mcr-comisca.org/sites/

all/modules/ckeditor/ckfinder/userfiles/files/ECVC Republica Dominicana 2012.pdf. Accessed 4 May 2017.

COPRESIDA. (2008). *Encuesta de vigilancia de comportamiento con vinculacion serologica en poblaciones vulnerables: Gay, trans y otros hombres que tienen sexo con hombres (GTH) trabajadoras sexuales (TRSX) y usuarios de drogas UD).* http://www.worldcat.org/title/encuesta-de-vigilancia-de-comportamiento-con-vinculacion-serologica-en-poblaciones-vulnerables-gay-trans-y-otros-hombres-que-tienen-sexo-con-hombres-gth-trabajadoras-sexuales-trsx-y-usuarios-de-drogas-ud-republica-dominicana-ano-2008/oclc/753988850. Accessed 4 May 2017.

Donastorg, Y., Barrington, C., Perez, M., & Kerrigan, D. (2014). *Abriendo Puertas*: Baseline findings from an integrated intervention to promote prevention, treatment and care among FSW living with HIV in the Dominican Republic. *PloS One, 9*(2), e88157. doi:10.1371/journal.pone.0088157.

Fleming, P. J., Barrington, C., Perez, M., Donastorg, Y., & Kerrigan, D. (2016). HIV testing, care, and treatment experiences among the steady male partners of female sex workers living with HIV in the Dominican Republic. *AIDS Care, 28*(6), 699–704. doi:10.1080/09540121.2016.1160027.

Foucault, M. (1978). *The history of sexuality: Volume 1: An introduction.* New York: Random House.

Ghimire, L., & Van Teijlingen, E. (2009). Barriers to utilisation of sexual health services by female sex workers in Nepal. *Global Journal of Health Science, 1*(1), 12–22. doi:10.5539/gjhs.v1n1p12.

Halperin, D. T., de Moya, E. A., Perez-Then, E., Pappas, G., & Garcia Calleja, J. M. (2009). Understanding the HIV epidemic in the Dominican Republic: A prevention success story in the Caribbean? *Journal of Acquired Immune Deficiency Syndromes, 51*(Suppl 1), S52–S59. doi:10.1097/QAI.0b013e3181a267e4.

Kennedy, C., Barrington, C., Donastorg, Y., Perez, M., Fielding-Miller, R., Mnisi, Z., Adams, D., Dlamini, B., Baral, S., Zulliger, R., & Kerrigan, D. (2013). *Exploring the positive health, dignity and prevention needs of female sex workers, men who have sex with men and transgender women in the Dominican Republic and Swaziland.* Baltimore: USAID | Project Search: Research to Prevention.

Kerrigan, D., Moreno, L., Rosario, S., & Sweat, M. (2001). Adapting the Thai 100% condom Programme: Developing a culturally appropriate model for the Dominican Republic. *Culture, Health & Sexuality, 3*(2), 221–240. doi:10.1080/13691050175015304 9.

Kerrigan, D., Moreno, L., Rosario, S., Gomez, B., Jerez, H., Barrington, C., Weiss, E., & Sweat, M. (2006). Environmental-structural interventions to reduce HIV/STI risk among female sex workers in the Dominican Republic. *American Journal of Public Health, 96*(1), 120–125. doi:10.2105/ajph.2004.042200.

Kerrigan, D., Wirtz, A., Baral, S., Decker, M., Murray, L., Poteat, T., Pretorius, C., Sherman, S., Sweat, M., Semini, I., N'Jie, N. D., Stanciole, A., Butler, J., Osornprasop, S., Oelrichs, R., & Beyrer, C. (2013). *The global HIV epidemics among sex workers.* Washington, DC: World Bank.

Kerrigan, D., Kennedy, C. E., Morgan-Thomas, R., Reza-Paul, S., Mwangi, P., Win, K. T., McFall, A., Fonner, V. A., & Butler, J. (2015). A community empowerment approach to the HIV response among sex workers: Effectiveness, challenges, and considerations for implementation and scale-up. *The Lancet, 385*(9963). doi:10.1016/S0140-6736(14)60973-9.

Kerrigan, D., Barrington, C., Donastorg, Y., Perez, M., & Galai, N. (2016). *Abriendo Puertas*: Feasibility and effectiveness a multi-level intervention to improve HIV outcomes among female sex workers living with HIV in the Dominican Republic. *AIDS and Behavior, 20*(9), 1919–1927. doi:10.1007/s10461-016-1376-z.

Link, B. G., & Phelan, J. (2014). Stigma power. *Social Science & Medicine, 103*, 24–32. doi:10.1016/j.socscimed.2013.07.035.

McClelland, L., Wanje, G., Kashonga, F., Kibe, L., McClelland, R. S., Kiarie, J., Mandaliya, K., Peshu, N., & Kurth, A. (2011). Understanding the context of HIV risk behavior among HIV-positive and HIV-negative female sex workers and male bar clients following antiretroviral therapy rollout in Mombasa, Kenya. *AIDS Education and Prevention, 23*(4), 299–312. doi:10.1521/aeap.2011.23.4.299.

Moreno, L., & Kerrigan, D. (2000). The evolution of HIV prevention strategies among female sex workers in the Dominican Republic. *Research for Sex Work, 3*, 8–10. doi:10.1007/s12119-015-9284-3.

Mountain, E., Mishra, S., Vickerman, P., Pickles, M., Gilks, C., & Boily, M. (2014a). Antiretroviral therapy uptake, attrition, adherence and outcomes among HIV-infected female sex workers: A systematic review and meta-analysis. *PloS One, 9*(9), e105645. doi:10.1371/journal.pone.0105645.

Mountain, E., Pickles, M., Mishra, S., Vickerman, P., Alary, M., & Boily, M. C. (2014b). The HIV care cascade and antiretroviral therapy in female sex workers: Implications for HIV prevention. *Expert Review of Anti-Infective Therapy, 12*(10), 1203–1219. doi:10.1586/14787210.2014.948422.

Murray, L. R., Lippman, S. A., Donini, A. A., & Kerrigan, D. (2010). 'She's a professional like anyone else': Social identity among Brazilian sex workers. *Culture, Health & Sexuality, 12*(3), 293–306. doi:10.1080/13691050903450122.

Parker, R., & Aggleton, P. (2003). HIV and AIDS-related stigma and discrimination: A conceptual framework and implications for action. *Social Science & Medicine, 57*(1), 13–24. doi:10.1016/s0277-9536(02)00304-0.

Peterson, N. A., & Hughey, J. (2004). Social cohesion and intrapersonal empowerment: Gender as moderator. *Health Education Research, 19*(5), 533–542. doi:10.1093/her/cyg057.

Rajchman, J. (1983). The story of Foucault's history. *Social Text, 8*, 3–24. doi:10.2307/466320.

Reay, G., Rankin, J. A., & Then, K. L. (2016). Momentary fitting in a fluid environment: A grounded theory of triage nurse decision making. *International Emergency Nursing, 26*, 8–13. doi:10.1016/j.ienj.2015.09.006.

Rowlands. (1997). *Questioning empowerment: Working with women in Honduras*. Oxford: Oxfam Publishing.

Scambler, G., & Paoli, F. (2008). Health work, female sex workers and HIV/AIDS: Global and local dimensions of stigma and deviance as barriers to effective interventions. *Social Science & Medicine, 66*(8), 1848–1862. doi:10.1016/j.socscimed.2008.01.002.

Shannon, K., Strathdee, S. A., Goldenberg, S. M., Duff, P., Mwangi, P., Rusakova, M., Reza-Paul, S., Lau, J., Deering, K., Pickles, M. R., & Boily, M. C. (2015). Global epidemiology of HIV among female sex workers: Influence of structural determinants. *The Lancet, 385*(9962), 55–71. doi:10.1016/S0140-6736(14)60931-4.

UNAIDS. (2013). *Epidemiological fact sheet on HIV and AIDS: Dominican Republic*. Geneva.

UNdata. (2016). *World statistics pocketbook: Dominican republic*. http://data.un.org/CountryProfile.aspx?crName=dominican%20republic. Accessed 21 Apr 2017.

WHO, UNFPA, UNAIDS, NSWP, & The World Bank. (2013). *Implementing comprehensive HIV/STI programmes with sex workers: Practical approaches from collaborative interventions*. Geneva: World Health Organization.

Zulliger, R., Barrington, C., Donastorg, Y., Perez, M., & Kerrigan, D. (2015a). High drop-off along the HIV care continuum and ART interruption among female sex workers in the Dominican Republic. *Journal of Acquired Immune Deficiency Syndromes, 69*(2), 216–222. doi:10.1097/qai.0000000000000590.

Zulliger, R., Maulsby, C., Barrington, C., Holtgrave, D., Donastorg, Y., Perez, M., & Kerrigan, D. (2015b). Retention in HIV care among female sex workers in the Dominican Republic: Implications for research, policy and programming. *AIDS & Behavior, 19*(4), 715–722. doi:10.1007/s10461-014-0979-5.

# Chapter 6
# Multi-level Responses to Multi-level Vulnerabilities: Creating an Enabling Environment for HIV Prevention for Girls in Botswana, Malawi, and Mozambique

**Carol Underwood, Jane Brown, and Hilary Schwandt**

## 6.1 Background

Of the estimated two million adolescents, or individuals aged 10–19, who were living with HIV in 2012, more than 80% lived in sub-Saharan Africa (UNICEF 2013a). Globally, adolescent girls continue to experience disproportionately high HIV rates compared to their male counterparts; in sub-Saharan Africa (SSA) the discrepancy is particularly dramatic with adolescent girls being two to five times more likely to be infected, continuing a trend that has been evident for more than a decade (Idele et al. 2014; Lake and Sidibé 2015; UNICEF 2013b). Tragically, the vital need for adolescent-centered programs and policies focused on the multifaceted vulnerabilities of girls is more urgent than ever (Idele et al. 2014: S152).

One such program, known as the Go Girls! Initiative (GG), was developed in 2008–2009 and implemented in 2010 to reduce adolescent girls' vulnerability to HIV. Informed by the understanding that girls' susceptibility is deeply entrenched within the families, communities, and societies in which they live, GG was designed in concordance with the social ecological framework (Bronfenbrenner 1979; Rose 1985; Fig. 6.1) that views individuals as nested or embedded within a system of socio-cultural relationships – families, social networks, communities, nations – that are influenced by and in turn influence their physical environments (Hawley 1950; Kincaid et al. 2006). Each of these contexts potentially influences, directly or indirectly, individual agency or the ability to engage in purposive action.

C. Underwood (✉)
Johns Hopkins Bloomberg School of Public Health, Baltimore, MD, USA
e-mail: carol.underwood@jhu.edu

J. Brown
Johns Hopkins Center for Communication Programs, Bloomberg School of Public Health, Baltimore, MD, USA

H. Schwandt
Fairhaven College, Western Washington University, Bellingham, WA, USA

 
D. Kerrigan, C. Barrington (eds.), *Structural Dynamics of HIV*, Social Aspects of HIV 4, DOI 10.1007/978-3-319-63522-4_6

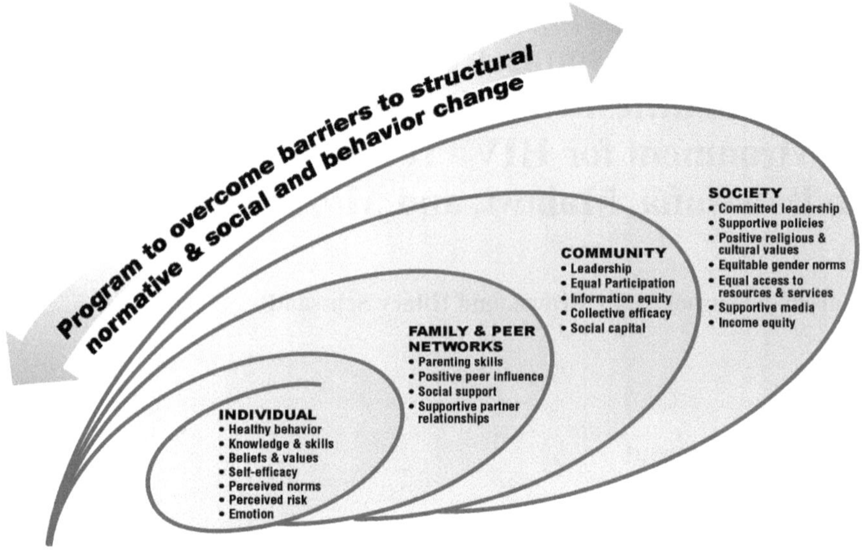


**Fig. 6.1** Social ecological framework for the Go Girls! Initiative (Underwood et al. 2008)

A review of the literature on adolescent girls' vulnerability to HIV (Underwood et al. 2008) was conducted to gain a fuller understanding of girls' susceptibility early in GG's developmental phase. The review found that the girls at increased risk of exposure to HIV were orphans (Birdthistle et al. 2008; Eaton et al. 2003), recent migrants (Mabala 2006; Rassjo et al. 2006), not in school (Gavin et al. 2006; Gregson et al. 2001; Obasi et al. 2001), marginalized or socially isolated (Campbell et al. 2005), and/or lived in impoverished conditions (Eaton et al. 2003; Hallman 2005; Machel 2001). Based on this literature review, GG adopted the following working definition of 'vulnerable girls' in the context of HIV risk: those who are *orphans, early school leavers, migrants, socially marginalized, live in impoverished conditions, and/or who lack close, trusting relationships with their parents* (Underwood et al. 2008).

We found no studies that examined girls' vulnerability to HIV through the eyes of community members; therefore, the definition required validation from community members themselves. To that end, a formative qualitative study was conducted.

## 6.2 Qualitative Research: Understanding Community Perspectives on Girls' Vulnerability to HIV

The formative qualitative study, which took place in 2008, comprised 35 focus group discussions (FGDs): 12 in Botswana, 12 in Malawi, and 11 in Mozambique. The FGDs were with young adolescent girls (ages 10–14), older adolescent girls (ages 15–19), adolescent boys (ages 15–19), adult women (ages 20–49), adult men (ages 20–49), and community elders (who were combined with the adult groups in Mozambique). A total of 143 female adolescents, 43 male adolescents, 150 female adults, and 90 male adults participated. The FGDs lasted approximately 2 h and were facilitated by same-age, same-sex peers, except for groups of young female adolescents, whose discussions were led by older teens.

The findings from the FGDs pointed to a widely, though not universally, shared understanding among participants that, while individual behaviors such as transactional and intergenerational sex heighten adolescents' risk, a complex constellation of socio-economic factors outside of girls' control was fueling the epidemic: specifically, inadequate adult-child communication, poverty, consumerism, underage access to alcohol, exploitation by their elders, and unsafe spaces, such as bars, schools (in some instances), and unmonitored routes within and between communities. Study interlocutors identified transactional and cross-generational sex, which they characterized as typically unprotected and often concurrent (more than one partner), as the nexus of HIV vulnerability among adolescent girls.

> When they leave [the bar] he takes her to a room, and if she starts complaining he tells her 'you can start paying my beers'. She has already drunk 4-5 beers, how will she pay back? She cannot ask for the money back home, because she is still underage, and she is scared of her dad, and so she accepts having sex with him, and without a condom, and hence sometimes, she can get infected. (Mozambique, peri-urban, adolescent boy 15–19 years)

For the most part, participants did not put the onus on girls; instead, they pointed to the abovementioned constellation of factors that combine in ways that make it difficult for girls to find safe passage into adulthood.

At the family level, participants suggested that some parents tried to advise their children on sensitive matters, such as transactional sex and concurrent sexual partnerships, while other parents remain reticent when faced with such conversations. Some parents believed sex was an inappropriate topic for parent-daughter communication and others felt that they were not sufficiently skilled to carry out such conversations. Additionally, several participants mentioned that some girls are 'stubborn' and unwilling to accept advice.

But not all participants blamed children or their modern ways for poor parent-child relationships. There was also the sense that parents themselves had abrogated their responsibilities, leaving their children alone and without adult supervision, or had failed to guide their children, as reflected in the following quotations.

> Parents do not have any time for their children; they leave the homes at six o'clock in the morning and only come back at night. Meanwhile the children go around as they please. The village administrators like the VDC [Village Development Committee] people give out warnings and yet they are the very ones who are actively involved in the bars. (Rural Botswana, adolescent boy 15–19 years)
>
> Our adolescent girls are at risk because we as parents are not giving these girls proper guidance. (Malawi, rural, opinion leader)

The influence of peers emerged as a largely negative phenomenon that contributes to girls' HIV-related vulnerability. Several groups talked about girls who actively pressure their female peers to engage in concurrent and transactional sex with older men for the explicit pursuit of material gain.

> I might be dating a person who doesn't have money and my friend will discourage that and would suggest that she will find me an older man who has a lot of money and as a result I end up dating him hence get infected because he has multiple partners. (Peri-urban Botswana, adolescent girl 15–19 years)

Others spoke of peer influence rather than peer pressure when they asserted that some girls seek transactional relationships as they strive for a modern social identity like other girls in their social networks.

> I think it's just because of the fact that girls like money. If she is asked to do something, as soon as she sees money she caves in and has sex and knows that if she lets go of the money then her friends will laugh at her when she eats cheaper food like samp [corn grits]. This will mean I have low self-esteem. Then in the end she reluctantly gives in even though she really did not mean to do so. Such is the temptation of money! (Rural Botswana, adolescent boy 15–19 years)

At the community level, participants identified a plethora of places where girls felt unsafe and very few where they felt safe. Girls believed they were at risk in a multitude of different environments, particularly in bars (as previously mentioned), but also in the market, rest houses, video houses, and unsupervised outdoor locations, which were depicted as unsafe places or places where girls have been assaulted, even raped.

> I would like to talk about Dwaru River, its unsafe because there are several trees and plantation of bananas. Men or boys can ambush you and rape you, even if you shout people cannot hear you. (Malawi, rural, adolescent girls aged 11–14)

Many of the groups talked about aggression and rape; tellingly, without mentioning that rapists were ever brought to justice.

Sexual exploitation by teachers was also mentioned as a real and present danger for school-going adolescents in Malawi and Mozambique, and, if to a lesser extent, in Botswana. As stated by a Malawian peri-urban, adolescent boy aged 15–19: 'There is no safety for girls at the school because they can be forced to have sex with their teachers, who will pass them if they sleep with him.'

One of the key societal/structural-level factors that came out in nearly all the FGDs was poverty and its effects on girls. In Malawi and Mozambique, both low-income countries, dire economic need was often considered the impetus for transactional sex as reflected in this quote from a Mozambican, peri-urban opinion leader: 'She has no food to eat. As a result, she will accept. She doesn't know if such man is HIV positive or negative. She just accepts without thinking of the consequences.'

Participants from Botswana, a middle-income country, tended to point to consumerism as a more important fact than economic exigencies as a dominant driver of transactional sex.

> In the olden days it did not matter whether one was poor or rich, but today we want high status, these are things we learn from television and emulate. The life we live changes by the day, and as it changes so do we. (Botswana, peri-urban woman 20–29 years)

There was also mention of economic exploitation as a threat to adolescent girls. Tragically, participants said that parents were known to coerce their daughters to have sex or to implicitly accept that sex would bring (buy) their daughters consumer goods they themselves could not afford.

> [Parents] tell her to go and do prostitution since there is nothing at home; therefore, she is forced to do sex or else she is chased out. The money raised is used to support the family. (Malawi, rural, pre-adolescent girl 10–14 years)
>
> The parents enjoy the material benefits brought by the children. .. Parents in Bluetown Village like classy stuff, they too are after money and they do not criticize their children but rather encourage them. (Botswana, peri-urban, adolescent boy 15–19 years)

On the legal front, study participants noted that extant laws and regulations, designed in principle to help protect adolescent girls – specifically those against child defilement, sexual coercion, rape, and under-age alcohol consumption – were rarely enforced, which represented a missed opportunity to protect adolescents. Participants reported that unregulated access to alcohol was readily available to underage girls across the three countries. Nearly every group mentioned that proprietors of bars and other alcohol outlets allowed underage adolescents to frequent their establishments where adolescents could consume and purchase spirits. Easy access to alcohol was identified as a key factor in girls' vulnerability. The relationship between alcohol and sexual risk behaviors was spoken of frequently in both sites in Botswana, the semi-urban area of Malawi, and both sites in Mozambique. According to the focus group discussants, alcohol disinhibition was a factor both in girls' attenuated decision-making capacity when they consumed alcohol and, whether they themselves drank or not, in increasing their risk of sexual harassment and rape by inebriated men.

> If you want some proof it is simple, you only have to go now to the bar and you will find 10-year-old girls completely drunk . . . (Mozambique, peri-urban, opinion leader)
>
> In this place even if one does not want to have sex, you can end up having it because you are drunk. (Malawi, rural, woman 20–49 years)
>
> These adolescent girls who go to bars get drunk, men harass and rape them, and this puts them at risk. (Botswana, rural, woman 20–49 years)

Although community members identified a wide range of factors that increase girls' vulnerability to HIV, and some expressed a feeling that these factors were difficult to change, most groups identified areas for interventions that could help bring about positive changes and create safer environments for female and male adolescents. All adult groups, as well as the adolescent groups, confirmed that communication between parents and daughters is very difficult. As a consequence, parents feel powerless and frustrated when it comes to guiding and protecting their daughters, and adolescents feel a lack of support from the adults in their lives. They called for programs to help adults communicate more effectively with their children.

Participants mentioned a range of additional actions that parents and the community could take to protect girls from HIV, including taking more responsibility to supervise and monitor girls' coming and goings, such as restricting them from establishments where alcohol is available. There were also calls for structural interventions to create an enabling environment for reducing HIV vulnerability, including more schools, easier access to schooling, improved security, enforcement of laws regarding child defilement, rape, and alcohol access, and better regulation of bars and video houses. Several groups suggested that girls need opportunities to earn money, such as through petty trade, sewing, or agricultural work, or access to microfinance, so that they will not be susceptible to men's advances (for a full exploration of the formative research, see Underwood et al. 2011.) These findings on the context of adolescent girls' HIV risk informed the design and implementation of the multifaceted, multilevel Go Girls! Program.

## 6.3 Program Design

### *6.3.1 Overview: The Go Girls! Approach*

As previously noted, GG was guided by the understanding that individuals are influenced by a system of socio-cultural relationships, including families, social networks, communities, and nations, so programs were designed to reach actors at all social ecological levels or, in the terms used for programmatic purposes, to work 'with the whole community' to prevent HIV among pre-adolescent and adolescent girls.

A key first step in the development of the program was to identify existing interventions upon which GG could build. A mapping exercise was conducted in each country to compile an inventory of interventions, services, and programs targeting girls, youth, or the broader communities, such as: youth-friendly health services, education, youth HIV programs, life skills, and economic empowerment programs, and identify potential implementation partners for the project. The findings highlighted that within HIV programs, there were few integrated models focused on girls or youth specifically; that economic empowerment programs targeted at youth were particularly lacking; and that micro-credit programs nearly unanimously did not give loans to girls under 18. This reinforced our assumptions that an integrated program would bring significant added value to the field and that inclusion of an economic component was essential. It also meant that GG would have to work with parents and adult guardians on the economic component since the funding agency did not allow direct payments, such as conditional cash transfers, to program participants. Findings from the mapping exercise were also used to select the intervention districts.

Eight separate, but overlapping, multilevel interventions, each with its own implementation guide and accompanying materials (available in a comprehensive toolkit at http://www.thehealthcompass.org/project-examples/go-girls-toolkit), were designed and implemented to simultaneously reach out to communities, leaders, teachers, parents/guardians, and adolescents themselves. Local partners who, for the most part, were already working in the selected GG districts and had relationships with the local communities implemented these interventions. They provided input into the program development and then were trained how to use the specific tools.

GG was implemented in a total of 16 sites: four communities in the Thyolo district of Malawi, four communities in the Francistown district of Botswana, and eight communities in Mozambique's Zambezia and Nampula provinces. The communities included equal numbers of both peri-urban and rural sites in each country. While the national HIV prevalence differs greatly between Botswana, Malawi, and Mozambique – the highest prevalence is found in Botswana and the lowest in Malawi – GG selected districts in each country with similar levels of high HIV prevalence: between 18 and 23% (BAIS III 2008; NSO and ORC Macro 2005; UNAIDS 2008). The program began in September 2009 and ended a year later in September 2010. The only program component implemented with a control group was the school intervention – as only half of the schools in the program communities received that intervention.

### 6.3.2 *Components and Tools*

GG comprised eight core activities (see Fig. 6.2), each with its own aforementioned guide, that together formed a comprehensive, multi-sectoral program targeting the whole community across the social ecological framework. Input was provided by local partners on drafts and through pre-tests. Throughout implementation, additional feedback was collected on the 'field test versions', which was incorporated into the finalized toolkit.

Three components aimed to influence the **societal/structural level**: (1) the school personnel (SP) training for teachers and school administrators that aimed to

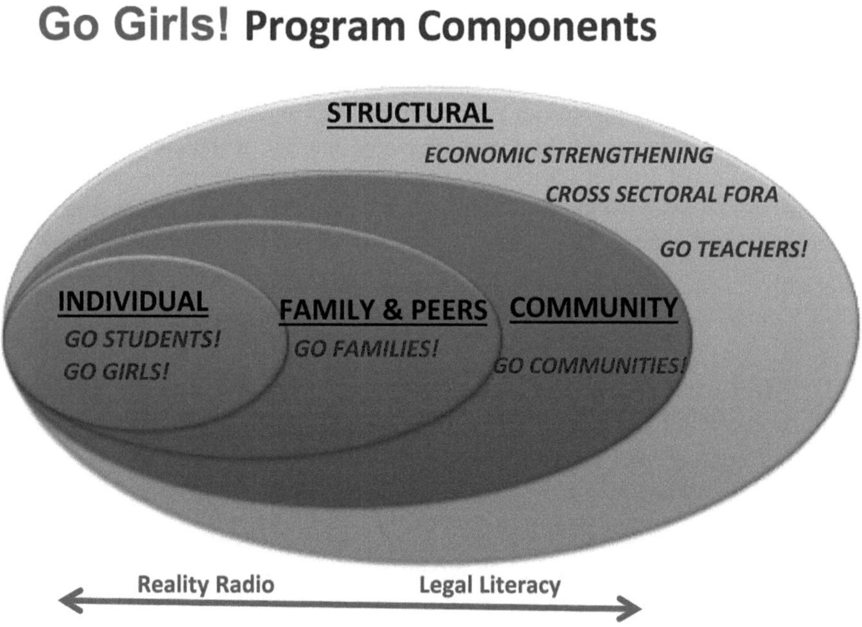


**Fig. 6.2** GG multi-level intervention components by social ecological levels

create safer school environments for girls (Gallant and Maticka-Tyndale 2004), (2) the economic strengthening (ES) component that was designed to improve access to financial resources previously unavailable to vulnerable adolescent girls and their families (Botswana and Malawi only) (Jukes and Bundy 2008; JHU/CCP 2010), and (3) the cross-sectoral fora (CSF) that brought leaders from various sectors together at the district level to give institutional support to the program. At the **community level**, community mobilization (CM) training gave community members – men and women alike, youth as well as adults – the skills to organize a collective response and motivate them to take action to safeguard adolescent girls (Bandura 1986). At the **family and social network levels**, the adult-child communication (ACC) component brought adults together to hone their skills to communicate with youth and increase their knowledge about how they could better nurture and positively influence the girls in their lives (Babalola et al. 2005; Fuglesang 1997). Finally, at the **individual level**, the community-based life skills (CBLS) program for girls who were out of school and the school-based life skills (SBLS) for boys and girls who were in school were designed to enhance HIV-related knowledge, build skills, and change social norms so as to enhance vulnerable girls' ability to avoid high-risk situations and behaviors (Gallant and Maticka-Tyndale 2004).

A reality radio program was designed to cut across all levels of the social ecological continuum and was aired in Malawi and Botswana. It provided listeners with information about key factors that contribute to girls' vulnerability; raised awareness about existing laws that are protective of girls but are often not enforced; and inspired communities to take collective action to make them safer and more protective for girls. Above all, it provided a forum for girls' voices so they could speak about their own experiences, something sorely lacking on the airwaves and in communities. A Listening Guide was developed for use by radio listening groups to further explore the themes of each broadcast in communities.

Content about existing laws and what communities and community leaders could do to ensure they were enforced was integrated into all of the GG interventions. GG's comprehensive approach ensured that reducing HIV vulnerability among girls was linked directly to the multi-level factors that put them at risk and held the whole community accountable for ensuring a safe and supportive environment in which girls can thrive.

## 6.4 Methods

### *6.4.1 Process and Impact Evaluations*

All GG intervention activities were monitored via an extensive process evaluation; after program completion, an endline survey was conducted with adolescent girls to evaluate the impact of the interventions. Between September and December of 2010, data were collected from girls aged 11 to 18 in the 16 communities through a post-intervention cross-sectional survey. All households in each community were first identified visually and then listed on a master list. Once the community listing exercise was complete, a random start was used to select households for study inclusion. If there was more than one eligible adolescent female at the household selected, the Kish grid, a table of random numbers, was utilized to select the respondent. The post-intervention survey included 404 Batswana, 414 Malawian, and 603 Mozambican adolescent girls ages 11–18.

## 6.5 Results

While the survey findings did point to some effects of the individual-level components of the intervention (see https://www.k4health.org/sites/default/files/Research Findings Report_English_Rev1-Approved.pdf), perhaps the most interesting results were related to the effects of the extra-individual level intervention components. In particular, the interpersonal component, Adult-Child Communication, and a structural-level component, School Personnel Training, had the most far-reaching effects. But also important were changes in legal literacy, which though measured at the individual level reflect perceptions about the broader community and society, as well as changes in community actions sparked by the community mobilization cycle that was integral to the GG program. We draw on data here from the endline survey and post-intervention qualitative work.

### *6.5.1 Adult Child Communication*

Conflicts between traditional and modern viewpoints, the failure of adults to supervise their children, and the lack of positive adult role models, all of which were identified as problems in the three countries during the formative research phase of GG, can damage the quality of adult-child relationships – relationships that are vital to adolescent wellbeing as the research previously cited demonstrates. To respond to this scenario, GG brought parents of adolescents together in small groups to learn about, and practice, how to talk to their children about sensitive subjects and how to strengthen their relationships. As a result of these efforts, parents reported improved relationships with their children, as did the adolescent girls.

In a post-intervention interview conducted in Botswana, one woman who participated in the adult-child program said:

> This program has helped me build a better relationship with my children. I used to be very strict with my children – I would beat them or yell at them. I attended the Go Girls! Adult Child Communication program and now I can sit with them and tell them that I love them. I can give them advice without beating them or yelling at them.

In Malawi, men are often reluctant to talk with their adolescent daughters because such communication is suspected of being sexually motivated. The fear of this kind of suspicion can lead fathers to withdraw from their daughters. Dickson, a father from Malawi, is a parent of two children, a boy and a girl. After participating in the Go Girls! Adult Child Communication sessions, he said:

> At first, it was difficult for me to talk to my daughter – I could only discuss sensitive issues with my son. Now, I am able to talk freely with my daughter, and my wife is now able to talk to my son. All of this is possible because of the Go Girls! Initiative.

We examined whether there was an association between adult participation in the adult-child communication intervention and an improvement in relationship between adults and children from the girl child's perspective – for both female and male caregivers. We found that girls whose closest female caregiver participated in the program were significantly more likely to indicate that their relationship had improved over the past 6 months than girls whose closest female caregiver did not participate in the program. In fact, over half of the respondents in all three countries indicated an improved relationship if their mother participated in the program (Botswana OR = 2.8; $p \leq 0.05$, Malawi OR = 10.5; $p \leq 0.001$, and Mozambique OR = 1.8; $p \leq 0.05$, data not shown).

As with the female caregivers, we found that girls whose closest male caregivers participated in the program were more likely to indicate that their relationship had improved over the past 6 months than girls whose closest male caregiver did not participate in the program. Between a third to nearly half of the girl respondents in all three countries indicated an improved relationship with their closest male caregiver if their male caregiver participated in the program (Botswana OR = 4.8; $p \leq 0.10$, Malawi OR = 5.1; $p \leq 0.001$, and Mozambique OR = 2.0; $p \leq 0.01$, data not shown).

Given that a close connection with an adult is associated with protective behaviors among youth (Bastien et al. 2011; WHO 2002), these findings suggest that the impact of this program with adults on the young girls in their lives might have been very beneficial on multiple levels for both the adults and the youth. It is also important to note that findings show improved relationships between girls and female caregivers and girls and male caregivers. Research often focuses on the gendered discussions between youth and adults – but this research suggests both female and male adult figures can have positive relationships with girls.

### 6.5.2 School Personnel Intervention

In the formative research, respondents identified teachers as contributing to girls' vulnerability to HIV through offers of favors in exchange for sex. The GG School Personnel Training was designed to address issues of girls' safety at school more broadly, but included the topic of teachers making inappropriate requests for sex from students. The adolescent girls' endline data were used to evaluate the GG School Personnel Intervention. In the multivariate, multilevel analysis, we examined the role of attending a school where the GG School Personnel Intervention was implemented and the outcome of whether teachers asked students for sex in exchange for favors. We found a significant reduction in the experience of having their teachers asking for sex in exchange for favors in Botswana comparing girls at GG intervention schools to those in non-intervention schools (OR = 2.6, $p < 0.0001$). The positive findings in Botswana were not echoed in Malawi and Mozambique, despite all three countries receiving the same program intervention. We reviewed all aspects of the program and evaluation upon discovering this unique finding to Botswana and came to a few potential conclusions. We first examined whether the training and/or facilitator in Botswana was superior to those in the other countries. We quickly deemed this possibility unlikely – as the facilitators in all three countries were experienced teachers and highly qualified to lead the training, the training materials were identical in all three locations, and there were other factors outside of the trainer's control that impacted the effect of the training. The other theory we considered is the difference in national income, and therefore, systems support for the educational system. Unlike Malawi and Mozambique, Botswana is a middle-income country. It is possible that the findings in Botswana are due to the fact that educators in Botswana feel more supported, as well as more accountable, to the educational system due to the strength of the system than do educators in Malawi and Mozambique. Therefore, when tasked with questioning their role in the education system and their ability to execute positive change for the students – there might have been more motivation among the educators in Botswana to actually do so, either due to the support of the system or the fear of retribution from the system as a result of failing to do so.

### *6.5.3 Legal Literacy*

Responses to questions about three laws – concerning rape, sex with minors, and restrictions of alcohol sales to minors – constitute the basis for the legal literacy score calculated in the context of GG at endline, which included questions about the laws as well as about whether or not the laws were enforced in their communities. Since legal issues were woven into many program components and a key aspect of Community Mobilization was to enable adults to come together to protect adolescent girls in their midst, in part through banding together to insist that laws on the books in their communities to protect adolescent girls be enforced, we anticipated that GG participants would be more knowledgeable about the laws and would also be more likely to state that such laws were enforced than non-participants. We found that adults who had been part of the GG program had higher legal literacy in all three countries even after holding SES variables constant (Botswana OR = 1.49 vs. 0.63; $p \leq 0.01$; Malawi OR = 1.08 vs. 0.73, $p \leq 0.05$; Mozambique OR = 3.00 vs. 1.95, $p \leq 0.001$, data not shown).

### 6.5.4 Community Mobilization

In each intervention community in all three countries, community members coalesced around Community Mobilization activities to enact local change to reduce girls' vulnerability to HIV. The Community Mobilization Facilitating Group went through a process of recognizing girls' vulnerability to HIV, identifying the root causes of this vulnerability, and calling for community action to address and reduce it. What follows are two examples of Community Mobilization activities – one in Botswana and the other in Malawi.

Some months after GG communication activities in a village in Botswana were well underway, an angry boyfriend killed his 17-year-old girlfriend, a type of killing that is common enough for the Batswana to have a name for it: 'passion killing'. Such killings occur when a disgruntled lover decides that the only way to resolve the situation – be it a case of infidelity, suspected infidelity, relationship dissolution, or another relationship issue – is to murder the loved one. Although the victim's mother in this case called the police immediately after the murder, it took them 2 h to respond, which caused her additional anxiety in an already stressful situation. In the past, she might have had no option but to accept a delayed response of the police. At the time of the incident the Community Mobilization Facilitating Group was active in the community. She turned to them for help. When the Facilitating Group received news of the murder, its members were angered by the police's delay in responding to the mother's call. They decided to visit the local police station commander to discuss the situation and to see if they could develop a feasible alternative way of handling such cases in the future. Unhappy with the performance of the police, the station commander asked the Facilitating Group to assist with the case – and with future work in the community.

A positive outcome arose from the tragic killing. The Facilitating Group, assisted by the victim's family, helped the police solve the case, and the guilty boyfriend was jailed. This led the police to invite the Facilitating Group to attend weekly meetings with them and community leaders, where the close collaboration could send a message to potential perpetrators and deter them from acting in ways that render girls vulnerable to HIV.

In Malawi, a factor that contributes to girls' HIV vulnerability is early marriage, which robs young girls of the opportunity to attend school and gain the skills and capacity to avoid HIV infection. As a young girl, Chimwemwe Banda[1] was abandoned by her mother and stepfather. Although she had an older sister to look after her, life was hard. The sisters had to struggle every day just to meet their basic needs, and there was not enough money for Chimwemwe to continue in school. These difficult circumstances compelled Chimwemwe to marry when she was only 15. However, she soon realized that marriage was not improving her situation as she had hoped.

[1] Pseudonym.

Chimwemwe's village Community Mobilization Facilitating Group recognized the detrimental effects of early marriage on girls and advocated delaying marriage as a strategy for maintaining girls' health and encouraging their educational pursuits. Understanding Chimwemwe's vulnerability, the team convened a meeting of all interested parties at the village headman's house to discuss her situation and officially dissolve the marriage.

As a result, Chimwemwe returned to school. When asked if her life improved, she affirmed that it is better now:

> I feel good about being back in school. If I had the opportunity to advise other girls, I would tell them not to marry early but to continue schooling because school is good. I am working hard at school every day so that I may have a brighter future.

## 6.6 Conclusions

An important focus of GG was structural level change – creating safer environments for girls – together with changes at other levels of the social ecological framework. Not surprisingly, therefore, some of the most important research findings reflect changes at extra-individual levels.

The findings show that, despite a short implementation period of 10 months or less, positive effects can be extended to girls when adults in their communities work together to create a more enabling environment for their health, well-being, and HIV prevention. For example, the fact that girls felt safer in schools where personnel had been through the GG program is evidence of structural-level effects. Additionally, when the adults in their lives gain communication skills, girls report higher quality relationships with their caretakers, which has been shown to be protective in relation to HIV outcomes. By weaving legal literacy into every GG component, legal literacy was higher among participants compared with non-participants. Additionally, community mobilization activities achieved profound changes in communities with regard to collectively responding to the vulnerability of girls and young women to HIV and other health risks, such as violence. Together, these findings demonstrate that interventions addressing the structural and social environment can have important effects on the well-being of adolescent girls. Additionally, because they are undertaken at a community-wide level, the potential for them to be sustained and institutionalized over time are greater than individual level change.

Yet, much remains to be done. The findings indicate that program-associated changes are incremental, uneven across countries and population groups, and do not always hold up after controlling for socioeconomic and vulnerability characteristics. Based on our experience with the GG program and evaluation, we have developed a number of recommendations for future programs to consider. Ideally, this program would be implemented for a 2–3 year period to reach as many community members as possible, to allow time for structural interventions to take hold, and to enable changes in social norms together with individual behavior change to reduce girls' vulnerability. It is our hope that the use of the program materials and toolkit will aid in enabling future programs with longer periods of implementation. We also learned from our experiences how important it is to introduce the project to the community through the local formal and informal leadership. This is so vital to a project's success, as the endorsement of leaders facilitates community engagement. Along these lines, it is important to encourage male involvement in program activities in order to strengthen full community engagement. At times, males, when hearing the project is about adolescent girls, tune out, as they feel girls' issues are in the female adult realm. In turn, the introduction of the project via community leadership along the framework of the social ecological model is particularly important for early and sustained adult male involvement. We also recommend phasing in the program components, leading with reality radio and next the community mobilization program component, reiterating information about HIV transmission and prevention in every project activity, and encouraging the community to engage with the judicial system to ensure that existing laws to protect girls are understood and enforced at all levels of the system.

These findings demonstrate the added value of multi-level programs but also point to some of the difficulties in implementation and evaluation. Increasingly, funders, programmers, and researchers alike are recognizing that social problems require a more nuanced and comprehensive response than most programs have incorporated in the past. Indeed, DREAMS (http://www.pepfar.gov/partnerships/ppp/dreams/), a program initiated in 2014, includes components that are very much in keeping with the GG approach. These components include: (1) school-based interventions to keep girls in school while working with teachers and school administers; (2) community mobilization to create safer communities; (3) programs for out-of-school girls to reduce their risks of contracting HIV; and (4) economic or employment opportunities. Thus, GG represented an important beginning – but it was only a beginning. It is hoped that the results reported herein may provide insight into how to design and implement future programming that will take us well beyond the beginning and into an era in which girls are no longer vulnerable.

## References

Babalola, S., Tambashe, B., & Vondrasek, C. (2005). Parental factors and sexual risk-taking among young people in Cote d'Ivoire. *African Journal of Reproductive Health, 9*(1), 49–65. doi:10.2307/3583160.

Bandura, A. (1986). *Social foundations of thought and actions: A social cognitive theory*. Englewood Cliffs: Prentice-Hall.

Bastien, S., Kajula, L. J., & Muhwezi, W. W. (2011). A review of studies of parent-child communication about sexuality and HIV/AIDS in sub-Saharan Africa. *Reproductive Health, 8*(1), 25. doi:10.1186/1742-4755-8-25.

Birdthistle, I. J., Floyd, S., Machingura, A., Mudziwapasi, N., Gregson, S., & Glynn, J. R. (2008). From affected to infected? Orphanhood and HIV risk among female adolescents in urban Zimbabwe. *AIDS, 22*(6), 759–766. doi:10.1097/QAD.0b013e3282f4cac7.

Botswana AIDS Impact Survey III (BAIS III). (2008). Gaborone, Botswana: NACA, CSO, UN, ACHAP, UNDP.

Bronfenbrenner, U. (1979). *The ecology of human development: Experiments by nature and design*. Cambridge, MA: Harvard University Press.
Campbell, C., Foulis, C. A., Maimane, S., & Sibiya, Z. (2005). The impact of social environments on the effectiveness of youth HIV prevention: A South African case study. *AIDS Care, 17*(4), 471–478. doi:10.1080/09540120412331319705.
Eaton, L., Flisher, A. J., & Aarø, L. E. (2003). Unsafe sexual behavior in South African youth. *Social Science & Medicine, 56*(1), 149–165. doi:10.1016/S0277-9536(02)00017-5.
Fuglesang, M. (1997). Lessons for life-past and present modes of sexuality education in Tanzanian society. *Social Science and Medicine, 44*(8), 1245–1254.
Gallant, M., & Maticka-Tyndale, E. (2004). School-based HIV prevention programmes for African youth. *Social Science & Medicine, 58*(7), 1337–1351. doi:10.1016/S0277-9536(03)00331-9.
Gavin, L., Galavotti, C., Dube, H., et al. (2006). Factors associated with HIV infection in adolescent females in Zimbabwe. *Journal of Adolescent Health, 39*(4), 596.e11–596.e18. doi:10.1016/j.jadohealth.2006.03.002.
Gregson, S., Waddell, H., & Chandiwana, S. (2001). School education and HIV control in sub-Saharan Africa: From discord to harmony? *Journal of International Development, 13*(4), 467–485. doi:10.1002/jid.798.
Hallman, K. (2005). Gendered socioeconomic conditions and HIV risk behaviors among young people in South Africa. *African Journal of AIDS Research, 4*(1), 37–50. doi:10.2989/16085900509490340.
Hawley, A. H. (1950). *Ecology: A theory of community structure*. New York: The Ronald Press Company.
Idele, P., Gillespie, A., Porth, T., Suzuki, C., Mahy, M., Kasedde, S., & Luo, C. (2014). Epidemiology of HIV and AIDS among adolescents: Current status, inequities, and data gaps. *JAIDS Journal of Acquired Immune Deficiency Syndromes, 66*(Suppl 2), S144–S153. doi:10.1097/qai.0000000000000176.
Johns Hopkins Bloomberg School of Public Health/Center for Communication Programs. (2010). *Strengthening economic opportunities for vulnerable girls and their families: programmatic recommendations*. JHSPH/CCP field report. Baltimore.
Jukes, M., & Bundy, D. (2008). Education and vulnerability: The role of schools in protecting young women and girls from HIV in Southern Africa. *AIDS, 22*(Suppl 4), S41–S56. doi:10.1097/01.aids.0000341776.71253.04.
Kincaid, D. L., Figueroa, M. E., Storey, J. D., & Underwood, C. R. (2006, October). *Attitude, ideation, and contraceptive behavior: The relationships observed in five countries*. In *Proceedings: World Bank Congress on Communication for Development*, Rome.
Lake, A., & Sidibé, M.. (2015). *To end the AIDS epidemic, start focusing on adolescents*. UNAIDS. http://www.unaids.org/en/resources/presscentre/featurestories/2015/february/20150217_oped_all-in. Accessed 21 Feb 2016.
Mabala, R. (2006). From HIV prevention to HIV protection: Addressing the vulnerability of girls and young women in urban areas. *Environment and Urbanization, 18*(2), 407–432. doi:10.1177/0956247806069624.
Machel, J. Z. (2001). Unsafe sexual behaviour among schoolgirls in Mozambique: A matter of gender and class. *Reproductive Health Matters, 9*(17), 82–90. doi:10.1016/s0968-8080(01)90011-4.
National Statistical Office (NSO) [Malawi], and ORC Macro. (2005). *Malawi demographic and health survey 2004*. Calverton: NSO and ORC Macro.
Obasi, A. I., Balira, R., Todd, J., et al. (2001). Prevalence of HIV and Chlamydia trachomatis infection in 15–19-year olds in rural Tanzania. *Tropical Medicine & International Health, 6*(7), 517–525. doi:10.1046/j.1365-3156.2001.00738.x.
Rassjo, E. B., Mirembe, F. M., & Darj, E. (2006). Vulnerability and risk factors for sexually transmitted infections and HIV among adolescents in Kampala, Uganda. *AIDS Care, 18*(7), 710–716. doi:10.1080/09540120500302934.
Rose, G. (1985). Sick individuals and sick populations. *International Journal of Epidemiology, 14*(1), 32–38. doi:10.1093/ije/14.1.32.

UNAIDS. (2008). *Report on the global AIDS epidemic*. Geneva: Joint United Nations Programme on HIV/AIDS.

Underwood, C., O'Brien, M., & Skinner, J. (2008). *Vulnerable girls and HIV in sub-Saharan Africa: A literature and program review* (Working Paper). Center for Communication Programs, Johns Hopkins Bloomberg School of Public Health. https://www.k4health.org/sites/default/files/GoGirls_Lit_Review-FINALMarch%2013%20-%202011.pdf

Underwood, C., Skinner, J., Osman, N., & Schwandt, H. (2011). Structural determinants of adolescent girls' vulnerability to HIV: Views from community members in Botswana, Malawi, and Mozambique. *Social Science & Medicine, 73*(2), 343–350. doi:10.1016/j.socscimed.2011.05.044.

UNICEF. (2013a). *Towards an AIDS-free generation – children and AIDS: Sixth stocktaking report, 2013* (pp. 26–27). New York: United Nations Children's Fund. http://www.unaids.org/sites/default/files/media_asset/20131129_stocktaking_report_children_aids_en_0.pdf.

UNICEF. (2013b). *UNICEF analysis of UNAIDS 2012 HIV and AIDS estimates*. New York: United Nations Children's Fund.

WHO. (2002). *Broadening the horizon: Balancing protection and risk for adolescents*. Geneva: World Health Organization.

# Part III
# Response

# Chapter 7
# Sustaining a Rights-Based Response to HIV in Brazil

**Laura Murray, Deanna Kerrigan, and Vera Paiva**

## 7.1 Introduction

The first cases of AIDS in Brazil were reported in the early 1980s and the epidemic continued to increase steadily until the mid 1990s (Szwarcwald et al. 2015). In 1992, the World Bank projected that 1.2 million people would be living with HIV in Brazil by 2000 (Brasil 2001). Instead, by 2000, the number of people living with HIV (PLHIV) was just over half what was originally predicted by the World Bank, a difference attributed to what came to be celebrated as the 'Brazilian Response to HIV' (Bastos et al. 2001; Berkman et al. 2005; Nunn 2009). A key foundation for this response was the constitutional guarantee to health enshrined in the country's 1988 Democratic Constitution. The social and political movements that fought for the end of the civil-military dictatorship guaranteed a significant group of social rights in the new constitution, two of which are especially relevant to this chapter: the organization of a Universal Health Care System (SUS – acronym in Portuguese) and the separation of Church and State. These two provisions provided a foundation during the first decades of the epidemic for an AIDS response based on human rights and implemented through a close partnership of health authorities and professionals with civil society organizations committed to decreasing stigma and discrimination among marginalized populations groups and guarunteeing universal access to testing and anti-retroviral therapy (ART).

L. Murray (✉)
Rio de Janeiro State University, Rio de Janeiro, Brazil
e-mail: laura.rebecca.murray@gmail.com

D. Kerrigan
Johns Hopkins Bloomberg School of Public Health, Baltimore, MD 21205, USA
e-mail: dkerrig1@jhu.edu

V. Paiva
University of São Paulo, São Paulo, Brazil
e-mail: veroca@usp.br



D. Kerrigan, C. Barrington (eds.), *Structural Dynamics of HIV*, Social Aspects of HIV 4, DOI 10.1007/978-3-319-63522-4_7

However, in 2016, the fundamental rights that made the response to HIV possible came under direct threat. Brazil faced its most conservative government since redemocratization, and after Congress voted to impeach the country's first female president in August, in December, the new administration proposed and Congress approved a constitutional amendment that reduces the state financial commitment to healthcare, paving the way for increased negligence and violations of the right to health.

Nevertheless, in its fourth decade, the government claims that the AIDS epidemic has stabilized, while many researchers and activists assert that AIDS incidence rates are actually growing (Grangeiro 2016). The overall national adult HIV prevalence in Brazil was most recently estimated to be 0.4% (Brasil 2015a), and remains concentrated in certain population groups such as men who have sex with men (MSM), sex workers, and people who use drugs (Brasil 2015a). Studies conducted between 2009 and 2013 estimate HIV prevalence to be 4.9% among female sex workers, 5.9% among people who use drugs, and 10.5% among MSM (Brasil 2015a). Of particular concern is a statistically significant increase in the AIDS cases reported among young men over the past decade. From 2005 to 2014, the AIDS detection rate more than tripled among all young men aged 15–19, in addition to an increase in the proportion of cases among young MSM during the same time period (Brasil 2015a).

These numbers are rising at a time of significant political turmoil and economic challenges in Brazil. The impeachment of Dilma Rousseff has been denounced – in Brazil and internationally – as a soft coup (Greenwald 2016). Different from countries like the United States, in Brazil, the federal government and, in particular, the political parties in power, wield a significant amount of influence in politics at all levels of government. For this reason, Dilma Rousseff's impeachment and the recent historical events that led to it, had, and will continue to have, far reaching effects on the country's public health system.

In this chapter, we look to the three presidential administrations that most affected Brazil's national response over the past decade: Fernando Henrique Cardoso (1994–2002), Luiz Ignacio da Silva Lula Inácio (popularly referred to as 'Lula') (2003–2010) and Dilma Rousseff (2011–2016), to discuss why and how the approach appears to have weakened over time and raise larger questions about the challenges of sustaining a rights-based response. We focus specifically on the 2010–2016 time-period, highlighting the major changes in Brazil's political landscape and how these changes have affected HIV prevention actions. A brief case study of the female sex worker movement illustrates how broader political changes affected one of the population groups that has been central to Brazil's response to HIV since the beginning. We conclude by offering thoughts on how to strengthen future actions to address HIV in Brazil by reinvigorating a rights-based agenda and creating a more strategic partnership between government and civil society.

## 7.2 Overview of Brazilian Response

Mobilization in response to the HIV epidemic in Brazil occurred in parallel to a larger, influential public health reform movement as part of the country's redemocratization process (Daniel and Parker 1991; Parker 2003). In the beginning of the epidemic, before the federal government became involved, responses were structured by the local historical and political context. In the territories such as São Paulo where the state and municipal governments were more democratic and established, even before the 1988 Constitution, health was valued as a right as was the participation of civil society members affected by the epidemic (Parker 2003; Teixeira 1997).

Civil society mobilizations around HIV in São Paulo were led by public health professionals and researchers dedicated to controlling the epidemic. The state was not only the site of the most reported AIDS cases but also the center of Brazil's recent gay liberation movement and dictatorship opposition. As Richard G. Parker notes, São Paulo's state government was 'perhaps uniquely willing to listen and respond to pressures coming from civil society' (Parker 2003: 147) given the sociopolitical context of that period. São Paulo was also home to Brazil's first state AIDS program, which was established in 1983, and the first non-governmental AIDS organization, the *Grupo de Apoio à Prevenção da AIDS-São Paulo* (Support Group for AIDS Prevention-São Paulo) (GAPA-SP), founded in 1985 (an organization that in 2016 is struggling due to a lack of funding).

The government in Rio de Janeiro was less responsive, though activism was also rising there. Herbert da Souza, known as 'Betinho', was the AIDS movement's most prominent leader. Betinho was a well-known sociologist and human rights activist in student movements against the dictatorship. He contracted HIV through a blood transfusion, as did his two brothers, the popular musician, Chico Mario, and the political cartoonist, Henfil. After his return from political exile in the early 1980s, he founded Rio de Janeiro's first AIDS NGO: the Brazilian Interdisciplinary AIDS Association (ABIA) in 1986. From very early on, Betinho advocated for a structural-, solidarity- and inclusion-based approach to HIV (de Souza 1994; Galvão 2008).

The National AIDS Program was established alongside the SUS in the late 1980s. Brazilian federal public health policies aimed to engage civil society organizations, as they were considered by the SUS principles to be the most efficient advocates for their constituencies. As such, from very early in the Program's existence, representatives of vulnerable population groups, including sex workers, were invited to participate in designing prevention actions for their peers. It is important to note that the extent to which social movements were included in the SUS largely depended on their institutional strength and ability to pressure the government. In this sense, the AIDS movement was in many ways an exception to other illnesses for its broad-reaching civil society response and success in both pressuring and collaborating with the government.

In the 1990s, the federal government supported policies that increased the visibility and voices of the people most affected by the epidemic. Yet, the fiscal and administrative nature of the federal government's AIDS policies in the 1990s under

Fernando Henrique Cardoso's administration (1994–2002) bypassed much of the state bureaucracy and transformed the relationship between NGOs and the government, both strengthening and proliferating AIDS NGOs throughout Brazil and moving towards a model of co-responsibility for the epidemic and its prevention (Galvão 2000; Parker 2002). In 1993, Brazil entered into a loan agreement with the World Bank (AIDS I 1994–1998) that funded the expansion of prevention initiatives increasingly focused on the relationship between poverty and HIV in addition to access to ART (Parker 2009). In 1996, the country began offering ART through the public health system and in 1998, Brazil entered into a second 4-year loan agreement with the World Bank. The conditions of the new agreement allowed for the continuation of the solidarity and human rights focus of earlier projects and instituted a policy that all prevention projects would be implemented directly by NGOs.

Brazil's ability to channel World Bank funding to rights-based HIV programming and strengthening of civil society at first might appear to contrast with the Bank's highly criticized projects in other contexts that reflected an agenda of neoliberalization and privatization (Pfeiffer and Chapman 2010). It is important to note, however, that both the decisions to make treatment available (Biehl 2006, 2009) and the ways in which World Bank resources were transferred to the local organizations through projects managed by UNESCO, rather than Brazil's decentralized health system, were consistent with broader neoliberal agendas. The World Bank allocated funds exclusively to primary prevention as they viewed spending on treatment as not cost-effective and explicitly prohibited it (meaning that the cost of HIV treatment was covered entirely by the Brazilian National Treasury) (Parker 2003; Galvão 2000). In addition, projects were implemented by NGOs under a neoliberal logic while decentralization attempted to construct and strengthen a state-run universal health care system. As Parker notes, the politics of the World Bank loan actually centralized funding and management, creating 'completely opposing philosophical trajectories in terms of confronting health' (Parker 2002: 33).

In her history of AIDS in Brazil, Jane Galvão (2000) refers to this phase as the 'dictatorship of projects', a time when NGOs wrote projects to meet funding demands, and started to become entangled in the management of specific projects in a way that changed their relationship to the epidemic, becoming, 'more aseptic and less activist' (p. 111). Galvão (2000) and Parker (2002) both note that this created a culture in which the responsibility for providing prevention services rested on NGOs who provided them on a short-term and project basis rather than permanent public health networks. Such policies diminished NGOs' potential as 'watchdogs' of AIDS policies and were denounced by many advocates as outsourcing through 'third-way' policies, similar to those being propagated in the United States and United Kingdom during this same time period (Muntaner et al. 2000).

The election of Luiz Ignacio da Silva Lula in 2002 ushered in a different kind of relationship between social movements and the government. For the populations that had supported him since his earlier days organizing for democracy, it also inaugurated an era of hope. Lula had been a labor union organizer and leader of the opposition to Cardoso's government, with a strong base among the Left and the poor. He founded the Workers Party (*Partido dos Trabalhadores* – PT) and symbolized a commitment to social activism and community organizing. Lula took office in 2003 and with his election, many activists from Brazil's women's, lesbian, gay, bisexual and transgender (LGBT), racial equality and AIDS movements took government office in Ministries and the newly established secretariats such as the Special Secretariat for Women's Policies (SPM) and Special Secretariat for Racial Equality.

Lula's government initially was active in addressing issues of income, racial, gender and sexuality inequalities and did so through tactics that included programs and plans designed at the federal level, involving large consultations in regional and national conferences with community-based organizations, civil society and social movements. Three programs were established through the Ministry of Health (MOH) and are of particular importance: *Brasil Sem Homophobia* (Brazil without Homophobia) (2004), the Integrated Plan to Confront the Feminization of the AIDS and STD Epidemics (2007), and the National Plan to Confront AIDS and STDS among MSM, Gays, and *Travestis* (2007). While *Brazil without Homophobia* focuses more on fighting violence and promoting LGBT citizenship with little focus on HIV specifically, the plans more directed at women and the MSM, gay and transgender communities contained a variety of specific recommendations and actions defined in partnership with the AIDS social movements.

Lula's government counted on the advocacy of civil society organizations to guarantee the implementation of these progressive programs and plans at the state and municipal level as the Ministry of Health decentralized its AIDS polices and actions through the first decade of 2000 (Rich 2013). Based on 17 months of fieldwork studying Brazil's AIDS bureaucracy from 2007 to 2010, Jessica Rich (2013) argues that progressive federal approaches to HIV treatment and prevention were initially maintained during decentralization due to the work of what she refers to as *activist bureaucrats* at the federal level who mobilized civil society groups to monitor and ensure the implementation of federal policies at the local level. Rich recognizes the diversity and inconsistency of state actors across contexts within Brazil, yet confirms the critical role that the federal government played in maintaining AIDS civil society organizations' activities and funding.

Decentralizing the AIDS response at the state and municipal level created new challenges for the governments that did not prioritize prevention and integral care for PLHIV. The AIDS movement remained deeply dependent on centralized federal programs where progressive thinking was more developed. At the same time, civil society groups increasingly faced institutional barriers as administrative burdens on NGOs increased due to the reporting requirements on funding received from state sources (IBISS 2007). The increased bureaucracy around NGOs' receiving and reporting on government funds post-2005 was in large part a backlash led by conservative opposition in the mass media and in Congress, referred to as the 'criminalization of social movements', that in addition to aggressive, directed fiscal oversight, also included violent police actions, threats and arrests (Filho and Frigo 2010). The increased fiscal oversight combined with the already complex municipal and state level paperwork processes for funding NGOs resulted in immense amounts of bureaucratic requirements and rules that crippled organizations and inhibited their ability to provide an effective response to HIV.

Brazil's economy and position in the global political landscape was also changing rapidly. In 2007, when Brazil was selected to be the host for the 2014 World Cup, the country was still being held up as an emerging global economic power. The economy weathered the 2008 international crisis, yet as will be further discussed below, decreases in the amount of international funding available overall had large effects on the sexual rights and AIDS movements in Brazil. As the country came to be seen as a middle-income country, large funders such as the World Bank, United States Agency for International Development (USAID) and the Ford Foundation either stopped funding AIDS and sexual rights initiatives entirely or significantly reduced their funding and presence in the country as they assumed that these issues were under control and government priorities. The first decade of 2000 thus ended with a large number of progressive plans and initiatives for HIV in place, yet many organizations were either on the brink of losing funding or lacking institutional structures to be able to pressure their municipal or state level governments to implement them. Finally, as we explore in more detail in the next section, Christian fundamentalists from the growing Evangelical movements were increasingly focused on converting new followers and seeking political office, disseminating their messages through their extensive TV and radio networks (Machado 2006). The Evangelical population expanded locally and regionally during Lula's two terms, reaching 22.2% of the country's population in 2010 (IBGE 2010), and forming a powerful Congressional lobby with 77 representatives. Despite these changes, the federal government maintained human rights actions and defended the separation between Church and State, political positions that started to erode throughout the years that followed.

## 7.3 Political Shifts and Weakening of the Response, 2010–2016

The 2010 election marked a large shift in the country's political landscape. Dilma Rousseff was Lula's hand-picked successor and easily won the 2010 election, defeating former Minister of Health Jose Serra. Her government largely continued Lula's economic and social policies, yet was fraught with splits among the diverse political parties and the increasing power of the Evangelical lobby within Congress. The large number of political parties in Brazil (there were 27 in 2010) meant that the governments in power had to make alliances and concessions if any legislation and government programs were to advance. In practice, this has increased widely publicized corruption scandals, and, in the case of Dilma, an arguably less radical and more sanitized approach to sexual politics than Lula's administration. One program that was frequently used as an example of the de-sexualized nature of Dilma's policies is the name for the country's maternal health program, 'The Stork Network' *(Rede Cegonha)*, which addresses reproductive health in a way that avoids debates about sexual rights and sexuality outside of maternity. Even more controversial, educational materials through the *Brazil without Homophobia* program were barred from distribution in the country's schools in 2011 and, 1 year later, a Carnival HIV prevention campaign for young gay men was suspended (Seffner and Parker 2016). During this time period, there was no significant federal investment in sustaining sexual and reproductive rights as an ethical horizon to public policies; morality and 'Christian values' occupied the center of political debates.

The AIDS movement in Brazil was vocal about the increasing power of the conservative Evangelical/Catholic lobby and what they perceived to be drastic changes in how the country was approaching HIV. One of the largest mobilizations against the shifts in Brazil's response happened in 2012 after Dr. Dirceu Grecco, the then Director of the Department of STD/AIDS and Viral Hepatitis (DDAVH), was asked what kept him up at night during a panel at the International AIDS Conference in Washington, D.C. and responded that 'he slept well' knowing that the epidemic in Brazil was under control. Activists from NGOs and academic institutions across the country organized a manifesto and blog called, 'What keeps us up at night' about the changes in the Brazilian response to AIDS. In their blog manifesto, they claimed that Dr. Grecco's statement, 'aside from incorrect, has undermined the national response, depoliticized the discussion and pushed away international investment' (*O que nos tira do sono* 2012).

This movement denounced that, despite a strong rhetorical support for rights-based interventions for key populations (sex workers, LGBT groups and adolescents), interventions targeting stigma and discrimination, human rights violations and other structural issues were declining in Brazil (Malta and Beyrer 2013). As the human rights language that had once made Brazil so widely recognized faded into the background, the federal government's campaigns became increasingly focused on HIV testing. Moreover, the expansion of religious fundamentalist movements within federal and state level governments led to recurrent waves of backlash in all matters related to gender and sexuality as health care and prevention policies begun to crawl backwards (Corrêa 2016). Health and educational policies of the previous decades were challenged and extracted from local policy plans and speaking about sexuality and prevention in schools was prohibited (Paiva and Silva 2015). State governments began rejecting harm reduction programs and instead, supporting compulsory drug rehab in 'therapeutic communities', many run by faith-based groups (Bastos 2013) and funded by the Ministry of Health starting in 2015.

AIDS activism continued, yet as indicated by a piece written for World AIDS Day in 2014 titled 'To end AIDS in Brazil', published by two prominent AIDS researchers and activists in São Paulo, Mario Scheffer and Caio Rosenthal, responsibility for HIV was increasingly decentralized and outsourced:

> In another improvised action, instead of SUS professionals being tasked with bringing the AIDS test to alternative locations in alternative hours, where vulnerable communities are, they decided to outsource it to NGOs and transform the AIDS diagnosis outside of health centers into an odd job. (Scheffer and Rosenthal 2014)

As Scheffer and Rosenthal's article emphasizes, rather than focusing on improving the structure of services and addressing multiple forms of stigma and discrimination, 'test and treat' is a continuation of the 'third way' policies established in the 1990s while also taking them a step further: members of vulnerable population groups are now *testing* their peers. A position and task that, as Scheffer and Rosenthal note, was previously reserved for public health professionals.

Starting in 2015, Brazil has been hard hit by an economic crisis that has aggravated setbacks in various social and human rights policies. As Richard G. Parker and Peter Aggleton argue (2014), 'test and treat' strategies offer material gains and are financially attractive both to governments and NGOs that face reduced budgets and pressure from international donors. The influence of the Evangelical lobbies on the federal, state and municipal level has also continued to increase and expand into the provision of health services. Conservative groups have been extremely successful in securing state funds, receiving public funding in 2015, for example, to place drug users in therapeutic communities to 'guarantee abstinence' without assuring a non-religious approach. Such programs were widely denounced for committing a series of egregious human rights violations including slave labor, keeping people in drug rehabilitation much longer than stipulated, violations of sexual and reproductive rights, isolation, imprisonment and physical violence, among others (Moncau 2013).

The economic crisis combined with the expansion of reactionary and far right social movements provided fertile ground for Dilma Roussef's impeachment proceedings in 2016. Michel Temer's interim entrance into the presidency was marked with the appointment of only white men (including several religious leaders and many ensnarled in corruption scandals) to his cabinet and the elimination of several ministries, including the Ministry of Women, Racial Equality, and Human Rights. For the first time since the installation of Brazil's democratic constitution, the country has a Minister of Health, Ricardo Barros, who publicly positioned himself against the SUS and in favor of expanding private health care plans (Colucci 2016). Not long after Barros' nomination, he prohibited the Department of STD/HIV and Viral Hepatitis from participating in the United Nations Special Session on HIV and AIDS (UNGASS). Fabio Mesquita resigned from his 3-year tenure as the Director of the Department after deciding that 'resisting from within the DDAHV would no longer be possible' (Agência de Notícias da Aids 2016).

In the following section, we explore the history of the female sex worker movement's response to HIV and their partnership with the federal government as a case study of how these political changes affected activism and prevention actions. Examples from the movement's beginnings and how the response evolved over time illustrate the broader political and economic dynamics discussed in the previous sections. The end of the section will bring the discussion back to 2016, and we will close with reflections on future directions.

## 7.4 Case Study: HIV Response with Sex Worker Rights Organizations

In the late 1980s, the recently formed National AIDS Program developed PREVINA, the first national HIV prevention program with sex workers, prisoners and drug users. Dr. Lair Guerra, the first Director of the National AIDS Program, invited sex worker activist and co-founder of the recently formed Brazilian Prostitute Network (RBP – acronym in Portuguese), Gabriela Leite, to Brasilia in the late 1980s to discuss the project. Dr. Guerra was part of a group of people from the sanitary reform movement that had taken jobs with the Ministry of Health during the redemocratization process and was directly engaging with civil society to develop a national response to the epidemic.

Despite a climate of broad civil society mobilization and the emerging female sex worker movement, Murray (2015) notes that the original project design of PREVINA presented a morally charged vision of prostitution and activities that were more clinical than community driven. Dialogue with the Brazilian Prostitute Network transformed the project into a groundbreaking initiative in terms of the civil society-government partnership and affirmative approach to sexuality and sex work (Murray 2015). The Institute for Religious Studies (ISER – acronym in Portuguese), where Gabriela Leite was working at the time, produced the material, *Fala Mulher da Vida* (Speak Woman of the Life) for the project (Fig. 7.1).

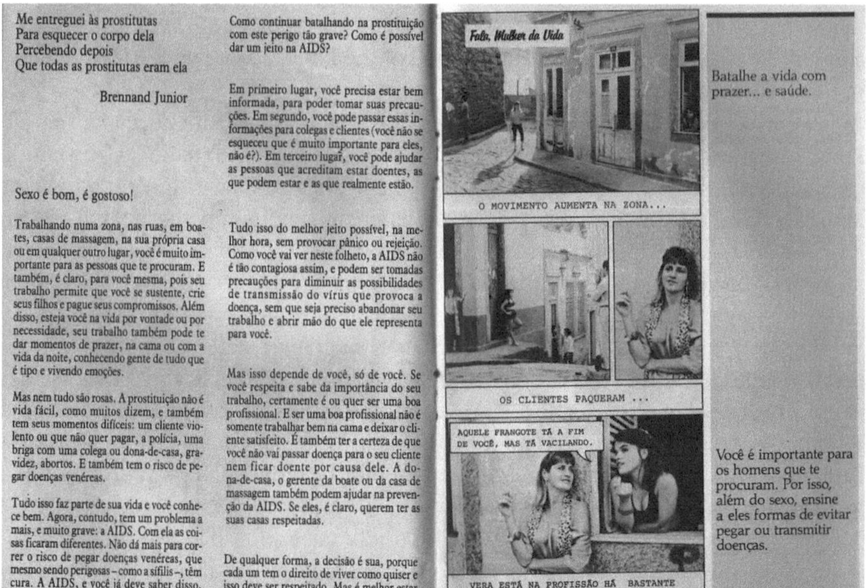
Me entreguei às prostitutas
Para esquecer o corpo dela
Percebendo depois
Que todas as prostitutas eram ela

Brennand Junior

Sexo é bom, é gostoso!

Trabalhando numa zona, nas ruas, em boates, casas de massagem, na sua própria casa ou em qualquer outro lugar, você é muito importante para as pessoas que te procuram. E também, é claro, para você mesma, pois seu trabalho permite que você se sustente, crie seus filhos e pague seus compromissos. Além disso, esteja você na vida por vontade ou por necessidade, seu trabalho também pode te dar momentos de prazer, na cama ou com a vida da noite, conhecendo gente de tudo que é tipo e vivendo emoções.

Mas nem tudo são rosas. A prostituição não é vida fácil, como muitos dizem, e também tem seus momentos difíceis: um cliente violento ou que não quer pagar, a polícia, uma briga com uma colega ou dona-de-casa, gravidez, abortos. E também tem o risco de pegar doenças venéreas.

Tudo isso faz parte de sua vida e você conhece bem. Agora, contudo, tem um problema a mais, e muito grave: a AIDS. Com ela as coisas ficaram diferentes. Não dá mais para correr o risco de pegar doenças venéreas, que mesmo sendo perigosas – como a sífilis –, têm cura. A AIDS, e você já deve saber disso, ainda não tem cura.

Como continuar batalhando na prostituição com este perigo tão grave? Como é possível dar um jeito na AIDS?

Em primeiro lugar, você precisa estar bem informada, para poder tomar suas precauções. Em segundo, você pode passar essas informações para colegas e clientes (você não se esqueceu que é muito importante para eles, não é?). Em terceiro lugar, você pode ajudar as pessoas que acreditam estar doentes, as que podem estar e as que realmente estão.

Tudo isso do melhor jeito possível, na melhor hora, sem provocar pânico ou rejeição. Como você vai ver neste folheto, a AIDS não é tão contagiosa assim, e podem ser tomadas precauções para diminuir as possibilidades de transmissão do vírus que provoca a doença, sem que seja preciso abandonar seu trabalho e abrir mão do que ele representa para você.

Mas isso depende de você, só de você. Se você respeita e sabe da importância do seu trabalho, certamente é ou quer ser uma boa profissional. E ser uma boa profissional não é somente trabalhar bem na cama e deixar o cliente satisfeito. É também ter a certeza de que você não vai passar doença para o seu cliente nem ficar doente por causa dele. A dona-de-casa, o gerente da boate ou da casa de massagem também podem ajudar na prevenção da AIDS. Se eles, é claro, querem ter as suas casas respeitadas.

De qualquer forma, a decisão é sua, porque cada um tem o direito de viver como quiser e isso deve ser respeitado. Mas é melhor estar informado para poder tomar uma decisão

Fala, Mulher da Vida

O MOVIMENTO AUMENTA NA ZONA...

OS CLIENTES PAQUERAM ...

AQUELE FRANGOTE TÁ A FIM DE VOCÊ, MAS TÁ VACILANDO.

VERA ESTÁ NA PROFISSÃO HÁ BASTANTE TEMPO. ELA É MUITO PROCURADA.

Batalhe a vida com prazer... e saúde.

Você é importante para os homens que te procuram. Por isso, além do sexo, ensine a eles formas de evitar pegar ou transmitir doenças.

**Fig. 7.1** The first two pages of the brochure Speak Woman of the Life developed for the PREVINA project by Gabriela Leite and Flavio Lenz. (Image is a scanned copy of the original)

The material is designed like a comic book with photos of actors, and accompanies a sex worker as she informs her colleagues and clients about how to protect themselves from HIV. Emblematic of the approach to prevention at the time, it discusses pleasure and the important role of sex workers as peer health educators.

The sex-positive approach to prevention and the protagonist role of sex workers in developing and implementing HIV programs were two of the defining features of the federally funded AIDS programs during the 1990s. Government AIDS programs and sex worker rights and AIDS advocacy organizations grew rapidly during this time period through financial support underpinned by the World Bank and international foundations. The rapid expansion of NGOs was sanctioned by the government: from 1993 through 1997, the National AIDS Program funded 564 projects with 181 AIDS NGOs nationally (Nunn 2009: 176), 52 of which were for male, female or transgender sex workers, with the majority (44) for female sex workers (Rossi 1998).

During the time period 1998–2003, the second World Bank loan funded even more projects with NGOs than AIDS I, with a total of 2163 projects with 795 organizations (Nunn 2009). *Esquina da Noite (Street Corner of the Night),* a national-level project implemented as part of the AIDS II World Bank loan, centered on expanding the number of sex worker-led organizations working in HIV prevention in rural areas and interior cities, where the epidemic was also spreading. The project spanned 50 municipalities throughout the country and was implemented at a time that the Ministry of Health (MOH) started to increasingly decentralize its actions. Given the climate of decentralization, *Esquina da Noite* focused its attention on forming strategic partnerships between sex worker organizations and state and municipal AIDS programs – a feat that Davida's newspaper, *Beijo da rua* [A Kiss from the street] identified at the time as one of the largest challenges to implementing the project's activities.

The principles of solidarity, respect and citizenship that Brazil became so well known for in its HIV programs made their way into the 2002 national prevention campaign, *Maria Sem Vergonha* (Maria Without Shame) that included radio spots and materials distributed in sex work establishments and points throughout Brazil. The image has Maria over a row of flowers called *sem vergonhas*, considered shameless because they will grow anywhere (Fig. 7.2). It was accompanied by a series of statements such as, 'No shame in being a prostitute' and 'No shame in valuing your work.' The Maria Without Shame campaign had even more relevance given its timing. It was launched the same year that the Ministry of Labor recognized *profissionais do sexo* [literally, sex professionals] as an official profession within the Classification System of Brazilian Occupations (CBO acronym in Portuguese) that qualify for federal government benefits such as retirement and government assistance in case of illness.

Two international events during the Lula administration had a profound symbolic effect on sex worker activism and HIV prevention. First, in 2005, as part of President Bush's Emergency Plan for AIDS Relief (PEPFAR), a contractual clause referred to as the 'anti-prostitution pledge' was introduced to all financial contracts involving US government funds. This stipulated that organizations must have a

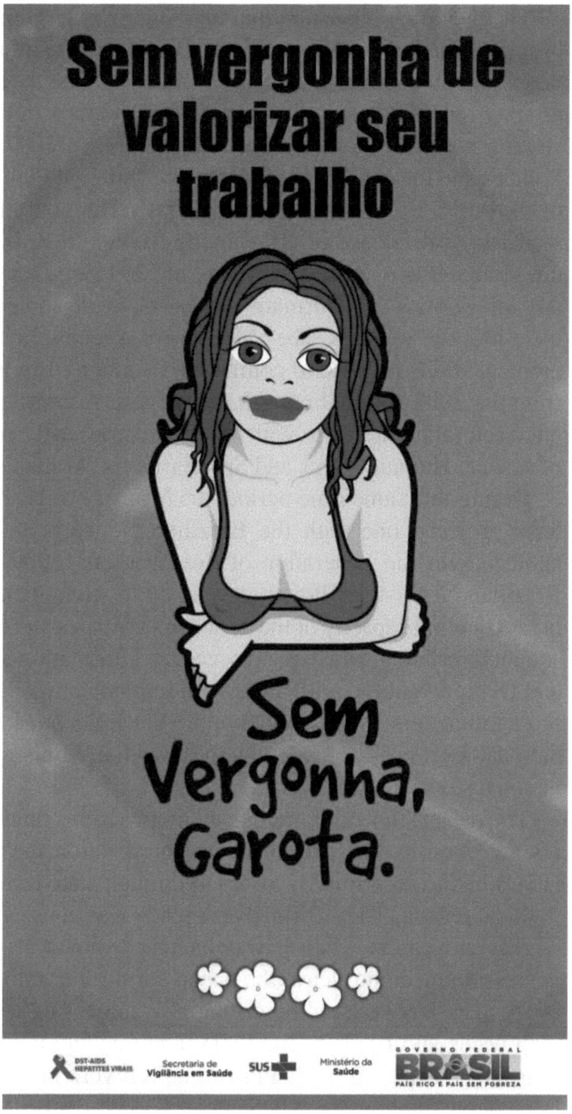


**Fig. 7.2** Maria Without Shame campaign material, re-released online in 2013, stating 'No shame to Value Your Work. Without Shame, Girl'. (Departamento de Vigilância, Prevenção e Controle das IST, do HIV/Aids e das Hepatites Virais 2017)

clause within their organizational statute explicitly opposing prostitution. In partnership with the Prostitute's Network, the Brazilian government refused to implement this mandate, eventually rejecting nearly US$40 million in HIV prevention funds that had been allocated to the country. Brazil's decision was heralded by the international community (Okie 2006) and applauded by sex worker activists globally. Second, UNAIDS held a Global Consultation on Sex Work in Rio de Janeiro in 2006 as part of its process to draw up global guidelines for member states to address HIV and sex work (Csete 2013). Subsequent meetings were held regionally, in Lima in 2007, and nationally again in Brazil in 2008 (Brasil 2008).

The National Consultation on STD/AIDS, Human Rights and Prostitution brought together leaders from the Brazilian Prostitute Network and the National Association of *Travestis* (ANTRA)[1] in 2008. The meeting resulted in the definition of sixty recommendations for moving forward a rights-based agenda of HIV prevention with sex workers. The year before, in 2007, the Secretariat of Women's Policies and the MOH had launched the 'Integral Plan to Confront the Feminization of the AIDS Epidemic and other STDs'. The goal of the plan was to address the increasing prevalence of HIV among women in Brazil and only mentioned prostitutes once. It was revised, however, in 2009 and a series of what were called, *agendas afirmativas*, or affirmative agendas, were included for specific populations, including sex workers. The 'Affirmative Agenda for Prostitutes' contained 34 recommendations on how to confront HIV among sex workers in Brazil, all adapted from the 2008 national consultation report. A cross-cutting issue was the need for intersectoral partnerships with other Ministries and Secretariats such as the Ministry of Justice, Human Rights and Secretariat for Women's Policies.

During this same time period, the Ministry of Health implemented two national level projects: one with the Brazilian Network of Prostitutes (2006–2008) and another with the Federation of Sex Workers (2009–2010). The project with the Brazilian Network of Prostitutes aimed to strengthen the network by building the organizational capacity of the network's affiliates and the project with the Federation sought to promote and expand access to information and advocacy in terms of STD and HIV prevention, with a focus on implementing the Integrated Plan to Confront the Feminization of the AIDS and STD Epidemic. As of 2016, this was the last national level project funded by the Brazilian Ministry of Health implemented by a national sex worker network.

The reasons for not funding any more actions on a national level with sex workers are twofold. On one hand, decentralization meant that government funds to NGOs had to be primarily awarded through state level bodies. Yet there was also a political reason. The Affirmative Agenda was considered to be a victory by the sex worker movement when it was launched, however, it did not *sair do papel* (an expression meaning 'leave the paper', or turning into action) (ABIA and DAVIDA 2013). The Network called on the government to support sex workers as women with needs and rights beyond HIV and this had not happened (Leite et al. 2015). Thus, in 2011, the Brazilian Prostitute Network made a decision to no longer apply for federal funding for AIDS projects. The decision was made at the Network's regional conference in Belém, in a statement that began with the phrase, 'We are professionals of sex, not the government'. The statement makes various references to the difficulties organizations encountered with state funding and reporting mechanisms and, while it recognizes the importance of the partnership with the National AIDS Program, it expresses the Network's dissatisfaction with the directions the Program was heading. In particular, the statement articulates a sense that

---

[1] *Travesti* is a gender subjectivity in Brazil (see Pelúcio 2009; Kulick 1998) that is distinct from the category of transvestite in English and references those who perform femininity in their daily livesand have not surgically altered their male sex.

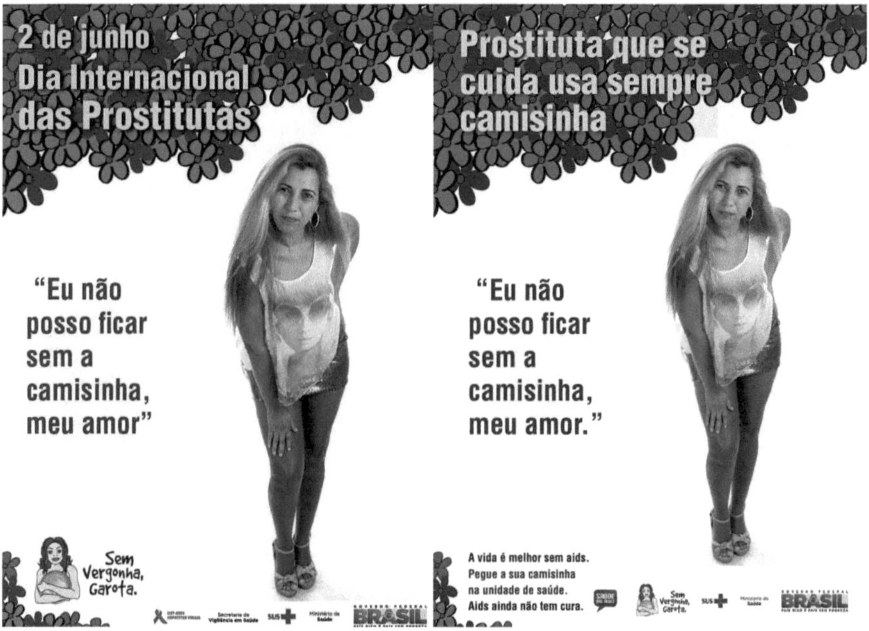


**Fig. 7.3** Original and altered campaign. The original campaign shows, in the bottom left corner, Maria Without Shame holding a condom, and saying, 'Without Shame Girl'. In the same place, the altered campaign states, 'Life is better without aids. Get your condom at the health center. Aids still doesn't have a cure'. Pictured is Cida Vieira. (Departamento de Vigilância, Prevenção e Controle das IST, do HIV/Aids e das Hepatites Virais 2013a, b)

the 'risk group' mentality that sex workers had fought so vehemently against in the late 1980s had returned through projects that 'reinforce prostitutes as spreaders of disease and distributors of condoms' (Leite et al. 2015: 18).

Two years later, the extent to which the MOH's approach to HIV prevention had changed became even clearer with the censorship of a campaign developed in a workshop with leaders from sex worker organizations throughout Brazil. The campaign, developed for International Sex Worker Rights Day on June 2nd, lasted less than 24 h online. The most controversial of the posters, which featured a sex worker with the sentence 'I'm happy being a prostitute', provoked immediate and angry reactions from conservatives in Brazil's Congress. The Director of the STD and HIV/AIDS Department was fired and the entire campaign was taken offline just 2 days after its release. An altered campaign was put up in its place and only the posters with phrases about condom use were retained. Figure 7.3 shows one of the original campaign posters alongside an altered version, and Fig. 7.4 displays two campaign posters that had not even been mentioned in the controversy yet were not re-released – one stating, 'Our biggest dream is that people see us as citizens' and the other, 'Not accepting people for the way they are is a form of violence'.

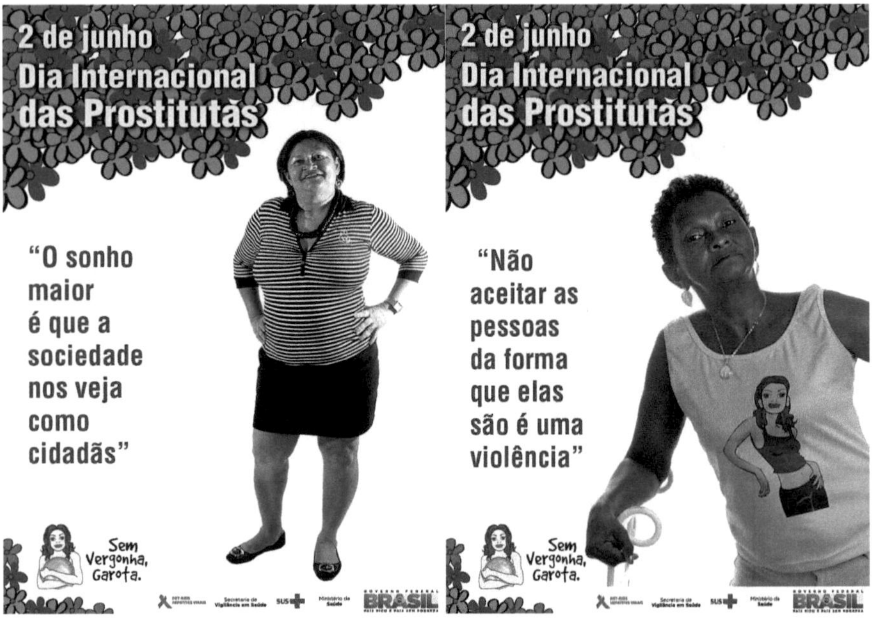


**Fig. 7.4** Original campaign removed by the Ministry of Health. Posters state, 'June 2: International Prostitutes Day' in upper left hand corner. *Left*: 'Our biggest dream is that society sees us as citizens' and *Right*: 'Not accepting people for the way they are is a form of violence'. Pictured are Nanci Feijó (*left*) and Jesus Marinho (*right*)

Although the Minister of Health at the time, Alexandre Padilha, expressed concern about the content (Rovai 2013), the official reason for taking down the campaign centered upon a technicality: the campaign had not passed through the appropriate bureaucratic channels for approval. The mass mobilization protesting the decision to dismantle the campaign disagreed. It was the third time in a year and a half that materials referring to HIV prevention and sexuality had been censored (a kit against homophobia designed for schools in 2011 and a Carnival campaign targeting young gays in 2012) and activists alleged that the reasons were paradoxically the same factors that the Brazilian response to HIV had previously been recognized for fighting against: stigma, censorship, and solely biomedical approaches to prevention. Sex worker organizations responded with strong statements and public actions (Fig. 7.5). Several organizations, including the Association of Prostitutes in Pernambucco (APPS) and the Brazilian Prostitute Network released public statements:

> We are positioning ourselves against the [state's] abusive attitude towards valuing prostitution as work, an aspect that constitutes one of main fights of the movement today in terms of reducing stigma against us and fundamentally diminishing our vulnerability to HIV and STD infection. **Once more, what was supposed to be a triumph for human rights has turned into a violation of those rights: the suspension of the right to affirm prostitution as a dignified and happy profession. – Association of Prostitutes in Pernambuco** [emphasis ours] (APPS in Murray 2015: 105)

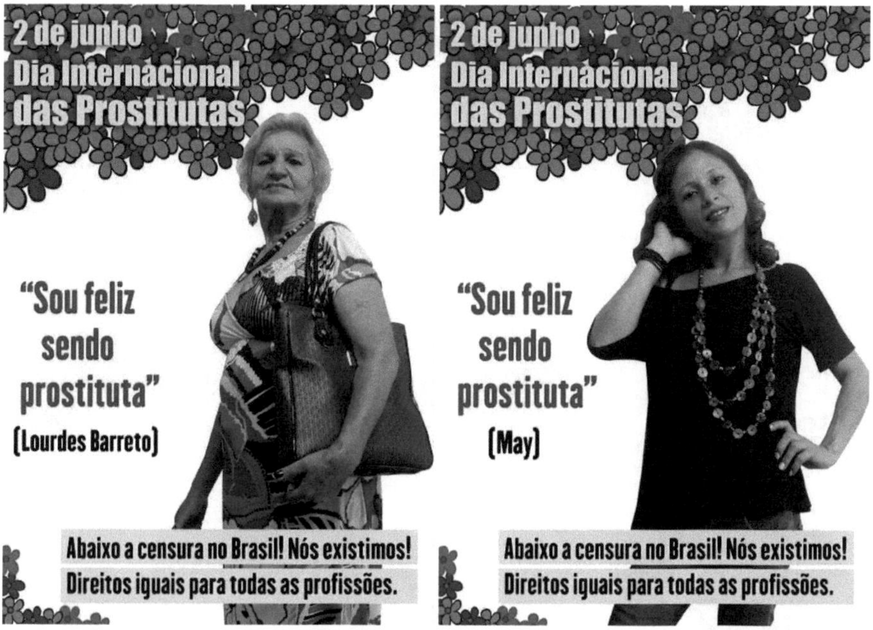


**Fig. 7.5** GEMPAC protest campaign posters stating (from *top* to *bottom*): 'June 2nd, International Prostitute Day' 'I'm happy being a prostitute'. And in *yellow*: 'Down with censorship in Brazil! We exist! Equal rights for all professions'. Downloaded from social media campaign. Pictured are Lourdes Barreto (*left*) and Maria Elias Silveira (*right*)

Several months after the campaign censorship, the MOH introduced *Live Better Knowing* [your HIV status], a 'test and treat' project directed at sex workers, MSM, and people who use drugs. The project caused sharp divisions within the Network because several organizations saw it as contrary to the clause of the Brazilian Prostitute Network's *Letter of Principles,* which repudiates the 'offering of exams and other medical procedures in locations where prostitution is practiced, except in cases that involve the general population'[2] (Leite et al. 2015: 19). The sex worker organizations that were critical of the project focused upon four, often overlapping, aspects (see Leite et al. 2015; Murray 2015). First, the authoritative way in which the project was perceived as having been developed and implemented. Second, the ethical issues involved in testing at sex workers' places of work. Third, the broader concerns associated with a biomedical emphasis in HIV prevention as opposed to community mobilization approaches in the past. And finally, perhaps the most prominent of the criticisms, that the NGOs were taking on a role (testing) that had previously belonged to – and should be of – the state.

[2]Although the Ministry of Health had been increasingly investing in testing since the rapid test became available in Brazil in 2005, oral tests were not yet developed, so the possibility that tests would be done by sex workers on other sex workers was not discussed.

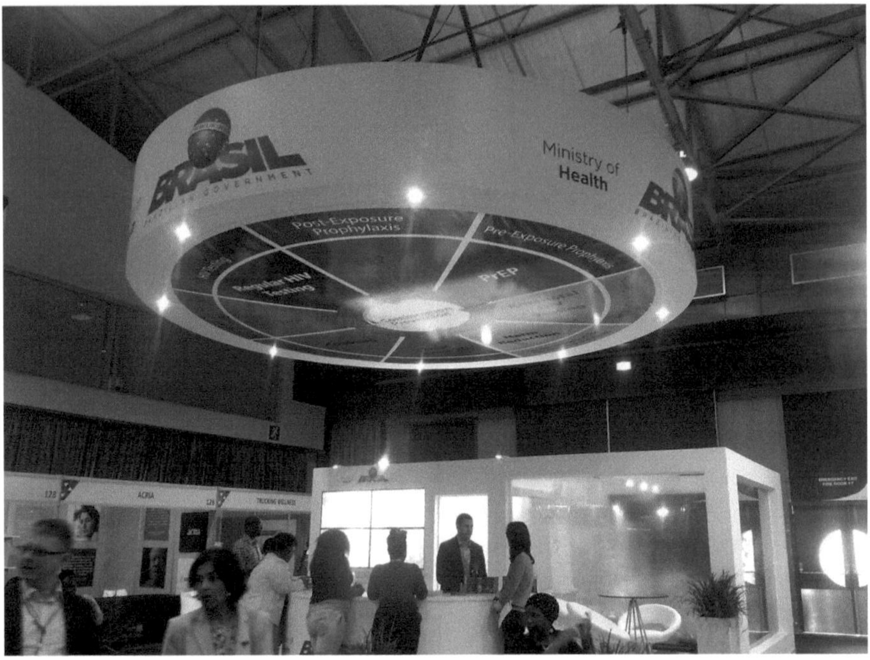


**Fig. 7.6** Brazilian Ministry of Health stand at the 2016 International AIDS Conference in Durban, South Africa (Photo by Laura Murray)

The *Live Better Knowing* project is emblematic of the AIDS Program's move away from social mobilization approaches and towards more biomedical projects focused on individual behaviors. Brazil's stand at the 2016 AIDS Conference in Durban is especially telling (Fig. 7.6). All of the 'Combination Prevention' methods in the wheel featured both in the pamphlet distributed (Fig. 7.7) and that loomed over the stand are individual interventions, the majority biomedical: post-exposure prophylaxis (PEP), pre-exposure prophylaxis (PrEP), treatment as prevention (TaSP), testing, and antenatal testing.[3] The only two not related in some way to medical interventions are condoms and harm reduction. In addition to the pamphlet with the prevention wheel, the stand only had postcards about condom use, and no mention of MSM, sex workers or the kinds of human rights focused, community mobilization projects that had made Brazil so well known and celebrated a decade earlier. Interestingly, next to South Africa, Brazil was the only other country to have a booth at the conference in the exhibition area, right behind all of the pharmaceutical companies and USAID/PEPFAR.

[3] It is important to note that this understanding of 'combination prevention' is fundamentally different from that originally intended by those who developed the concept to refer to tailored and context specific responses to the epidemic that combine biomedical, behavioral and structural approaches (see Hankins and de Zalduondo 2010).

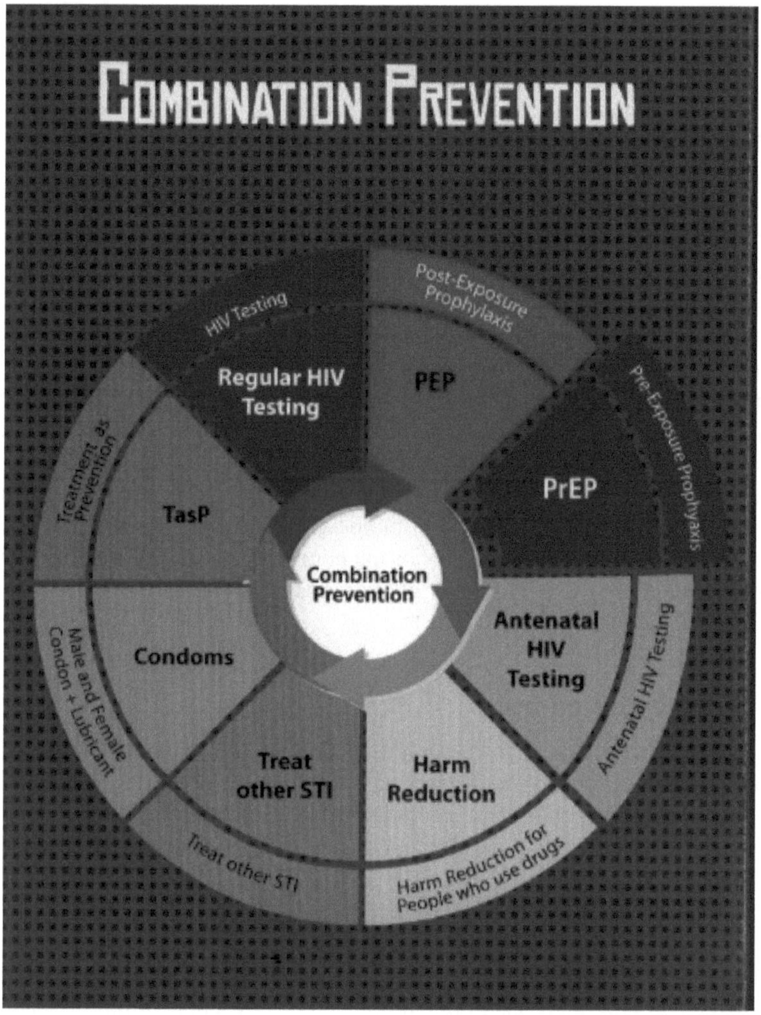


**Fig. 7.7** Page of pamphlet: 30 Years of HIV/AIDS Response in Brazil 2016

The protagonist role that sex workers held in the PREVINA project was not present in the MOH's combination prevention model as disseminated at the 2016 AIDS Conference. In accordance with a 2015 Ministry report, the model 'offers a variety of prevention commodities and services and its users can chose and combine the prevention methods that best meet their situation of vulnerability' (Brasil 2015b: 45). Rather than designing materials and programs, vulnerable population groups like sex workers are consumers of prevention commodities. Language about stigma, discrimination, and sex virtually disappear within this model. Rights are reduced to the right to choose a method.

The HIV response with sex workers arguably reached its peak in 2002 when both the social movement and the federal AIDS program were strong. While the development of the diverse plans and programs during Lula's administration had a strong symbolic effect and reflected participatory processes, challenges posed by decentralization and the increasing power of Evangelical fundamentalists made implementing them nearly impossible as fewer and fewer Ministries and secretariats were willing to defend sex worker rights. Parallel to these processes, biomedical approaches such as PreP, TaSP, and 'test and treat' gained steam on the global health landscape (Nguyen et al. 2011) providing programmatic justification, and funding, for a shift in approaches.

The neoliberal groundwork had been laid during Fernando Henrique Cardoso's administration in terms of shifting responsibility from the state to NGOs to provide prevention services. However, the shift from condom use and community mobilization (methodologies that required discussions of sexuality and stigma to be successful) to testing, transforms activists into health professionals and NGOs into health services. The history of the relationship between the sex worker movement and Ministry of Health has had loud and public conflicts, yet it is the government's silence surrounding the human rights of the populations most affected by HIV that is currently deafening as this chapter goes to press.

## 7.5 Future Directions

Historical processes are constantly in flux, yet at the time of writing this chapter, the very backbone of Brazil's democracy, the 1988 Constitution, is under threat. In December of 2016, Congress passed a constitutional amendment that will freeze the health and education budgets for 20 years, a disaster for the SUS (Dias 2016). The project was the subject of large street protests, occupations of more than 1000 schools throughout Brazil, teachers' strikes, heavily criticized by the country's top universities and scholars (Reis 2016) and the subject of a strong statement from UN officials denouncing the constitutional amendment as 'condemning a generation' and as an 'affront to human rights' (Melo 2016). The SUS, built from civil society mobilizations, has always been cornerstone to the AIDS response; when it is threatened, the response as a whole is threatened.

Human rights approaches to health depend on the principles of community participation and input to monitor accessibility, acceptability and the quality of services. As we could observe in AIDS activism in Brazil, vulnerable population groups were crucial to holding governments responsible and managers accountable – two key principles of human rights-based approaches to health (Gruskin et al. 2007). Brazil was a leader in incorporating a human rights approach into HIV prevention, as the sex work case study shows here. At a time when this approach has been incorporated into the international system, with groups such as the World Health Organization endorsing structural approaches and decriminalization of sex work as a way to fight HIV (WHO 2012), Brazil is going in the opposite direction.

The Brazilian experience thus raises extremely important and complex questions for thinking more broadly about how to sustain human rights-based responses to HIV driven by communities but with true (i.e. financial and social) commitment from the state, including: How should the relationship between state institutions and non-state institutions be constructed to ensure both autonomy and partnership?; What does country ownership mean for the Brazilian response in a 'divided country'?; How can Brazil's AIDS activist, practitioner and scholarly communities (re) construct the principles of solidarity, citizenship and respect in the current socio-economic and political environment?; Are consultative and representative roles for vulnerable population groups enough to guarantee a truly rights-based approach?

In our final paragraphs, we begin to think about these very difficult questions. Certainly, the role of NGOs must involve ensuring government accountability to fund and implement HIV programming and services that are constitutional rights of its citizens. At the same time, NGOs must also maintain the autonomy necessary to take a protagonist role in designing the kinds of HIV preventions they see as being most important for their constituents. Brazil's response was built through collaborations with everyone from the Catholic Church to the porn industry (Murray et al. 2011). This sort of wide reaching mobilization is needed once again.

Further research bringing together the diverse actors and spheres that made the 'Brazilian Response to HIV' possible is also needed. Sex workers frequently cite the 2002 study conducted with the MOH, that evaluated peer-led and implemented HIV programs, as an example of the kind of research they see as needing to be done (Brasil 2004). Participatory in nature from the very beginning, these sorts of projects not only produce reliable data, but more importantly are ways for communities that are so researched to lead research about themselves. Two research interventions in Brazil, the *Encontros* Project (Lippman et al. 2012) and the *Princesinha* Project (Benzaken et al. 2007), both conducted outside of major urban centers (in the Pantanal and Amazon respectively), found that buy-in from local government officials and participatory intervention approaches involving a wide range of local stakeholders – from cultural producers to health care providers – had effects on reducing sexually transmitted infection incidence and increasing condom use. Similar models of collaborative research projects can be found in Brazilian studies with religious communities (Paiva et al. 2010) and high school students (Paiva 2003), even in context of backlash. The challenge, as this chapter and subsequent research on the *Encontros* intervention have shown (Murray 2015), is sustaining such meaningful engagement and public policies over time as political and economic contexts drastically change.

Finally, rather than extensive consultations and meetings, we also see a need for solidarity between key populations and with broader social movements. Rather than just being consulted, it its crucial that these groups are given the financial resources and support they need to be able to develop and define their responses and priorities. Although there were many consequences to the NGO boom in the 1990s, one of the positive aspects frequently cited by sex worker organizations is how they felt that they had the autonomy they needed to grow their organizations and define their HIV prevention actions. We know both from experience and research that this sort of protagonist role is the backbone to any successful and sustainable response to HIV (Kerrigan et al. 2015; WHO 2012). Yet in the current scenario in Brazil, with many NGOs demobilized, it is increasingly important that there is support across social movements, especially women's movements in the case of sex workers, and broader human rights' movements for the larger conversations about HIV prevention and treatment. It was this type of wide mobilization across the health, political activist and religious sectors that built the response. At a time when democracy is threatened once again, it is even more critical to politicize solidarity, resist fundamentalist backlash and radicalize, rather than extinguish, human rights-based approaches. As a 2016 protest slogan states: *'nenhum direito a menos'* ( not a single right less).

## References

ABIA & DAVIDA. (2013). *Analysis of prostitution contexts in terms of human rights, work, culture, and health in Brazilian Cities*. Rio de Janeiro: ABIA. www.sxpolitics.org/ptbr/wp-content/uploads/.../analise_contexto_abia-davida.pdf. Accessed 28 Apr 2017.

Agência de Notícias da Aids (2016). Diretor do Departamento de Aids, Fábio Mesquisa, pede demissão por incompatibilidade com atual governo. http://agenciaaids.com.br/home/noticias/noticia_detalhe/24907%23.V05FnvkrLIU. Accessed 10 Dec 2016.

Bastos, F. (2013). Against the tide: Current perspectives in Brazilian drug policy. *Cadernos de Saúde Pública, 29*(2), 216–218. doi:10.1590/s0102-311x2013000200002.

Bastos, F., Kerrigan, D., Malta, M., Carneiro-da-Cunha, C., & Strathdee, S. (2001). Treatment for HIV/AIDS in Brazil: Strengths, challenges, and opportunities for operations research. *AIDScience, 1*(15). http://www.aidscience.com/Articles/aidscience012.asp.

Benzaken, A., Paiva, V., Galban-Garcia, E., & Sarinha, J. (2007). Community-based intervention to control STD/AIDS in the Amazon region, Brazil. *Revista de Saúde Pública/Journal of Public Health, 41*, 118–126.

Berkman, A., Garcia, J., Munoz-Laboy, M., Paiva, V., & Parker, R. (2005). A Critical Analysis of the Brazilian response to HIV/AIDS: Lessons learned for controlling and mitigating the epidemic in developing countries. *American Journal of Public Health, 95*(7), 1162–1172. doi:10.2105/ajph.2004.054593.

Biehl, J. (2006). Pharmaceutical governance. In A. Petryna, A. Lakoff, & A. Kleinman (Eds.), *Global pharmaceuticals: Ethics, markets, practices* (pp. 206–239). Durham: Duke University Press.

Biehl, J. (2009). *Will to live: AIDS therapies and the politics of survival*. Princeton: Princeton University Press.

Brasil (2001). *Implementation and monitoring report – AIDS II – December 1988–May 2001*. World Bank Loan BIRD 4392/BR, 2001.

Brasil (2004). Avaliação de efetividade das ações de prevenção dirigidas as profissionais do sexo, em três regiões brasileiras. Brasília: Ministério da Saúde – Programa Nacional de DST/AIDS. http://www.aids.gov.br/publicacao/2008/avaliacao-da-efetividade-das-acoes-de-prevencao-dirigidas-profissionais-do-sexo-em-t

Brasil. (2008). *Consulta nacional sobre DST/AIDS, direitos humanos e prostituição*. Brasília: Ministério da Saúde - Departamento de DST/Aids e Hepatites Virais.

Brasil. (2015a). *Boletim epidemiologico - AIDS e DST, Ano IV, No. 1*. Brasília: Ministério da Saúde. http://www.aids.gov.br/sites/default/files/anexos/publicacao/2015/58534/boletim_aids_11_2015_web_pdf_19105.pdf. Accessed 28 Apr 2017.

Brasil. (2015b). *The Brazilian response to HIV and AIDS: Global AIDS response progress eporting (GARPR)*. Brasilia: Ministério da Saúde – Departamento de DST/Aids e Hepatites Virais.

Colucci, C. (2016, May 17, 2016). Tamanho do SUS precisa ser revisto, diz novo Ministro da Saúde. *Folha de São Paulo*. http://www1.folha.uol.com.br/cotidiano/2016/05/1771901-tamanho-do-sus-precisa-ser-revisto-diz-novo-ministro-da-saude.shtml.

Corrêa, S. O. (2016). The Brazilian response to HIV and AIDS in troubled and uncertain times. In A. Basthi, R. Parker, & V. Terto Júnior (Eds.), *Myth v reality: Evaluating the Brazilian response to HIV in 2016* (pp. 7–15). Rio de Janeiro: Brazilian Interdisciplinary AIDS Association (ABIA)/Global AIDS Policy Watch (GAPW).

Csete, J. (2013). Victimhood and vulnerability: Sex work and the rhetoric and reality of the global response to HIV/AIDS. In L. Murthy (Ed.), *The business of sex* (pp. 45–80). New Dehli: Zubaan.

Daniel, H., & Parker, R. (1991). *AIDS: A terceira epidemia (ensaios e tentativas)*. São Paulo: Iglu.

de Souza, H. (1994). *A Cura da AIDS/The Cure of AIDS* (bilingual ed.). Rio de Janeiro: Relumé Dumará.

Departamento de Vigilância, Prevenção e Controle das IST, do HIV/Aids e das Hepatites Virais (2013a). [Original campaign image]. www.aids.gov.br. Accessed 1 June 2013.

Departamento de Vigilância, Prevenção e Controle das IST, do HIV/Aids e das Hepatites Virais (2013b). [Altered campaign image]. www.aids.gov.br. Accessed 8 June 2013.

Departamento de Vigilância, Prevenção e Controle das IST, do HIV/Aids e das Hepatites Virais (2017). Profissionais de Sexo – Sem vergonha garota você tem profissão. http://www.aids.gov.br/campanhas/2002/38289. Accessed 28 Apr 2017.

Dias, B. (2016). Golpe fatal: PEC 55 é aprovada em meio a manifestações e brutal repressão policial. https://www.abrasco.org.br/site/noticias/movimentos-sociais/golpe-fatal-pec-55-e-aprovada-em-meio-a-manifestacoes-e-brutal-repressao-policial/24431/. Accessed 15 Dec 2016.

Filho, A. S. E., & Frigo, D. (2010). A luta por direitos e a criminazlização dos movimentos sociais: A qual Estado de Direito serve o sistema de justiça? http://terradedireitos.org.br/2010/05/10/a-luta-por-direitos-e-a-criminalizacao-dos-movimentos-sociais-a-qual-estado-de-direito-serve-o-sistema-de-justica/. Accessed 28 Apr 2017.

Galvão, J. (2000). *AIDS no Brasil: A agenda de construção de uma epidemia* (Vol. 34). Rio de Janeiro: ABIA/Editora.

Galvão, J. (2008). Betinho: A celebration of a life in Brazil. In D. Perlman & A. Roy (Eds.), *The practice of international health* (pp. 231–243). Oxford: Oxford University Press.

Grangeiro, A. (2016). From stabilization to reemergence: Challenges for confronting the HIV/AIDS epidemic in its fourth decade in Brazil. In A. Basthi, R. Parker, & V. Terto Júnior (Eds.), *Myth vs. reality: Evaluating the Brazilian response to HIV in 2016* (pp. 16–21). Rio de Janeiro: Brazilian Interdisciplinary AIDS Association (ABIA)/Global AIDS Policy Watch (GAPW).

Greenwald, G. (2016, June 30). Major new Brazil events expose the fraud of Dilma's impeachment – and Temer's corruption. *The Intercept*. https://theintercept.com/2016/06/30/major-new-brazil-events-expose-the-fraud-of-dilmas-impeachment-and-temers-corruption/.

Gruskin, S., Mills, E., & Tarantola, D. (2007). History, principles, and practice of health and human rights. *The Lancet, 370*(9585), 449–455. doi:10.1016/s0140-6736(07)61200-8.

Hankins, C. A., & de Zalduondo, B. O. (2010). Combination prevention: A deeper understanding of effective HIV prevention. *AIDS, 24*(Suppl 4), S70–S80. doi:10.1097/01.aids.0000390709.04255.fd.

IBISS (Instituto Brasileiro pró-Sociedade Saudável do Centro-Oeste). (2007). *Trançando redes*. Campo Grande: IBISS.

IBGE (Instituto Brasileiro de Geografia e Estatística) (2010). Censo Demográfico. http://www.ibge.gov.br/home/estatistica/populacao/censo2010/default.shtm. Accessed 30 Oct 2011.

Kerrigan, D., Kennedy, C., Morgan-Thomas, R., Reza-Paul, S., Mwangi, P., Win, K. T., McFall, A., Fonner, V. A., & Butler, J. (2015). A community empowerment approach to the HIV response among sex workers: Effectiveness, challenges, and considerations for implementation and scale-up. *The Lancet, 385*(9963), 172–185. doi:10.1016/s0140-6736(14)60973-9.

Kulick, D. (1998). Travesti. Chicago: University of Chicago Press.

Leite, G., Murray, L. R., & Lenz, F. (2015). The Peer and Non-peer: The potential of risk management for HIV prevention in contexts of prostitution. *Revista Brasileira de Epidemiologia, 15*(Suppl 1), 7–25. doi:10.1590/1809-4503201500050003.
Lippman, S., Chinaglia, M., Donini, A., Kerrigan, D., Reingold, A., & Diaz, J. (2012). Findings from Encontros: A multi-level STI/HIV intervention to increase condom use, reduce STI, and change the social environment among sex workers in Brazil. *Sexually Transmitted Diseases, 39*(3), 209–216. doi:10.1097/OLQ.0b013e31823b1937.
Machado, M. d. D. C. (2006). *Política e religião: A participação dos evangelicos nas eleições*. Rio de Janeiro: Editora FGV.
Malta, M., & Beyrer, C. (2013). The HIV epidemic and human rights violations in Brazil. *Journal of the International AIDS Society, 16*, 18817. doi: http://dx.doi.org/10.7448/IAS.16.1.18817.
Melo, D. (2016). Toda uma geração está condenada diz relator da ONU sobre a PEC 55. *Carta Capital*. http://www.cartacapital.com.br/politica/toda-uma-geracao-esta-condenada-diz-relator-da-onu-sobre-a-pec-55. Accessed 16 Dec 2016.
Moncau, G. (2013). Nem comunidades, nem terapeuticas. *Caros Amigos*. http://www.carosamigos.com.br/index.php/politica/1263-nem-comunidades-nem-terapeuticas. Accessed 16 Mar 2016.
Muntaner, C., Lynch, J., & Davey Smith, G. (2000). Social capital and the third way in public health. *Critical Public Health, 10*(2), 107–124. doi:10.1080/713658240.
Murray, L. R. (2015). *Not fooling around: The politics of sex worker activism in Brazil*. PhD Dissertation in the Sociomedical Sciences Department, Columbia University, New York.
Murray, L. R., Garcia, J., Munoz-Laboy, M., & Parker, R. (2011). Strange bedfellows: The Catholic Church and Brazilian National AIDS Program in response to HIV/AIDS in Brazil. *Social Science and Medicine, 72*(6), 945–952. doi:10.1016/j.socscimed.2011.01.004.
Nguyen, V.-K., Bajos, N., Dubois-Arber, O'Malley, J., & Pirkle, C. M. (2011). Remedicalizing an epidemic: From HIV treatment as prevention to HIV treatment is prevention. *AIDS, 25*, 291–293. doi:10.1097/QAD.0b013e3283483697.
Nunn, A. (2009). *The politics and history of AIDS treatment in Brazil*. New York: Springer.
Okie, S. (2006). Fighting HIV: Lessons from Brazil. *New England Journal of Medicine, 354*(19), 1977–1981. doi:10.1056/NEJMp068069.
O que nos tira o sono (2012). *Manifesto*. Oquenostiraosono.tumblr.com/manifesto. Accessed 20 Feb 2013.
Paiva, V. (2003). Beyond magic solutions: Prevention of HIV and AIDS as a process of psychosocial empancipation. *Saúde para Debate, 27*, 192–203.
Paiva, V., Garcia, J., Munoz-Laboy, M., Santos, A., & Terto Júnior, V. (2010). Religious communities and HIV prevention: An intervention-study using human rights based approach. *Global Public Health, 5*(3), 280–294. doi:10.1080/17441691003677421.
Paiva, V., & Silva, V. (2015). Facing negative reactions to sexuality education through a multicultural human rights framework. *Reproductive Health Matters, 23*(46), 96–106. doi:10.1016/j.rhm.2015.11.015.
Parker, R. (2002). Estado e sociedade em redes: Descentralização e sustentabilidade das ações de prevenção das DST/AIDS. In R. Parker, V. Terto Jr., & M. C. Pimenta (Eds.), *Aprimorando o debate: Respostas sociais frente a AIDS: anais do seminario: principios possiveis para as respostas ao HIV/AIDS?* (pp. 31–36). Rio de Janeiro: ABIA.
Parker, R. (2003). Building the foundations for the response to HIV/AIDS in Brazil: The development of HIV/AIDS policy, 1982–1996. *Divulgação em Saúde para Debate, 27*, 143–183.
Parker, R. (2009). Civil society, political mobilization, and the impact of HIV scale-up on health systems in Brazil. *Journal of Acquired Immune Deficiency Syndromes, 52*(1), S49–S51. doi:10.1097/QAI.0b013e3181bbcb56.
Parker R, & Aggleton P. (2014). Test and treat from a human rights perspective. GAPW Bulletin, No. 1, 16–23. Rio de Janeiro: ABIA/GAPW. http://gapwatch.org/news/articles/test-and-treat-from-a-human-rights-perspective/118
Pelucio, L. (2009). *Abjeção e desejo: Uma etnografia travesti sobre o modelo preventivo de aids*. Sao Paulo: Editora Annablume.

Pfeiffer, J., & Chapman, R. (2010). Anthropological perspectives on structural adjustment and public health. *Annual Review of Anthropology, 39*, 149–165. doi:10.1146/annurev.anthro.012809.105101.

Reis, V. (2016). Alerta: PEC 55 vai desmantelar o SUS e agravar as desigualdades. https://www.abrasco.org.br/site/noticias/sistemas-de-saude/alerta-pec-55-vai-desmantelar-o-sus-e-agravar-as-desigualdades/24465/. Accessed 16 Dec 2016.

Rich, J. A. J. (2013). Grassroots bureaucracy: Intergovernmental relations and popular mobilization in Brazil's AIDS policy sector. *Latin American Politics and Society, 55*(2), 1–24. doi:10.1111/j.1548-2456.2013.00191.x.

Rossi, L. (1998). *Prevencao das DST/Aids e a prostitucao feminina no Brasil*. Brasília: Ministeiro de Saude: Coordenacao Nacional de DST e Aids.

Rovai, R. (2013). Padilha explica por que não permitiu campanha 'sou feliz sendo prostituta'. http://revistaforum.com.br/blogdorovai/2013/06/11/padilha-explica-porque-nao-permitiu-o-sou-feliz-sendo-prostituta/. Accessed 26 June 2013.

Scheffer, M., & Rosenthan, C. (2014). Para acabar com Aids no Brasil. *Folha de Sao Paulo*. http://www1.folha.uol.com.br/opiniao/2014/12/1555175-mario-scheffer-e-caio-rosenthal-para-acabar-com-a-aids-no-brasil.shtml. Accessed 27 Apr 2017.

Seffner, F., & Parker, R. (2016). The neoliberalization of HIV prevention in Brazil. In A. Basthi, R. Parker, & V. Terto Júnior (Eds.), *Myth vs. reality: Evaluating the Brazilian response to HIV in 2016* (pp. 22–30). Rio de Janeiro: Brazilian Interdisciplinary AIDS Association (ABIA)/ Global AIDS Policy Watch (GAPW).

Szwarcwald, C., Pascom, A. R., & Souza Junior, P. (2015). Estimation of the HIV incidence and of the number of people living with HIV/AIDS in Brazil, 2012. *Journal of AIDS & Clinical Research, 6*(3), 430. doi:10.4172/2155-6113.1000430.

Teixeira, P. R. (1997). Políticas públicas em AIDS. In R. Parker (Ed.), *Políticas, instituições e AIDS: Enfrentando a epidemia no Brasil* (pp. 43–68). Rio de Janeiro: Jorge Zahar/ABIA.

WHO. (2012). *Prevention and treatment of HIV and other sexually transmitted diseases for sex workers in low and middle income countries*. Agency Report. World Health Organization. http://apps.who.int/iris/bitstream/10665/77745/1/9789241504744_eng.pdf?ua=1. Accessed 15 Mar 2016.

# Chapter 8
# Structural Approaches Are Building Power: South Africa's National HIV Response Among Female Sex Workers (1990–2016)

**Daniel M. Woznica, Anna M. Leddy, and Tim Lane**

## 8.1 Introduction

South Africa is unique among southern and eastern African nations for having concentrated HIV epidemics among key populations such as men who have sex with men (MSM) and female sex workers (FSW) before its high-prevalence general population epidemic took off. As in Europe, the Americas, and Australia, HIV in South Africa first was detected clinically most often among MSM (Jochelson et al. 1991). However, by 1991, South African clinicians were diagnosing HIV among FSW and men with no apparent history of same-sex sexual partners (Jochelson et al. 1991). As HIV cases began appearing among women and men with no apparent participation in sex work, male same-sex sexual activity, or injection drug use, it became clear that a generalized, heterosexually transmitted epidemic similar to those throughout the eastern and southern African region was taking root in South Africa. While the impact of the missteps and misuse of science in South Africa's national generalized epidemic response during early post-apartheid years has been previously researched (Chigwedere et al. 2008), less well-understood is how national political discourse among the scientific community, government actors, and civil society contributed to the erasure of MSM and FSW from the national HIV agenda – an erasure that is all the more remarkable given South Africa's comparatively favorable legal, human rights, and civil society contexts for an effective response among these groups.

Following on a previous analysis of the history of South Africa's national HIV response among MSM (Lane 2009), this chapter reviews the history of South

D.M. Woznica (✉) • A.M. Leddy
Johns Hopkins Bloomberg School of Public Health, Baltimore, MD, USA
e-mail: dwoznic1@jhmi.edu

T. Lane
University of California, San Francisco, San Francisco, CA, USA

 
D. Kerrigan, C. Barrington (eds.), *Structural Dynamics of HIV*, Social Aspects of HIV 4, DOI 10.1007/978-3-319-63522-4_8

Africa's national HIV response among FSW. We frame our analysis using Campbell and Cornish's writing on community mobilization as a third 'generation' approach to HIV (Campbell and Cornish 2010). From this vantage point, we review the literature on South Africa's national response to HIV among FSW between 1990 and 2016. We show how a pattern of delays characterized scientists', governmental, and much of civil society's responses to the epidemic among FSW. Typically, these responses paired awareness and peer education approaches with ineffectual calls for sex work decriminalization, prompting limited action and meeting continued setbacks. We find further evidence of this same pattern through a document analysis of the country's HIV National Strategic Plans. We then identify a rupture in the South African national response to HIV among FSW: the 2016 National Sex Worker HIV Plan, which adopts a multi-level peer education and community mobilization approach. To better understand the background to this change, we present a case study of how the South African sex worker rights organization, SWEAT, and the related sex worker rights movement, Sisonke, mobilized South African sex workers into a nationwide movement. In the end, we argue that public health researchers and practitioners can learn crucial lessons from the history of South Africa's national HIV response among FSW. In short, FSW have extended national HIV awareness peer education approaches as well as calls for sex work decriminalization into a broad-based movement that affirms sex workers' identities, proclaims their rights to social and economic capital, and is now building power.

## 8.2 Conceptual Framework: Campbell and Cornish on Community Mobilization

Campbell and Cornish's writing on community mobilization provides an overarching framework for this chapter. Specifically, their conceptual framework of successive 'generations' of approaches to HIV/AIDS management (Campbell and Cornish 2010) denotes useful terminology for describing the history of the South African national response to HIV among FSW. Briefly, their first three 'generations' of approaches are: HIV awareness; peer education; and community mobilization. Awareness approaches focus on individuals' health education, information, and risk perception. Peer education approaches shift focus toward interpersonal influences; accordingly, they hold that peers access hard-to-reach groups, normatively influence them, and bridge individual knowledge-action-practice gaps. Community mobilization approaches encompass peer education, but in contrast with some peer education methods, focus on participant empowerment. Community mobilization approaches additionally emphasize building social capital and creating safe spaces for dialogue.

With Campbell and Cornish's conceptual framework about community mobilization as a third 'generation' in mind, we now turn to a literature review of the history of South Africa's national HIV response among FSW.

## 8.3 A Pattern of Delays: The Scientific, Government, and Civil Society Response to HIV Among FSW, 1990–2016

Initially, the South African national HIV response among FSW was characterized by a scientific discourse that treated FSW as an auxiliary problem to the larger issue of male labor migrants driving the epidemic's spread (Jochelson et al. 1991). As the end of apartheid ushered in both new urban policing strategies and a human rights-based constitutional framework, the country's transitional government fleetingly considered decriminalization as part of a crime management strategy that also prevented HIV; this strategy resonated with calls for decriminalization from an incipient sex worker rights movement (Wojcicki 2003). But in the decade that followed, high-level political decisions as well as setbacks in the courts relegated sex workers to the periphery, despite ongoing calls for decriminalization from researchers, the Department of Health, and sex workers themselves (Crowe 1997; Richter 2008; Scheibe et al. 2016). Mounting anxieties around the sex trade in the build-up to the 2010 World Cup led to a short-lived move to decriminalize sex work that again produced little change (Richter 2008). The following section briefly reviews this history.

One of the earliest scientific studies to draw attention to HIV among FSW in South Africa – Jochelson's 'Human Immunodeficiency Virus and migrant labor in South Africa' (Jochelson et al. 1991) – presented HIV among 'women dependent on prostitution' as a national crisis insofar as mineworkers who visited FSW in urban areas could spread HIV across the country. This narrative was partly deduced from Sydney Kark's 1949 research on syphilis among migrant mine workers returning home and partly induced from early records showing HIV transmission rates to be highest among White homo-/bisexual males and Black heterosexual males and females (Jochelson et al. 1991). Because Kark's influential study implicated apartheid-era economic and historical factors in the distribution of sexually transmitted infections by mineworkers, what came to be termed the 'male-migrant-infector' model was widely adopted by scholars seeking a counterpoint to then-prevalent and often biased or even racist narratives about non-Western, 'African' patterns of transmission (Hunter 2010). Missing from this scientific narrative were the effects of unemployment, changing marital rates, and women's own migration on the growing HIV epidemic (Hunter 2007).

Against the backdrop of this scientific discourse came two nascent government and civil society responses to female sex work that focused alternately on crime and human rights but converged at least initially on the common cause of decriminalization. First, massive urban in-migration at the end of apartheid forced the creation of new policing strategies that could manage crime with limited resources (Wojcicki 2003). Attuned to this need, in 1993, the Human Sciences Research Council published a report on sex work and HIV that presented decriminalization of sex work as a strategy to reduce demand on overburdened police forces; 1 year later, the national Safety and Security Minister and the Gauteng Minister for Safety and Security were at the head of a government sex work decriminalization effort (Wojcicki 2003). At the same time, the new South Africa's human rights-based constitutional framework and the concurrent growth of the international sex worker rights movement facilitated the formation of sex worker advocacy groups, including Sex Worker Education and Advocacy Taskforce (SWEAT) in Cape Town in 1994 (Wojcicki 2003). This group began as a safe sex education initiative, but soon was advocating on behalf of sex workers' legal and human rights and issuing calls for decriminalization.

With scientific evidence of the significance of HIV among sex workers and a push for decriminalization from both government and the sex work sector, an overall national response to HIV among FSW emerged that promoted awareness and peer education approaches coupled with support for legal reform. In 1997, following a pilot study led by AMREF (African Medical Research Foundation) South Africa, the national AIDS control program director rolled out truck firm awareness and sex worker peer education campaigns and, in a press release, voiced support for decriminalization of sex work through the courts (Crowe 1997). Intervention and rapid assessment studies continued to make the case for prevention of HIV among FSW through programs at mines and at truck stops (Ramjee and Gouws 2002; Williams et al. 2003). Meanwhile, at a Reproductive Health & HIV Research Unit conference in 2001, Minister of Health Manto Tshabalala-Msimang declared, 'The Department of Health and NGOs [non-governmental organizations] are fully supporting the process of reforming the law on sex work' (Richter 2008).

But while scientists, NGOs, and the health department were pairing awareness and peer education approaches with support for decriminalization, national elections and the Constitutional Court dealt major blows to legal reform that persist to this day. In 1998, the African National Congress (ANC) deemed the issue of sex work too sensitive for its platform and pushed it to after the 1999 elections (Richter 2008). Legal advocacy groups moved to the courts, but in 2002 the Constitutional Court affirmed the criminalization of sex work and brothel-keeping in *Jordan vs State*; other challenges and law reform efforts met with prolonged delays (Richter 2008). To date, the South African Law Reform Commission's charge to provide recommendations on sex work has been ongoing for over 15 years (Scheibe et al. 2016). Sex work remains a criminal act in South Africa.

For a brief time, the buildup to the 2010 World Cup brought with it elevated concerns about sex work's impact on the HIV epidemic and an array of moratorium proposals that again fell by the wayside. In 2007, the National Police Commissioner called for legalization of sex work during the World Cup; in 2008, Durban's municipal manager proposed creating red-light districts in the city during the event (Richter 2008). Media reports in the months immediately prior to the Cup sensationalized the risk of HIV spreading through as many as 40,000 foreign sex workers entering the country, purportedly to capitalize on the high volume of visiting male soccer fans (Delva et al. 2011). Subsequent research found no evidence of changes in rates of sex work (Richter et al. 2012). No legal reforms resulted.

## 8.4 The Sex Work Sector Demands Change: From the National Strategic Plans to the National Sex Worker HIV Plan

Bringing together the various scientific, state, and civil society responses (at least pro forma), the South African National Strategic Plans (NSPs) between 1994 and 2012 reflect the above pattern of delays. South Africa's first strategic plan in 1994 calls for decriminalization and the 2000–2005 plan calls for investigation into legal reform (Scheibe et al. 2016), while the 2007–2011 plan calls for decriminalization (National Department of Health 2007) and the 2012–2016 plan recommends an 'enabling legal framework' (South African National AIDS Council [SANAC] 2012). The plans pair these continued calls for legal reform with awareness and peer education approaches. The 2007–2011 plan states an intention to create a supportive legal environment for marginalized populations through development and distribution of informational materials; the plan outlines a prevention package for sex workers that consists of testing, condoms, sexually transmitted infection (STI) awareness, and 'information on gender rights' (National Department of Health 2007). The 2012–2016 plan recommends targeted prevention toward sex workers at brothels and on the street, as well as a broad swathe of legal and health care changes with 'sex-worker involvement' (SANAC 2012).

But where the NSPs reflect the overall pattern of delays previously outlined, the drafting of the National Sex Worker HIV Plan signals a rupture in the history of South Africa's national response to HIV among FSW. Launched in 2016 with support from research institutions and NGOs and a foreword by the Minister of Health, this comprehensive, multi-level plan outlines a six-package intervention strategy comprising of sex workers' peer education, health care, psychosocial services, human rights, social capital building, and economic empowerment (SANAC 2016). The plan includes guiding principles for peer education, a call for social mobilization that promotes sex workers' sense of collective identity, and a detailed plan for achieving sex worker human rights and justice literacy (SANAC 2016). In terms of legal reform, the plan makes a clear call for securing commitment for decriminalization from the Department of Justice and Constitutional Development.

What produced this rupture from past approaches? In part, the explanation is top-down: the initial draft of the 2012–2016 NSP included a call for the South African national government to table a bill to decriminalize sex work by mid-2013 (Richter and Chakuvinga 2012), but after this language was removed prior to the plan's launch a compromise was made between the South African National AIDS Council (SANAC) and its Sex Work Sector to draft a separate Sex Worker NSP (Scheibe et al. 2016). Notwithstanding these high-level actions, bottom-up processes also contributed significantly to the Sex Work Sector being able to demand change in this way. To better understand these bottom-up processes, we now turn to a case study of the history of two of the groups involved with drafting the plan: the South African sex worker rights organization, SWEAT, and the sex worker rights movement, Sisonke.

## 8.5 Case Study: History of the Sex Worker Rights Organization, SWEAT, and the Sex Worker Rights Movement, Sisonke

The Sex Worker Education and Advocacy Taskforce (SWEAT) is a community-based registered non-profit organization that provides HIV prevention, care, and human rights services to FSW on a national level. Sisonke ('togetherness') is the national sex worker movement, which emerged from SWEAT. Sisonke was started by sex workers, is led by sex workers, and is for sex workers. The SWEAT organization and members of the Sisonke movement work together to provide health and human rights services to sex workers in South Africa and help mobilize sex workers to advocate and fight for their human rights, including a life free of violence and exploitation, equal access to health care and other social services, decent working conditions, and the right to work, which includes the decriminalization of sex work.

### *8.5.1 The Beginning of SWEAT*

Founded in 1994, SWEAT began as a safe sex education program for adult sex workers in Cape Town, in affiliation with the Triangle Project, an LGBT rights organization (then known as the AIDS Support and Education Trust) (Mgbako 2016). In 1996, SWEAT broke away from the Triangle Project and became its own official nonprofit organization (SWEAT 2016).

### *8.5.2 Transition from Education to Rights-Based Focus*

Through their work with FSW, SWEAT organizers became increasingly aware of the structural barriers to HIV prevention that sex workers face, including stigma and discrimination, limited access to health care, violence, and other human rights abuses (Mgbako 2016). It soon became clear that HIV prevention education, alone, would not be effective in reducing HIV acquisition and transmission among this population (Mgbako 2016). As a consequence, SWEAT expanded their services to embody a more comprehensive approach founded on the principles of community mobilization and human rights. In particular, SWEAT launched their mobile outreach program, which provides actual health and legal services in addition to HIV prevention education, as well as a new initiative to advocate for the decriminalization of sex work in South Africa.

SWEAT's mobile outreach program offers free health and human rights services to sex workers on the street and in bars, clubs, and brothels in Cape Town (SWEAT 2016). The health services provided through the mobile caravans include free HIV testing, pap smears, and screenings for tuberculosis (TB) and STIs. A vital component of the outreach program are the peer educators, who are former or current FSW and are trained to provide their FSW colleagues with information about HIV prevention (i.e. condom demonstrations, condom negotiation skills, etc.) and sex worker rights, among other topics. Additionally, peer educators encourage their sex worker colleagues to test for HIV every 3 months in the mobile clinic, and support those who test positive in linking to care. Finally, FSW who access the mobile caravan are provided with male and female condoms, lubricant, brochures on health and human rights, as well as referrals to partner organizations including the Women's Legal Centre, which provides FSW with paralegals and offers legal advice.

In 2000, SWEAT also began strongly advocating for the decriminalization of sex work in South Africa. As part of this effort, SWEAT has actively engaged sex workers around the country to mobilize and advocate for the decriminalization of sex work (SWEAT 2016). These efforts, along with the mobile outreach, provided sex workers with opportunities to come together, learn and strategize about ways to access their health and human rights, and ultimately set the stage for a larger sex worker-led movement that advocates for sex worker rights.

### *8.5.3 The Birth of Sisonke*

Sisonke is the national sex worker-led movement in South Africa, which was founded by sex workers attending a SWEAT conference in Cape Town in 2003. Sisonke was founded on the recognition that the movement that SWEAT started in South Africa would only truly take flight if sex workers started organizing themselves and came together to fight for their human rights (Mgbako 2016).

### *8.5.4 SWEAT and Sisonke's Programs and Activities*

Sisonke joined forces with SWEAT to create a comprehensive package of services for FSW in South Africa, founded on the principles of community mobilization. In addition to the mobile outreach already being conducted by SWEAT, Sisonke and SWEAT have teamed up to engage in the following activities: offering a 24/7 helpline, conducting creative space workshops, advocacy, as well as forming partnerships with key stakeholders and conducting sensitivity trainings with them. Each of these activities is described in detail below.

#### 8.5.4.1 24/7 helpline

SWEAT and Sisonke partner to provide a 24-h hotline where sex workers can call for counseling and referrals to services they need. Some of the calls the helpline receives are related to police abuse, violence from clients or partners, and need for legal advice, especially if FSW have been arrested. The helpline staff refer FSW to relevant partner organizations including the Women's Legal Centre for legal advice and support, the South African College of Applied Psychology (SACAP) for counseling services, and other organizations for food and accommodations (SWEAT 2015).

#### 8.5.4.2 Creative Space Workshops

Sisonke and SWEAT also launched Creative Space Workshops, which are safe places where sex workers can convene to discuss the issues they face and brainstorm strategies to overcome them. Workshops are led by peer educators and cover topics such as condom negotiation skills, HIV, gender, and human rights (SWEAT 2015). In an effort to provide more holistic support for sex workers, Sisonke and SWEAT also offer workshops on leadership skills, substance abuse, family planning, fatherhood and parenting courses, training in beadwork, hairdressing, as well as business development and financial management. Importantly, the topics of each workshop are shaped by the needs expressed by the sex workers themselves, and are meant to acknowledge all aspects of individuals' identities – not just their work and HIV status (SWEAT 2015). These workshops serve as a space where sex workers can gain practical skills to improve their livelihood, build a strong and cohesive community, and come together as one voice and mobilize to fight for their health and human rights.

#### 8.5.4.3 Advocacy

SWEAT and Sisonke work together to mobilize sex workers to fight for their rights. This includes their continued effort to decriminalize sex work through marches, protests, and coalition building. Additionally, in 2009 SWEAT launched a group litigation against the Cape Town police, in response to routine arbitrary arrests of sex workers in the city. As part of this process, a group of sex workers publicly protested outside of the high court, advocating for their right to work without fear of police abuse, harassment, and arbitrary arrest. The court ruled in favor of SWEAT, and an interdict ordered the Cape Town Police to refrain from arresting FSW without prosecution following arrest (SWEAT 2016).

#### 8.5.4.4 Partnership with Key Stakeholders and Sensitivity Trainings

Additionally, SWEAT and Sisonke have also built relationships and made alliances with key stakeholders including the police and health care providers. For example, they invite police and health care providers to Creative Space workshops to listen to sex workers share stories about the challenges they face, and conduct trainings to sensitize police and health care providers to sex worker rights and the unique needs of this community (SWEAT 2015). The aim of these activities is to have allies within these important institutions to advocate for and protect the rights and health of sex workers (SWEAT 2015).

### 8.5.5 *Funding from the Global Fund for National Expansion of SWEAT's Programs*

In 2010, the Global Fund to Fight TB, HIV and Malaria awarded SWEAT funding, through the National AIDS Convention of South Africa (NACOSA), to coordinate the expansion of their programs at the national level (Rangasami et al. 2013; SWEAT 2015). During Phase I of this program, SWEAT partnered with eight organizations in eight sites (both urban and rural) throughout the country and trained peer educators in each location to rollout the services and programs offered by SWEAT and Sisonke in Cape Town (Rangasami et al. 2013). The midterm evaluation of this initiative revealed that the SWEAT program had positive influences on HIV knowledge and condom use behaviors among FSW, but also demonstrated the need for further resources and programs to improve FSW engagement in HIV prevention (SWEAT 2015).

In Phase II of this program, SWEAT received additional funding to further expand their program to include 19 organizations and 560 peer educators in 74 sites around the country. This large network of implementers was re-branded as the Red Umbrella Programme (Impact Consulting 2016). Evidence from the evaluation of Phase II suggests that the Red Umbrella Programme has made an important difference in the lives of South African FSW. Specifically, the results of the Phase II evaluation revealed significant reductions in violence against FSW, compared to Phase I (Impact Consulting 2016). Qualitative evidence indicates that FSW are more likely to seek legal services and feel better equipped to avoid and/or respond to violent situations as a result of participation in the Red Umbrella Programme (Impact Consulting 2016). HIV care and treatment outcomes also improved in Phase II, compared to Phase I. For example, the Phase II evaluation revealed significant increases in condom use (Impact Consulting 2016). This finding is supported by qualitative evidence, which suggests that FSW feel better able to demand condom use after participating in the Red Umbrella Programme (Impact Consulting 2016). Qualitative evidence also revealed that more FSW have initiated ART since the end of Phase I, and that FSW attribute this increase to peer navigator support for accessing and staying engaged in HIV care and treatment services. Finally, qualitative results indicate that FSW perceive there to be less community stigma towards FSW as a result of the Red Umbrella Programme (Impact Consulting 2016).

### 8.5.6 *Reasons for the Red Umbrella Programme's Success*

As described above, the Red Umbrella Programme, along with SWEAT and Sisonke, has made a tangible difference in the lives of FSW in South Africa. Arguably one of the main reasons for this program's success is SWEAT's acknowledgement of the importance and necessity of a rights-based, community empowerment approach early on. The adoption of such an approach allowed sex workers to claim ownership of the program and create a strong sense of shared social identity around a common cause to raise awareness about and fight for their health and human rights. Ultimately, SWEAT's efforts, along with the Sisonke movement, drew attention to the fact that the high rates of HIV among FSW could never be truly addressed without addressing their marginalization and limited access to health services and human rights. With a growing movement, the government could not turn a blind eye, and was forced to acknowledge the needs of this community.

It is also important to recognize that SWEAT and Sisonke bridged to a larger global sex worker-rights movement, which included similar rights-based community mobilization approaches toward HIV prevention. These programs and movements included Sonagachi and Avahan in India, Encontros in Brazil, and *Compromiso Colectivo* in the Dominican Republic, among others (Basu et al. 2004; Jana et al. 2004; Kerrigan et al. 2006, 2015; Laga et al. 2010; Lippman et al. 2012). Such programs have also demonstrated the positive influence rights-based community empowerment approaches have on HIV prevention outcomes (Blankenship et al. 2008; Kerrigan et al. 2015; Kuhlmann et al. 2014; Lippman et al. 2012; Reza-Paul et al. 2008; Vejella et al. 2015). It is likely that the global movement towards such approaches to HIV prevention among sex workers, and the mounting evidence of their success, is what garnered the support of the Global Fund to fund the expansion of SWEAT's Red Umbrella Programme. With funding from an international donor to support their cause, and backing from a global movement of sex workers, activists, and scientists, SWEAT and Sisonke were better able to gain the attention of the government and build the power necessary to put their issues on the national AIDS agenda.

## 8.6 Structural Approaches Are Building Power: Insights on Community Mobilization from the History of South Africa's National Response to HIV Among FSW

For much of the South African HIV epidemic, FSW were marginalized from the national HIV response. Scientists, the national government, and much of civil society responded to HIV among FSW with limited awareness and peer education approaches paired with calls for decriminalization that met continued delays. But with the launch of the South African National Sex Worker HIV Plan in 2016, the South African Sex Work Sector demanded change. The Sex Work Sector was able to create this rupture in part because organizations like SWEAT and Sisonke had mobilized sex workers into a national movement. It is to this last point, on the transition toward a third 'generation' of community mobilization approaches to HIV (Campbell and Cornish 2010), that we now turn for our conclusion. To anchor our discussion, we focus on key insights and questions related to three concepts: identity, social capital, and power.

A first insight from the history of community mobilization by FSW in South Africa is that self-identification, both in the sense of autonomous self-determination and in the sense of identification with a larger group, is an essential pre-requisite for community mobilization. SWEAT and Sisonke's creative space workshops explicitly allowed for sex workers' self-expression of identity. Such self-identification is necessary to prevent 'essentialist assumptions about community and identity' (Campbell 2014) from threatening the creation of authentic community. At the same time, self-identification with the particular community mobilizing is also essential. The National Sex Worker HIV Plan defines sex workers as 'self-identified adult male, female, and transgender sex workers' (SANAC 2016). Identification by group members *as* group members ensures the formation of shared social identity.

A second insight from the history of community mobilization by FSW in South Africa is that the purpose of building social capital is not to supplant accountability from the state but to demand it. In one sense, the strategies through which SWEAT and Sisonke built social capital – creating a helpline and connecting with a global sex worker movement, among others – provided self-support within and across borders. But ultimately, as seen in the National Sex Worker HIV Plan, the South African sex worker movement was concerned with securing rights from the state. It should be axiomatic in future community mobilization work that the purpose of building social capital is in the end to achieve state-level changes to the policies and programs that impact populations' health. As Campbell writes:

> … 'in the final instance', the state has a role to play in programs of redistribution and health service provision in protecting the health of the most marginalized – and…co-ordinated national movements, backed up by local-global alliances, may often have an important role to play in pressurizing states, and global economic actors, to create contexts where it is possible for the most marginalized to be healthy. (Campbell 2014: 57).

A final insight is that empowerment in community mobilization has less to do with achieving 'power over' and more to do with building 'power with' (Glanz et al. 2008). Undoubtedly mobilization by SWEAT and Sisonke against police abuse and harassment was inseparable from resistance to deeply entrenched systems of subordination and othering. At the same time, the end goal in community mobilization cannot be just to achieve 'power over' agents of oppression, a 'win' that by definition reproduces the power binary of over/under (Campbell 2014). A 'power with' approach, seen in FSW partnership-building with health care providers and police, seeks to achieve power through simultaneously building power inside communities and strategically allying with powerful actors outside of them. 'Power with' should be a modus operandi for community mobilization approaches with marginalized populations. Research with FSW in other countries has begun to explore implications of this approach (Blanchard et al. 2013).

With these insights in mind, questions remain for future research into community mobilization by FSW in South Africa and key populations in general. First, when it comes to matters of identity, how can researchers more effectively document multiple experiences of oppression? Intersectionality theory recognizes that individuals have multiple overlapping identities (i.e. sex, gender, sexual orientation, race, class, etc.), and that these identities intersect with macro-level factors (i.e. sexism, transphobia, homophobia, racism, classism, etc.) to shape individuals' lived experiences (Bowleg 2012; Crenshaw 1991). For example, studies from South Africa have demonstrated that transgender sex workers experience more violence than their cisgender female counterparts (Impact Consulting 2016) and are excluded from support services when their gender identities are seen as illegitimate (Samudzi and Mannell 2016). Given that FSW in South Africa often belong to multiple groups experiencing oppression, and that there is a general lack of data on key populations in South Africa other than MSM and FSW, it is imperative to further research and develop programs and policies that address key populations' intersecting identities and the multiplicative experiences of oppression associated with these intersections.

Second, when it comes to questions of social capital, how can we better contribute to closing the gap between social capital and material deprivation in the context of extreme economic inequality? 'Linking social capital' has been used to describe connection to the social institutions that can meaningfully redress material impoverishment, such as linkage to state-sanctioned economic support (Muntaner et al. 2000). Previous research in this area has highlighted the need to examine whether social capital alone can truly mediate pathways between economic inequality and health (Muntaner et al. 2000; Hawe and Shiell 2000). South Africa is frequently ranked as having among the world's highest income inequality by the Gini coefficient: does building bonding and bridging social capital in this context ultimately link to material empowerment? If so, how? And how does this, in the end, improve health? These are pressing questions to explore.

Finally, when it comes to questions of power, how can we write definitions of power that recognize South African and other Global South intellectual traditions? Recent student-led uprisings at South African universities, in addition to calling for changes in university representation and reduced fees (#RhodesMustFall, #FeesMustFall), have demanded 'epistemological diversity' that explicitly decolonizes academic disciplines' theoretical approaches ('Work stream on curriculum transformation at the University of Pretoria' n.d.). We have sought to problematize notions of 'power over' using conceptions of 'power with'. How might our own definitions of power in community mobilization be transformed and improved by incorporating a full, inclusive set of epistemological approaches, such as Steve Biko's conception of Black Consciousness (Biko 2015), the experiences of Florence Mkhize, Lillian Ngoyi, and other women in planning the 1956 Women's March, and more? In the end, re-conceptualizing power might be one of the most difficult tasks for us as public health researchers and practitioners; it might also be one of the most important.

## References

Basu, I., Jana, S., Rotheram-Borus, M. J., Swendeman, D., Lee, S. J., Newman, P., & Weiss, R. (2004). HIV prevention among sex workers in India. *Journal of Acquired Immune Deficiency Syndromes, 36*(3), 845–852. doi:10.1097/00126334-200407010-00012.

Biko, S. (2015). *I write what i like: Selected writings*. Chicago: The University of Chicago Press.

Blanchard, A. K., Mohan, H. L., Shahmanesh, M., Prakash, R., Isac, S., Ramesh, B. M., Bhattacharjee, P., Gurnani, V., Moses, S., & Blanchard, J. F. (2013). Community mobilization, empowerment and HIV prevention among female sex workers in South India. *BMC Public Health, 13*, 234. doi:10.1186/1471-2458-13-234.

Blankenship, K. M., West, B. S., Kershaw, T. S., & Biradavolu, M. R. (2008). Power, community mobilization, and condom use practices among female sex workers in Andhra Pradesh, India. *AIDS, 22*(Suppl 5), S109–S116. doi:10.1097/01.aids.0000343769.92949.dd.

Bowleg, L. (2012). The problem with the phrase women and minorities: Intersectionality – an important theoretical framework for public health. *American Journal of Public Health, 102*(7), 1267–1273. doi:10.2105/AJPH.2012.300750.

Campbell, C. (2014). Community mobilisation in the 21st century: Updating our theory of social change? *Journal of Health Psychology, 19*(1), 46–59. doi:10.1177/1359105313500262.

Campbell, C., & Cornish, F. (2010). Towards a 'fourth generation' of approaches to HIV/AIDS management: Creating contexts for effective community mobilisation. *AIDS Care, 22*(Suppl. 2), 1569–1579. doi:10.1080/09540121.2010.525812.

Chigwedere, P., Seage, G. R., III, Gruskin, S., Lee, T. H., & Essex, M. (2008). Estimating the lost benefits of antiretroviral drug use in South Africa. *JAIDS Journal of Acquired Immune Deficiency Syndromes, 49*(4), 410–415. doi:10.1097/qai.0b013e31818a6cd5.

Crenshaw, K. W. (1991). Mapping the margins: Intersectionality, identity politics, and violence against women of color. *Stanford Law Review, 43*, 1241–1299. doi:10.2307/1229039.

Crowe, S. (1997). South Africa revolutionises HIV prevention and education strategies. *Lancet, 349*(9062), 1377. doi:10.1016/s0140-6736(05)63225-4.

Delva, W., Richter, M., De Koker, P., Chersich, M., & Temmerman, M. (2011). Sex work during the 2010 FIFA World Cup: Results from a three-wave cross-sectional survey. *PloS One, 6*(12), e28363. doi:10.1371/journal.pone.0028363.

Glanz, K., Rimer, B. K., & Viswanath, K. (2008). *Health behavior and health education: Theory, research, and practice*. Hoboken: Wiley.

Hawe, P., & Shiell, A. (2000). Social capital and health promotion: A review. *Social Science & Medicine, 51*(6), 871–885. doi:10.1016/s0277-9536(00)00067-8.

Hunter, M. (2007). The changing political economy of sex in South Africa: The significance of unemployment and inequalities to the scale of the AIDS pandemic. *Social Science & Medicine, 64*(3), 689–700. doi:10.1016/j.socscimed.2006.09.015.

Hunter, M. (2010). Beyond the male-migrant: South Africa's long history of health geography and the contemporary AIDS pandemic. *Health & Place, 16*(1), 25–33. doi:10.1016/j.healthplace.2009.08.003.

Impact Consulting. (2016). *Creating safe spaces: Evaluation of the red umbrella sex work programme*. http://www.nacosa.org.za/wp-content/uploads/2016/07/CREATING-SAFE-SPACES-Evaluation-of-the-Red-Umbrella-Sex-Work-Programme-web.pdf. Accessed 4 May 2017.

Jana, S., Basu, I., Rotheram-Borus, M. J., & Newman, P. A. (2004). The sonagachi project: A sustainable community intervention program. *AIDS Education and Prevention, 16*(5), 405–414. doi:10.1521/aeap.16.5.405.48734.

Jochelson, K., Mothibeli, M., & Leger, J. P. (1991). Human immunodeficiency virus and migrant labor in South Africa. *International Journal of Health Services, 21*, 157–173. doi:10.2190/11ue-l88j-46hn-hr0k.

Kerrigan, D., Moreno, L., Rosario, S., Gomez, B., Jerez, H., Barrington, C., et al. (2006). Environmental–structural interventions to reduce HIV/STI risk among female sex workers in the Dominican Republic. *American Journal of Public Health, 96*(1), 120–125. doi:10.2105/AJPH.2004.042200.

Kerrigan, D., Kennedy, C. E., Morgan-Thomas, R., Reza-Paul, S., Mwangi, P., Thi Win, K., McFall, A., Fonner, V., & Butler, J. (2015). A community empowerment approach to the HIV response among sex workers: Effectiveness, challenges, and considerations for implementation and scale-up. *Lancet, 385*(9963), 172–185. doi:10.1016/s0140-6736(14)60973-9.

Kuhlmann, A. S., Galavotti, C., Hastings, P., Narayanan, P., & Saggurti, N. (2014). Investing in communities: Evaluating the added value of community mobilization on HIV prevention outcomes among FSWs in India. *AIDS and Behavior, 18*(4), 752–766. doi:10.1007/s10461-013-0626-6.

Laga, M., Galavotti, C., Sundaramon, S., & Moodie, R. (2010). The importance of sex-worker interventions: The case of Avahan in India. *Sexually Transmitted Infections, 86*(Suppl. 1), i.6–i.7. doi:10.1136/sti.2009.039255.

Lane, T. (2009). From social silence to social science: HIV research among township men who have sex with men in South Africa. In V. Reddy, T. Sandfort, & L. Rispel (Eds.), *Social silence to social science. Same-sex sexuality, HIV & AIDS and gender in South Africa* (pp. 66–79). Cape Town: HSRC Press.

Lippman, S. A., Chinaglia, M., Donini, A. A., Diaz, J., Reingold, A., & Kerrigan, D. L. (2012). Findings from encontros: A multilevel STI/HIV intervention to increase condom use, reduce STI, and change the social environment among sex workers in Brazil. *Sexually Transmitted Diseases, 39*(3), 209–216. doi:10.1097/OLQ.0b013e31823b1937.

Mgbako, C. A. (2016). *To live freely in this world: Sex worker activism in Africa*. New York: New York University Press.

Muntaner, C., Lynch, J., & Smith, G. D. (2000). Social capital and the third way in public health. *Critical Public Health, 10*(2), 107–124. doi:10.1080/713658240.

National Department of Health. (2007). *HIV & AIDS and STI strategic plan for South Africa 2007–2011*. http://data.unaids.org/pub/externaldocument/2007/20070604_sa_nsp_final_en.pdf. Accessed 4 Apr 2017.

Ramjee, G., & Gouws, E. (2002). Prevalence of HIV among truck drivers visiting sex workers in KwaZulu-Natal, South Africa. *Sexually Transmitted Diseases, 29*(1), 44–49. doi:10.1097/00007435-200201000-00008.

Rangasami, J., Boshoff, N., & Konstant, T. (2013). Beginning to build the picture: South African national survey of sex worker knowledge, experiences and behaviour. http://www.sweat.org.za/wp-content/uploads/2016/02/National-Sex-Workers-Programme-Evaluation.pdf. Accessed 12 May 2017.

Reza-Paul, S., Beattie, T., Syed, H. U., Venukumar, K. T., Venugopal, M. S., Fathima, M. P., Raghavendra, H. R., Akram, P., Manjula, R., Lakshmi, M., Isac, S., Ramesh, B. M., Washington, R., Mahagaonkar, S. B., Glynn, J. R., Blanchard, J. F., & Moses, S. (2008). Declines in risk behaviour and sexually transmitted infection prevalence following a community-led HIV preventive intervention among female sex workers in Mysore, India. *AIDS, 22*(Suppl. 5), S91–S100. doi:10.1097/01.aids.0000343767.08197.18.

Richter, M. (2008). Sex work, reform initiatives and HIV/AIDS in inner-city Johannesburg. *African Journal of AIDS Research, 7*(3), 323–333. doi:10.2989/AJAR.2008.7.3.9.656.

Richter, M., Luchters, S., Ndlovu, D., Temmerman, M., & Chersich, M. F. (2012). Female sex work and international sport events – no major changes in demand or supply of paid sex during the 2010 soccer world cup: A cross-sectional study. *BMC Public Health, 12*, 763. doi:10.1186/1471-2458-12-763.

Richter, M., & Chakuvinga, P. (2012). Being pimped out – how South Africa's AIDS response fails sex workers. *Agenda, 26*(2), 65–79.

Samudzi, Z., & Mannell, J. (2016). Cisgender male and transgender female sex workers in South Africa: Gender variant identities and narratives of exclusion. *Culture, Health & Sexuality, 18*(1), 1–14. doi:10.1080/13691058.2015.1062558.

Scheibe, A., Richter, M., & Vearey, J. (2016). Sex work and South Africa's health system: addressing the needs of the underserved. *South African Health Review, 2016*(1), 165–178.

SANAC. (2012). *National strategic plan on HIV, STIs and TB, 2012–2016*. South African National AIDS Council. http://sanac.org.za//wp-content/uploads/2015/11/National-Strategic-Plan-on-HIV-STIs-and-TB.pdf. Accessed 4 Apr 2017.

SANAC. (2016). *The South African national sex worker HIV plan, 2016–2019*. South African National AIDS Council. http://sanac.org.za/wp-content/uploads/2016/03/South-African-National-Sex-Worker-HIV-Plan-2016-2019-FINAL-Launch-Copy....pdf. Accessed 4 Apr 2017.

SWEAT (2015). *Good practice guide to integrated sex worker programming: Based on the experiences of the red umbrella programme*. http://www.sweat.org.za/wp-content/uploads/2016/02/Good-practice-guide-1.pdf. Accessed 4 Apr 2017.

SWEAT (2016). *History timeline*. http://www.sweat.org.za/who-we-are-2/who-we-are-2/

Vejella, S., Patel, S. K., Saggurti, N., & Prabhakar, P. (2015). Community collectivization and consistent condom use among female sex workers in southern India: Evidence from two rounds of behavioral tracking surveys. *AIDS and Behavior, 20*(4), 778–787. doi:10.1007/s10461-015-1171-2.

Williams, B. G., Taljaard, D., Campbell, C. M., Gouws, E., Ndhlovu, L., Van Dam, J., Carael, M., & Auvert, B. (2003). Changing patterns of knowledge, reported behaviour and sexually transmitted infections in a South African gold mining community. *AIDS, 17*(14), 2099–2107. doi:10.1097/00002030-200309260-00011.

Wojcicki, J. M. (2003). The movement to decriminalize sex work in Gauteng Province, South Africa, 1994–2002. *African Studies Review, 46*(3), 83–109. doi:10.2307/1515043.

Work stream on curriculum transformation at the University of Pretoria. (n.d.). *Draft framework document: Reimagining curricula for a just university in a vibrant democracy*. http://www.up.ac.za/media/shared/9/HumPdf%20docs/up-curriculum-transformation-framework-final--draft_23may2016_1.zp89110.pdf. Accessed 9 Dec 2016.

# Chapter 9
# Structural Factors and the National HIV/AIDS Strategy of the USA

**Ronald O. Valdiserri, Catherine H. Maulsby, and David R. Holtgrave**

## 9.1 Introduction

Structural factors are those environmental influences and contextual circumstances that influence health-related behaviors and outcomes (see Blankenship et al. 2006). Even in the initial months of the AIDS epidemic in the United States of America (USA), prior to the discovery of the human immunodeficiency virus (HIV), structural factors were thought to be mediators of the risk of acquiring the disease, particularly laws and policies that could influence the behaviors and practices of gay men and people who inject drugs. Granted, many of the earliest examples of actions taken in response to this deadly new disease were based on uncertainty, fear and stigma – rather than evidence or proven public health practices. Arguably, legislative and policy interventions that prohibited the use of US federal government funds to support needle and syringe exchange programs (Valdiserri 2013), closed gay bathhouses (Burris and Gostin 2003) and limited the scope of Federally funded risk-reduction efforts and written prevention materials, for fear of 'promoting' homosexuality, (Lawrence 1987) may have done more to facilitate the transmission of the virus than to interrupt its spread.

After more than three decades of dealing with the HIV epidemic not enough has been done to eliminate AIDS-related ignorance and stigma – either nationally or elsewhere. But we have made considerable progress in our understanding of the *positive* contributions that structural interventions can make toward reducing the transmission of HIV and in promoting healthy outcomes for those who are living with the infection. Hard-won experience has come to show the limitations of embracing a rigid, monolithic approach to the HIV epidemic and the necessity of flexible, interdisciplinary approaches that incorporate individual, community and structural interventions and responses (Valdiserri 2011). This evolution in perspec-

R.O. Valdiserri (✉) • C.H. Maulsby • D.R. Holtgrave
Johns Hopkins Bloomberg School of Public Health, Baltimore, MD, USA
e-mail: rvaldis1@jhu.edu



D. Kerrigan, C. Barrington (eds.), *Structural Dynamics of HIV*, Social Aspects of HIV 4, DOI 10.1007/978-3-319-63522-4_9

tive parallels similar developments in thinking about how best to address the social and structural factors fueling other persistent health disparities among vulnerable racial/ethnic and other minority groups (Braverman et al. 2011).

When the United States of America's first-ever comprehensive, national HIV/AIDS strategy was released in July 2010 (White House Office of National AIDS Policy 2010a), it delineated three key goals: reduce new HIV infections, increase access to care and improve health outcomes for people living with HIV, and reduce HIV-related disparities and health inequities. A fourth cross-cutting operational goal called for a more coordinated national response to the epidemic. An accompanying document, 'The Federal Implementation Plan,' outlined the specific steps required of US Federal departments to achieve these goals (White House Office of National AIDS Policy 2010b).

Rather than representing an entirely new approach to HIV prevention, treatment and care, the US National HIV/AIDS Strategy (NHAS) outlined 'top line priorities' – informed by cutting-edge science and on-the-ground community perspectives – that would 'move the nation forward in responding to the domestic HIV epidemic' (2010a: 3). An explicit, fundamental tenet of the strategy was the necessity of deploying a combination of effective, evidence-based interventions including individual, community and structural approaches. A 'better understanding of network, social and structural factors' influencing disease risk was deemed essential to achieve NHAS goals since, in disproportionately affected communities, 'individual risk reduction interventions alone will not meaningfully reduce HIV incidence' (Millet et al. 2010: S146). An updated version of the strategy, released in 2015, continued to call for the adoption of 'structural approaches to reduce HIV infections and improve health outcomes in high risk communities' (White House Office of National AIDS Policy 2015: 40).

## 9.2 Framing the Social and Structural Factors That Influence HIV Outcomes

There are a number of ways to describe the social and structural factors that influence HIV risk and HIV health outcomes (Auerbach et al. 2011; Poundstone et al. 2004; Sweat and Denison 1995). All of these frameworks share features in common, most notably the fundamental understanding that health is determined by a complex interplay of biology, behavior, environment and social context. In our assessment of the NHAS's approach to the structural elements and social drivers that mediate HIV-related health outcomes in the USA, we focus on two major domains: environment and social context. In this framing, we define environment as comprised of the resources and opportunities that can impact health, specifically: access to necessary HIV-related clinical services, access to essential HIV prevention services, and stable housing and economic security. We use the construct of social context to account for societal and cultural factors that influence the uptake of the aforementioned health-influencing resources and opportunities. Specifically, when considering the impact of social context on HIV-related health outcomes, we focus exclusively on the concept of HIV-related stigma (Mahajan et al. 2008) as an overarching frame for our discussion.

Utilizing the broad taxonomy referenced above, in this chapter we review the major structural interventions called for in the initial 2010 release of the NHAS and its subsequent 2015 update, describe what, if any, actions have been undertaken in response and identify issues and areas where additional science, resource and/or policy development are required to advance national HIV prevention and treatment goals. Throughout this chapter, we strive to examine these topics using select examples that highlight the HIV epidemic among Black men-who-have-sex-with-men (MSM), the community in the USA that is currently most disproportionately affected by the HIV epidemic (Maulsby et al. 2014). It should be noted that the scope of this chapter precludes a comprehensive review of every structural and social factor capable of influencing HIV-related health outcomes in the USA. Those highlighted were deemed by the authors to be especially germane to achieving the NHAS goals.

## 9.3 Environmental Factors

### *9.3.1 Access to Necessary Health Care Services*

Promoting access to quality care for those infected with HIV is not only necessary to ensure improved health outcomes, it is also an essential means of preventing further transmission of HIV (Cohen et al. 2011). Admittedly, there are various components that contribute toward achieving successful and consistent healthcare access; these components reflect consumer, provider, delivery system and situational influences. Among these, healthcare insurance coverage is one of the more potent variables in the healthcare access equation. Although the USA supports an extensive 'safety net' program for uninsured and underinsured persons living with HIV, the Ryan White HIV/AIDS Program (RWHAP), some analysts have opined that 'the program is inadequately funded to effectively address the increasing number of patients who rely on these services' (Mugavero et al. 2011: S241). Thus, the NHAS's recognition that the Affordable Care Act (ACA) would 'expand access to insurance coverage for people living with HIV' and 'provide a platform for improvements in health care coverage and quality' (White House Office of National AIDS Policy 2010a) can be considered among the most substantial of the structural interventions identified in the national plan.

Enacted in March 2010, one of the major objectives of this sweeping health care reform legislation was to 'bring the security of health insurance to uninsured Americans' (Shaw et al. 2014: 75), in large part through the expansion of Medicaid eligibility.[1] Because of the disproportionate burden of HIV among low-income pop-

[1] Prior to the passage of the Affordable Care Act, eligibility for the US Medicaid program was based on a number of factors including: income, household size, disability and family status. Prior

ulations, Medicaid expansion was anticipated to result in a major positive impact on healthcare access for persons living with HIV (Martin and Schackman 2012). However, as a consequence of legal challenges, a US Supreme Court ruling in 2012 essentially made Medicaid expansion a state decision (Shaw et al. 2014). As of March 2016, 32 states, including the District of Columbia, had opted to expand Medicaid coverage so that many more low-income Americans would have access to health insurance; nineteen states – many located in the southeastern USA – have opted not to expand Medicaid at the present time (Kaiser Family Foundation 2016). Snider et al. (2014) estimated that 'nearly 115,000 uninsured, low-income adults living with HIV would be eligible for insurance coverage through the ACA Medicaid expansion,' but that half of these persons were living in states that were not planning to expand Medicaid coverage (Snider et al. 2014).

Will the ACA's impact on improving access to HIV care mean that there will no longer be a need for the RWHAP and other categorical 'safety net' programs (Cahill et al. 2015)? This question has been of paramount importance in the arena of US domestic HIV/AIDS policy ever since the passage of the ACA and is currently under active study. One recent analysis by Berry and his colleagues (2016) compared healthcare coverage for HIV provider visits before and after ACA implementation in states that expanded Medicaid and those that did not. Among 28,734 people living with HIV followed in the expansion states of California, Oregon and Maryland, half 'shifted to Medicaid' while in the non-expansion states (Texas and Florida), reliance on the RWHAP 'remained constant' (Berry et al. 2016: 2), leading the authors to conclude that 'in the first half of 2014, the ACA did not eliminate the need for RWHAP safety net provider visit coverage' (Berry et al. 2016: 2). Another significant consideration when addressing this question is the fact that important services like case management and treatment adherence counseling – vital to ensuring that clients remain engaged in HIV care and routinely provided to those enrolled in the RWHAP – are not typically covered by insurance plans (Kates 2013; Eaton and Mugavero 2016). This reality may, in part, explain the higher rates of retention and viral suppression seen among RWHAP clients when compared to overall national estimates (Doshi et al. 2015).

As stated earlier, a variety of factors can influence access to consistent HIV clinical care, for example, housing instability, transportation challenges, competing personal priorities, mental health issues and provider attitudes. Nevertheless, issues arising from insufficient health insurance are frequently cited as one of the major barriers to consistent HIV care (Yehia et al. 2015). Data from 19 US jurisdictions revealed that among 153,581 Black people living with HIV (PLHIV) in 2010 'males had a lower prevalence than females of linkage to care, retention in care, ART (antiretroviral therapy) prescription and viral suppression' (Whiteside et al. 2014: 88). Black MSM living with HIV had a somewhat lower rate of retention in HIV care (46.3%) compared to black men infected with HIV through heterosexual sex

---

to the ACA, people living with HIV had to manifest end-stage disease (i.e. AIDS) to be considered eligible for Medicaid. For states that have opted to expand Medicaid eligibility under the ACA, household income is now the only qualification.

(48.4%) (Whiteside et al. 2014). Another analysis looked at retention in HIV care among all MSM who were living with diagnosed HIV as of December 31, 2010 and found that 'Black/African American MSM had the lowest levels of care compared with MSM of all other race/ethnicities', i.e., 37% viral suppression among Black MSM compared to 43.9% among whites (Singh et al. 2014: 832). A more recent study reviewed trends in consistent retention in HIV care from 2011 through 2013, finding that African Americans were less likely to be retained in HIV care compared to other racial/ethnic groups and that Black MSM had lower rates of consistent retention in HIV care (35%) compared to Black men and women infected through heterosexual contact – 37.3% and 44.9%, respectively (Dasgupta et al. 2016: 80).

### *9.3.2 Access to HIV Prevention Services as a Function of Funding Availability*

Reducing the incidence of HIV infection in the USA requires access to effective HIV prevention services available at a scale commensurate with the burden of viral transmission. The NHAS embraces the notion that 'effective prevention should involve multiple interventions to reduce risk behavior, reduce opportunities for transmission and lower biological susceptibility of transmitting or acquiring infection' (Millet et al. 2010: S144). As is the case with access to HIV clinical services, many factors influence access to HIV prevention services. Perhaps the most obvious of these is the need for adequate resources to support the development and implementation of prevention services that are tailored to the needs and preferences of the communities being served. In both the original NHAS and in the 2015 update, major emphasis is placed on allocating prevention funding to reflect the current epidemiology of the US HIV epidemic and supporting cost-effective, scalable interventions that serve hard-hit communities.

In June 2011, the Centers for Disease Control and Prevention (CDC) announced a major change in how it would allocate nearly $360 million in HIV prevention funding to state and local health departments (Centers for Disease Control and Prevention 2011). Re-directing the allocation of federal HIV prevention resources, both in terms of geography and by giving preference to the highest-impact interventions, epitomizes a system-wide, structural response to the NHAS's call to 'intensify HIV prevention efforts in the communities where HIV is most heavily concentrated' (White House, Office of National AIDS Policy 2010a: 8). Prior to this change, HIV prevention funding allocations to health departments were based on AIDS case numbers; this new 'high-impact approach to HIV prevention' distributes funds based on the number of people reported to be living with an HIV diagnosis in each jurisdiction, a better measure of current disease burden since not all people living with HIV have progressed to AIDS (Centers for Disease Control and Prevention 2011). The new approach also requires that at least 75% of core funding be directed to the following 'high-impact' activities: HIV testing, comprehensive prevention for PLHIV, condom distribution and policy initiatives that seek to 'align structures, policies and regulations to enable optimal HIV prevention, care and treatment' (Centers for Disease Control and Prevention 2011: 3). In part, this change was made because many previously funded HIV prevention interventions, while evidence-based, were 'not reaching the majority of people most likely to acquire or transmit HIV and some were not cost-effective' (Purcell et al. 2016: 8).

Ongoing evaluation will be necessary to determine whether this shift in resource allocation and change in prevention focus will result in decreased HIV incidence. However, because the *total* amount of federal HIV prevention resources allocated to health departments did not substantially increase, many jurisdictions experienced a decrease in their annual federal HIV prevention funding as a result of the new funding formula. In 2013, the National Alliance of State and Territorial AIDS Directors (NASTAD) reported that while 30 jurisdictions saw an increase in federal HIV prevention funding as a result of the change in CDC policy, 29 experienced a decrease (NASTAD 2013). In its report, NASTAD noted that 'funding decreases have driven health departments to make tough choices around cutting programs for low prevalence populations, such as rural communities' (2013: 3). Iowa, for example, had its federal HIV prevention budget decreased by more than half as a result of the new policy, raising concerns among state leaders about their ability to provide adequate access to HIV testing and other key prevention services – especially for populations not easily reached in clinical settings (Elmer 2012).

Allocating prevention resources to those jurisdictions with the greatest HIV burden may be consistent with the dictates of the NHAS but it will not resolve the problem of unmet need across all jurisdictions – especially in light of the fact that the total federal HIV prevention investment has not been increased, only reapportioned. In an analysis published following the release of the NHAS, Holtgrave (2010) estimated that an additional prevention investment of over $2 billion would be necessary to achieve the NHAS goals and, in a subsequent modeling analysis, he and his colleagues noted that 'without expansion of diagnostic services and of prevention services for people living with HIV, scaling up coverage of HIV care and treatment alone in the USA, will not achieve the incidence and transmission rate reduction goals of the NHAS' (Holtgrave et al. 2012: 1365). The association between investment and population health outcomes is evidenced in a study of state-level spending trends over the period of 2000–2009, which found that 'states with higher spending on social services and public health per person in poverty had significantly lower HIV and AIDS case rates and fewer AIDS deaths' (Talbert-Slagle et al. 2016: 657).

HIV prevention needs are especially pronounced among Black MSM. Matthews et al. calculated a staggering annual estimate of HIV incidence of 4.16% among Black MSM based on data from six published studies (2016) and, according to the CDC, young Black MSM account for more new HIV infections in the USA than any other subgroup by race, ethnicity, age and sex (Centers for Disease Control and Prevention 2015a). Despite well-documented need, allotment of HIV prevention services targeted to MSM, including Black MSM, has not typically matched the scope of the problem. An analysis of CDC-funded HIV prevention allocations to state and local health departments for the year 2010 found that 'the proportion of allocations for MSM was much lower than the proportion of reported diagnoses among MSM' (Centers for Disease Control and Prevention 2012a: 11). While MSM accounted for 61% of reported HIV diagnoses in 2010, the analysis indicated that, on average, health departments reported only 19% of HIV testing funds and 28% of health education/risk reduction funds were allocated to MSM (CDC 2012a). Another appraisal of unaddressed need can be found in a quantitative estimation of unmet HIV service needs for HIV infected Black MSM living in 2011, reckoning that among 195,313 Black MSM living with HIV in the USA, over 50,000 had not yet been diagnosed (Holtgrave et al. 2014).

Although stigma and other social drivers have undoubtedly contributed to suboptimal prevention outcomes among populations of MSM, we cannot ignore the impact of chronically underfunded HIV prevention services (Valdiserri 2016). The consequences of underfunding are likely manifest in the outcomes of a 2012–2013 state/MSA/county-level analysis showing that 'HIV infection is hyperendemic among MSM in many areas of the USA, particularly in the South' (Rosenberg et al. 2016: e22). While advocacy to increase appropriations is an obvious response to the reality of gaps in HIV prevention and care services for Black MSM and other vulnerable populations, public health leaders must also ensure that existing resources are being targeted to communities and populations in greatest need and that the interventions being employed are scientifically sound, cost effective and culturally acceptable to the intended recipients. The focus on high-burden communities and jurisdictions does not negate the responsibility of 'appropriately responding to HIV among groups that represent a small share of both the population and of HIV infections' (White House, Office of National AIDS Policy 2015: 19). Thus, it remains imperative that we continue to monitor surveillance and other data sources to promptly respond to emerging trends in HIV incidence and deploy existing prevention resources accordingly.

### *9.3.3 Access to HIV Prevention Services as a Function of Policy*

While adequate fiscal resources are necessary to support HIV prevention services, budget alone, does not determine access. Policy, in its many manifestations, can often be the decisive factor in determining the availability of needed prevention services. Nowhere is this more evident than in the example of access to needle and syringe services for people who inject drugs (PWID). Organized needle exchange programs (NEP) started among PWIDs in Amsterdam in the early 1980s and in the USA a handful of pragmatic public health leaders called for similar efforts at about the same time (Valdiserri 2003). But these appeals faced formidable barriers. In addition to strong public opinion that perceived syringe exchange programs as encouraging illicit drug use, in 1981, when AIDS was first described, almost every state in the USA had laws criminalizing the possession and distribution of needles and syringes for the use of injecting illicit drugs (Bramson et al. 2015). Since that time a number of states have changed their laws to authorize syringe exchange programs and/or to exclude syringes from the definition of drug paraphernalia for those participating in syringe exchange programs; however, some states still ban the practice (Public Health Law Research 2016).

An equally daunting policy obstacle was instituted in 1988 when the US Congress enacted a specific prohibition to the use of federal funds to support NEPs (Weinmeyer 2016). Congressional action temporarily lifted the ban in 2010, but by 2012 it was back in place (Weinmeyer 2016). The ban was effectively lifted again, in 2016 (Ungar 2016), largely in response to an outbreak of HIV in rural Indiana among persons sharing syringes to inject the prescription opioid oxymorphone (Conrad et al. 2015). At the time the outbreak was first reported, Indiana was 'one of twenty-five states where it's illegal to purchase syringes without a prescription and where state law does not explicitly authorize needle-exchange programs' (Strathdee and Beyrer 2015: 398). Shortly after the outbreak was recognized, the governor of Indiana declared a public health emergency and sanctioned a short-term needle exchange program (Rudavsky 2015).

When the NHAS was first released in 2010, it unequivocally identified access to sterile needles and syringes as a 'scientifically proven' prevention intervention for PWID (White House Office of National AIDS Policy 2010a: 16) calling for the CDC and the Substance Abuse and Mental Health Services Administration (SAMHSA) to develop guidance for 'evidence-based comprehensive prevention, including syringe-exchange and drug treatment programs, for injection drug users' (White House Office of National AIDS Policy 2010b: 13). A telephone survey of 187 syringe exchange programs conducted during the first year that the ban was lifted, in 2010, reported that only three programs were receiving federal funds to support their needle exchange prevention activities and that while many other programs anticipated seeking federal funding for their NEP activities, they were concerned about experiencing barriers in light of necessary federal requirements (Green et al. 2012).

Although there is no one approach to dealing with the complex issues surrounding substance use and addiction, access to sterile injection equipment for PWID has been shown to be a scientifically sound (see, for example Abdul-Quader et al. 2013) and cost effective (Nguyen et al. 2014) strategy to prevent the transmission of HIV. For this reason, the updated NHAS released in 2015 advised that 'providing new, sterile syringes and other injection equipment to persons who inject drugs should be part of a comprehensive HIV prevention strategy' (White House Office of National AIDS Policy 2015: 21).

As stated above, The Consolidated Appropriations Act of 2016 includes language that allows US states and localities the opportunity to use federal funds to support certain components of NEP under limited circumstances (The Congress of the United States of America 2015). However, jurisdictions must first demonstrate that they are experiencing or are at risk for significant increases in hepatitis infections or an HIV outbreak due to injection drug use by providing data and other quantitative evidence to CDC for review; furthermore, the prohibition against using federal funds to purchase actual syringes and needles for NEPs remains in place (US Department of Health and Human Services 2016). The 2016 partial lifting of the ban on the use of federal funds to support access to syringe services was generally viewed in a positive light by most prevention advocates (Gorman 2016). Nevertheless, the ability to legally prohibit – or limit – funding of certain prevention interventions, even when they've been shown to be effective, demonstrates that policy, and policymakers, can have a profound impact on access to needed HIV prevention services.

### *9.3.4 Stable Housing and Economic Security*

Across a spectrum of health threats, stable housing and economic security are increasingly recognized as essential ingredients for the assurance of healthy outcomes for individuals, families and communities (see, for example, Robert Wood Johnson Foundation 2013; Stahre et al. 2015). The observation that HIV disease has a disproportionate impact on populations beset by homelessness, unemployment and poverty is not a new one. In fact, recognizing the 'intertwined and mutual enhancing health and social problems facing the urban poor,' Singer coined the term 'syndemics' in the early 1990s to describe the pernicious way that HIV interacts with existing threats to health and social well-being among our most vulnerable populations (Singer 1994: 933).

Singer's observations continue to hold true. A review of 152 studies representing 139,757 PLHIV found that 'lack of stable, secure adequate housing is a significant barrier to consistent and appropriate medical care, access and adherence to antiretroviral medications, sustained viral suppression and risk of forward transmission' (Aidala et al. 2016: e1). Data from a large sample of heterosexual men and women living in 24 US cities found that 'HIV prevalence was higher among persons with lower socioeconomic status' leading the investigators to suggest that 'poverty-related factors might account for some of the racial/ethnic disparities in HIV prevalence observed nationally' (Denning et al. 2011: 1048). And in an analysis of 1,553 Black MSM enrolled across six US cities in an HIV prevention trial, researchers determined that men who were newly diagnosed with HIV infection 'were significantly more likely than uninfected peers to be unemployed' (Mayer et al. 2014).

Access to stable housing and economic security are acknowledged as important to maintaining health in both the 2010 and 2015 versions of the NHAS. The 2010 NHAS specifically called for an increase in the percentage of RWHAP clients who have permanent housing from 82 to 86%; this target was noted to be an inclusive proxy for efforts to expand housing supports 'to all needy people living with HIV' (White House Office of National AIDS Policy 2010a: 21). In 2015, the indicator was changed to consider all persons in HIV medical care (i.e., not just those in the RWHAP) and focused more narrowly on homelessness rather than housing instability: 'Reduce the percentage of persons in HIV medical care who are homeless to no more than five percent, from the baseline of 7.7 percent' (White House Office of

National AIDS Policy 2015: 53). The 2015 NHAS noted that 'the percentage of persons in HIV medical care who were homeless in 2012 (8.3%) did not meet the annual target (7.4%) and increased rather than decreased' (White House Office of National AIDS Policy 2015: 53). There are no specific targets for employment or economic security cited in either the 2010 or the 2015 NHAS – although both documents give mention of the importance of employment initiatives for PLHIV.

Admittedly, housing status and economic security are huge, interrelated issues that can impact health outcomes through a complex array of intermediary factors that encompass physical, mental, emotional, environmental and situational variables. Adding to this complexity is the fact that research on structural interventions addressing these two fundamental needs has been modest, at best. Two published randomized controlled trials (Buchanan et al. 2009; Wolitski et al. 2010) have demonstrated that the receipt of housing assistance along with other supportive services can improve health outcomes among PLHIV. However, investigators have cautioned that additional research is urgently needed 'to examine different models and levels of housing assistance, to inform the development of housing interventions' (Aidala et al. 2016: e18). Even less studied is the specific impact of steady employment and economic security on HIV risk and HIV-related health outcomes – although increasingly, 'precarious employment' is recognized as an important social determinant of health (Benach et al. 2014). Consider recent US experience during the 'Great Recession' (2007–2009). While not specific to HIV or any other disease state, a comprehensive review of over 80 studies found that the recession was associated with negative health-related sequelae, including increasing morbidity, in the USA and other developed nations; effects were especially pronounced among racial/ethnic minorities (Margerison-Zilko et al. 2016). And structural equation modeling of the responses from over 2500 persons recruited from AIDS service organizations supported the hypothesis that vocational rehabilitation services 'had a significant direct effect on reducing health-risk behaviors, increasing access to care and increasing job support services' (Conyers and Boomer 2014: 1208).

Responding to a Congressional directive, in 2015, the US Government Accountability Office (GAO) published a review of how well federal programs funded by the US Department of Housing and Urban Development (HUD) and the Health Resources and Services Administration (HRSA) were meeting the housing needs of PLHIV (US Government Accountability Office 2015). The report noted that in response to the National HIV/AIDS Strategy both HUD and HRSA 'have made formal and informal efforts to collaborate by sharing information related to housing for persons with HIV' (2015: 35). But the analysis also documented the following shortcomings: (1) HUD's estimate of housing needs of PLHIV is 'not reliable' because grantees fail to use a standardized methodology to calculate unmet need; (2) the statutory formula used to calculate HOPWA ('Housing Opportunities for Persons with AIDS') awards 'does not effectively target funds' because it relies on cumulative AIDS cases rather than the number of persons living with HIV; and

(3) HRSA's failure to require grantees to maintain current data on clients' housing status may limit its ability to monitor NHAS' housing goals (US Government Accountability Office 2015: 11).

Even in the face of incomplete data, it is clear that much more must be done to address the housing and employment needs of PLHIV and those at increased, ongoing risk of infection. A 2011 survey of 89 agencies providing housing services to PLHIV across 32 US states found housing to be the highest ranked among the top 5 service priorities, and employment and vocational assistance among the highest ranked unmet service needs (Lennon et al. 2013). Some broad-thinking providers have even called for the US Medicaid program to 'allow capital funding for supportive housing' as a strategy to improve care and reduce costs for homeless Medicaid recipients (Doran et al. 2013: 2375).

While they may not rise to the level of fully developed structural interventions, steps have been taken at the federal level to address the issue of employment/economic security for persons living with HIV. In July 2015, HUD announced a new training curriculum developed in collaboration with the US Department of Labor's (DOL) Office of Disability Employment Policy (US Department of Housing and Urban Development 2015). The curriculum, *Getting to Work*, targets housing and service providers and provides basic information about employment services for PLHIV and how best to access them. These efforts build-off of the work of Martin and his colleagues who demonstrated, using a randomized clinical trial study design, that 'theoretically-based workforce-reentry assistance programs can assist disabled people living with HIV in their return-to-work efforts' (Martin et al. 2012: 280).

Understanding the health and social consequences of unemployment and underemployment is an emerging subject of research in the investigation of social determinants that affect health (Benach et al. 2014). A broader focus that views health as more than just the absence of disease can be seen in programs and interventions aimed at improving mental health and employment outcomes among Black gay men living with HIV as a cross-cutting strategy to improve adherence and other health outcomes (Hergenrather et al. 2013). Another example of the move toward emphasizing employment as a component of health for persons living with or at risk for HIV can be found in a national demonstration project for MSM of color funded at the end of fiscal year 2015 (Centers for Disease Control and Prevention 2015b). The purpose of this demonstration project is to support health departments in the development of functional collaboratives with a broad range of organizations so as to provide a comprehensive array of medical, behavioral and social services to MSM of color, whether infected with or at risk for HIV infection. In addition to housing, job counseling and employment services are cited as among the necessary social services that must be provided, by the collaborative, to men served by the program.

## 9.4 Social Context

### *9.4.1 HIV-Related Stigma*

More and more, stigma is coming to be acknowledged as an important factor influencing population health, especially for racial/ethnic, sexual, and other minority groups (Hatzenbuehler et al. 2013). Newer conceptualizations of stigma have moved beyond an 'excessively individual focus' to a construct that is more 'sociological' in perspective, defining stigma as 'the co-occurrence of labeling, stereotyping, separation, status loss and discrimination in a context in which power is exercised' (Hatzenbuehler et al. 2013: 813). Hatzenbuehler and his colleagues (2013) argue that stigma influences health through both psychological and structural pathways and that its impact on coping behaviors, social relationships and resources – among other domains – qualifies it as a major determinant of population health. HIV-related stigma provides a compelling example of the pernicious interplay of multiple dimensions in the production of sub-optimal health outcomes. In addition to the stigma attached to a serious, incurable (albeit now treatable) disease, we must also acknowledge the added contributions of racism, sexism, homophobia, transphobia and judgmental values directed toward the poor and PWID – to name several of the more obvious factors that can contribute to undesirable HIV-related health outcomes (Mahajan et al. 2008; Valdiserri 2002).

In its 2010 release, the NHAS stated that 'working to end stigma and discrimination against people living with HIV is a critical component of curtailing the epidemic' (White House Office of National AIDS Policy 2010a: 36). The plan called for the following actions to reduce stigma and discrimination against PLHIV: engage communities to affirm support for PLHIV, promote public leadership of PLHIV, promote public health approaches to HIV prevention and care and strengthen the enforcement of civil rights laws. The 2015 NHAS reiterated this call to action and pointed out that, the year before, the Department of Justice (DOJ) had released a best practices document for states wishing to reform their HIV-specific criminal statutes to bring them in line with scientifically supported evidence describing HIV transmission risk. To wit, DOJ observed that 'many of these state laws criminalize behaviors that the CDC regards as posing either no or negligible risk for HIV transmission even in the absence of risk reduction measures' (US Department of Justice 2014).

Other US federal actions have taken place in proactive response to HIV-related stigma. Notably, in July 2012, the CDC launched 'Let's Stop HIV Together', a multi-level (i.e., local, national and social media) marketing campaign to combat HIV stigma by disseminating positive images of PLHIV along with their loved ones (Centers for Disease Control and Prevention 2012b). Granted, this particular approach to stigma reduction is more cognitive in nature, striving as it does to increase acceptance of and empathy for PLHIV (see Mahajan et al. 2008). However, one might argue that an indirect by-product of marketing campaigns like 'Let's Stop AIDS Together' is to support empowerment of people living with HIV, especially those who have been newly diagnosed and are still coming to terms with the realities of their illness. The campaign remains active at the time of writing, but outcome evaluation data are not available to evaluate its impact on specific health outcomes.

For many at risk for or living with HIV, homophobia is a potent contributor to HIV-related stigma. A study of 1,154 Black MSM, recruited from New York City and Philadelphia, found that men who had experienced homophobic events in the past 12 months were more likely to engage in sexual behaviors that increased their risk of acquiring or transmitting HIV (Jeffries et al. 2013). A 2013 analysis of 4,098 HIV uninfected MSM recruited from a large MSM social and sexual networking site found that men living in states with a higher measured level of structural sexual stigma (i.e. structural stigma related to sexual orientation) were more likely to report increased sexual risk behavior, decreased awareness and use of antiretroviral chemoprophylaxis and decreased comfort discussing sexual health issues with their providers, compared to men who lived in states with a lower measured level of structural sexual stigma (Oldenburg et al. 2015). Qualitative interviews with 28 young (aged 13–29 years) MSM living with HIV – two-thirds of whom were Black – not only documented the pervasive existence of HIV-related stigma in their subjects' daily lives but also found that stigma is often internalized, where it may contribute to unhealthy behaviors and poor health outcomes (Jeffries et al. 2015). Another qualitative study of 20 HIV positive Black MSM from Chicago (aged 23–58 years) found that 'HIV-related stigma was considered a significant barrier to candid discussion about HIV with family, friends and sexual partners' (Bird and Voisin 2013: 2197).

Given the evidence linking homophobia and homonegativity (Jeffries and Johnson 2015) with unhealthy behaviors related to HIV acquisition/transmission, it seems logical to ask whether recent structural changes in the USA legalizing same sex marriage (Liptak 2015) might contribute toward reducing negative attitudes about same gender loving persons and, as such, improve health outcomes – for HIV as well as other threats to well-being. While this question has not been definitively answered, preliminary evidence is both intriguing and hopeful. A population-based telephone survey of 2,881 gay men from San Francisco, Los Angeles, Chicago and New York, conducted between November 1996 and January 1998 revealed that 'men with domestic partners were significantly less likely to have had two or more male sex partners, to have had a 'one-night stand,' or to have had unprotected anal intercourse with a male non-primary partner than men with non-domestic primary partnerships or those with no steady partner' (Klausner et al. 2006: 141). A comparison of health care use and expenditures among 1,211 gay and bisexual men in Massachusetts following the enactment of same sex marriage laws in 2003 found that the mean number of medical care and mental health visits decreased significantly in the 12 months following legalization of same-sex marriage: a decrease from 5.00 to 4.67 medical care visits ($p = 0.05$) and a decrease from 24.72 to 22.20 mental health visits ($p = 0.03$) (Hatzenbuehler et al. 2012: 285). The authors hypothesized that reduced stressors related to sexual minority status, resulting from the affirmation of same-sex marriage, might explain these findings (Hatzenbuehler et al. 2012). Consistent with this hypothesis, an analysis published shortly before the Supreme Court ruling legalizing gay marriage across the USA found that same-sex couples living in states with legally sanctioned marriage had ‘higher levels of self-assessed health’ compared to those living in states with antigay marriage constitutional amendments (Kail et al. 2015: 1104).

Legalizing gay marriage, salubrious though it may be, will not erase homophobia nor address all of the facets of HIV-related stigma facing same gender loving men. Unraveling the impact of HIV-related stigma on health outcomes for populations at risk for or living with HIV will require investment in additional structural approaches. In a multi-year review of interventions to reduce HIV-related stigma and discrimination, Stangl and her colleagues (2013) recognized progress but noted the critical need for novel interventions that target multiple domains of stigma and operate at the individual, community and population levels. To maximize outcomes, these interventions must be theoretically sound and informed by the perspectives of knowledgeable providers and the intended recipients. For example, reflecting on their experiences of providing public health services to Black MSM, health department and community leaders surveyed from nine states and the District of Columbia opined that ‘stigma…prevented Black MSM from mobilizing and engaging in community-building activities’ (Wilson and Moore 2009: 1020). Another study, an ethnographic survey of 31 Black MSM recruited from the New York City area, revealed pervasive instances of community-based homophobia in school, at places of worship, from law enforcement officials – even from family members (Garcia et al. 2015). After interviewing 17 community stakeholders and observing participants at 8 community-based organizations, the investigators concluded that ‘safe spaces’ where Black MSM could meet to connect, socialize and support one another were an important resource for promoting empowerment and supporting community mobilization (Garcia et al. 2015).

Safe spaces present a promising structural approach to minimize community and institutional sources of stigma that can impede community mobilization and interfere with positive HIV health outcomes for Black and other MSM populations. Besides providing a supportive environment, these spaces can offer protected opportunities for the receipt of necessary prevention and care services delivered by culturally competent, non-judgmental staff. In North Carolina, for instance, the state Department of Health and Human Services has implemented a Safe Spaces intervention for MSM, including Black MSM, as a way to provide social support and culturally relevant HIV prevention and care services to MSM (personal communication, Dr. Timothy Harrison, Office of HIV/AIDS and Infectious Disease Policy, US Department of Health and Human Services, August 24, 2016). Current technologies offer additional opportunities to support virtual community empowerment. A pilot study found that a ‘mobile phone-optimized online intervention’ for young Black MSM and Black transgender women helped to improve social support and reduce social isolation by providing ‘a safe space in which HIV-positive and HIV-negative young Black MSM and transgender women can explore their opinions, feelings, and perhaps even prejudices in dialogue with their peers’ (Hightow-Weidman et al. 2015: 495).

For the foreseeable future, at least, stigma and discrimination will continue to impact our efforts to achieve the goals of the NHAS. To make progress, we must commit to identifying and supporting effective and reproducible stigma-reduction strategies that address the needs of Black MSM and other similarly vulnerable populations.

## 9.5 Conclusion

While we acknowledge movement toward achieving the goals of the US National HIV/AIDS Strategy, prudence dictates that we also recognize those instances where progress has been insufficient (Bonacci and Holtgrave 2016). Furthermore, we must concede that there is no, one single explanation for why we may fail to realize adequate reductions in HIV incidence, timely diagnosis of HIV infection and consistent engagement with stable, high-quality, systems of comprehensive care. But mounting evidence suggests that structural and social factors are important contributors to these suboptimal outcomes (Valdiserri 2014) and this chapter has endeavored to describe how the US National HIV/AIDS Strategy directs us to address these impediments.

Throughout this assessment it has become apparent that our success in reaching an AIDS-free generation in America is dependent, in large part, on our collective commitment to actively mediate those structural factors and social drivers that impact HIV-related health outcomes. This will require new ways of thinking about the intersections between health and society and novel interventions that transcend single disciplines and strictly biomedical approaches. Consider, for example, the intriguing state-level association of higher spending on social services and public health and lower HIV and AIDS case rates and reduced AIDS deaths (Talbert-Slagel et al. 2016). Or think about how racism, homophobia, financial hardship and lack of social support interact and are associated with high risk sexual behaviors for Latino and Black MSM (Ayala et al. 2012). These complex relationships underscore the fact that individual behaviors and actions take place within a larger, dynamic milieu of powerful structural forces and as such, call for interventions that embrace a definition of health that extends far beyond the mere absence of disease.

In thinking about how best to develop effective interventions and promulgate policies that respond proactively to the non-biologic determinants shaping HIV-related health outcomes, the paradigm of systems science may be particularly relevant. Many public health challenges, including the HIV epidemic, can be described in the context of dynamic complex systems (Luke and Stamatakis 2012). Systems science posits that in complex systems, multiple disparate elements can interact to produce outcomes that differ from the effects of individual elements and can change in response to changing circumstances (Luke and Stamatakis 2012: 358). Apropos of efforts to improve HIV-related health outcomes for Black MSM, a systems science perspective *mandates* that we address 'upstream factors' that contribute to poor HIV outcomes, including social disadvantage and social inequity (Bharmal et al. 2015). Investing in longitudinal research that can collect data both on health outcomes and social factors (Bharmal et al. 2015) will enable the development and testing of interventions that can improve the health of our most vulnerable populations and make the vision of the US National HIV/AIDS Strategy a reality:

> The United States will become a place where new HIV infections are rare and when they do occur, every person, regardless of age, gender, race/ethnicity, sexual orientation, gender identity or socio-economic circumstance, will have unfettered access to high quality, life-extending care, free from stigma and discrimination (White House, Office of National AIDS Policy 2010a: iii)

## References


Abdul-Quader, A. S., Feelemyer, J., Modi, S., Stein, E. S., Briceno, A., Semaan, S., et al. (2013). Effectiveness of structural-level needle/syringe programs to reduce HCV and HIV infection among people who inject drugs: A systematic review. *AIDS and Behavior, 17*(9), 2878–2892. doi:10.1007/s10461-013-0593-y.

Aidala, A. A., Wilson, M. G., Shubert, V., Gogolishvili, D., Globerman, J., Rueda, S., et al. (2016). Housing status, medical care, and health outcomes among people living with HIV/AIDS: A systematic review. *American Journal of Public Health, 106*(1), e1–e23. doi:10.2105/AJPH2015.302905.

Auerbach, J. D., Parkhurst, J. O., & Caceres, C. F. (2011). Addressing social drivers of HIV/AIDS for the long terms response: Conceptual and methodological considerations. *Global Public Health, 6*(Suppl. 3), S293–S309. doi:10.1080/17441692.2011.594451.

Ayala, G., Bingham, T., Kim, J., Wheeler, D. P., & Millett, G. A. (2012). Modeling the impact of social discrimination and financial hardship on the sexual risk of HIV among Latino and Black men who have sex with men. *American Journal of Public Health, 102*(S2), S242–S249. doi:10.2105/ajph.2011.300641.

Benach, J., Vives, A., Amable, M., Vanroelen, C., Tarafa, G., & Muntaner, C. (2014). Precarious employment: Understanding an emerging social determinant of health. *Annual Review of Public Health, 35*, 229–253. doi:10.1146/annurev-publhealth-032013-182500.

Berry, S. A., Fleishmann, J. A., Yehia, B. R., Cheever, L. W., Hauck, H., Korthuis, P. T., et al. (2016). Healthcare coverage for HIV provider visits before and after implementation of the Affordable Care Act. *Clinical Infectious Diseases, 63*(3), 387–395. doi:10.1093/cid/ciw278.

Bharmal, N., Derose, K. P., Felician, M., & Weden M. M. (2015). *Understanding the upstream social determinants of health* (Rand Health Working Paper. WR-1096-RC). Available at: www.rand.org/content/dam/rand/pubs/working_papers/WR1000/WR1096/RAND_WR1096.pdf

Bird, J. D., & Voisin, D. R. (2013). 'You're an open target to be abused': A qualitative study of stigma and HIV self-disclosure among black men who have sex with men. *American Journal of Public Health, 103*(12), 2193–2199. doi:10.2105/ajph.2013.301437.

Blankenship, K. M., Friedman, S. R., Dworkin, S., & Mantell, J. E. (2006). Structural interventions: Concepts, challenges and opportunities for research. *Journal of Urban Health, 83*(1), 59–72. doi:10.1007/s11524-005-9007-4.

Bonacci, R. A., & Holtgrave, D. R. (2016). Evaluating the impact of the US National HIV/AIDS Strategy, 2010–2015. *AIDS and Behavior, 20*(7), 1383–1389. doi:10.1007/s10461-016-1416-8.

Bramson, H., Des Jarlais, D. C., Arasteh, K., Nugent, A., Guardino, V., Feelemyer, J., & Hodel, D. (2015). State laws, syringe exchange, and HIV among persons who inject drugs in the United States: History and effectiveness. *Journal of Public Health Policy, 36*(2), 212–230. doi:10.1057/jphp.2014.54.

Braverman, P. A., Egerter, S. A., Woolf, S. H., & Marks, J. S. (2011). When do we know enough to recommend action on the social determinants of health? *American Journal of Preventive Medicine, 40*(1S1), S58–S66. doi:10.1016/j.amepre.2010.09.026.

Buchanan, D., Kee, R., Sadowski, L. S., & Garcia, D. (2009). The health impact of supportive housing for HIV-positive homeless patients: A randomized controlled trial. *American Journal of Public Health, 99*(S3), S675–S680. doi:10.2105/ajph.2008.137810.

Burris, S., & Gostin, L. O. (2003). The impact of HIV/AIDS on the development of public health law. In R. O. Valdiserri (Ed.), *Dawning answers: How the HIV/AIDS epidemic has helped to strengthen public health* (pp. 96–117). New York: Oxford University Press.

Cahill, S. R., Mayer, K. H., & Boswell, S. L. (2015). The Ryan White HIV/AIDS Program in the age of health care reform. *American Journal of Public Health, 105*(6), 1078–1085. doi:10.2105/ajph.2014.302442.

Centers for Disease Control and Prevention. (2011). *CDC's new high-impact approach to HIV prevention funding for health departments: Advancing the National HIV/AIDS Strategy*. Program Backgrounder. http://www.cdc.gov/hiv/pdf/prevention_programs_healthdepts.pdf. Accessed 10 May 2016.

Centers for Disease Control and Prevention. (2012a). *HIV prevention funding allocations at CDC-funded state and local health departments, 2010*. http://www.cdc.gov/hiv/pdf/research/testing_prevention_funding.pdf. Accessed 11 May 2016.

Centers for Disease Control and Prevention. (2012b). *New CDC campaign fights stigma and apathy fueling HIV epidemic*. NCHHSTP Press Release. www.cdc.gov/nchhstp/newsroom/2012/letsstophivtogether2012-pressrelease.html. Accessed 22 June 2016.

Centers for Disease Control and Prevention. (2015a). *HIV among gay and bisexual men*. CDC Fact Sheet. https://www.cdc.gov/nchstp/newsroom/docs/factsheets/cdc-msm-508.pdf. Accessed 30 May 2016.

Centers for Disease Control and Prevention. (2015b). Health department demonstration projects for comprehensive prevention, care, behavioral health, and social services for men who have sex with men of color at risk for and living with HIV infection: CDC-RFA-PS15-1509. Funding Opportunity Announcement. http://www.cdc.gov/hiv/funding/announcements/ps15-1509/. Accessed 4 May 2016.

Cohen, M. S., Chen, Y. Q., McCauley, M., Gamble, T., Hosseinipour, M. C., Kumarasamy, N., et al. (2011). Prevention of HIV-1 infection with early antiretroviral therapy. *New England Journal of Medicine, 365*(6), 493–505. doi:10.1056/nejmoa1105243.

Congress of the United States of America. (2015). *Consolidated Appropriations Act, 2016*. https://www.congress.gov/114/bills/hr2029/BILLS-114hr2029enr.pdf. Accessed 7 June 2016.

Conrad, C., Bradley, H. M., Broz, D., Buddha, S., Chapman, E. L., Galang, R. R., et al. (2015). Community outbreak of HIV infection linked to injection drug use of oxymorphone – Indiana, 2015. *Morbidity and Mortality Weekly Report, 64*(16), 443–444.

Conyers, L., & Boomer, K. B. (2014). Examining the role of vocational rehabilitation on access to care and public health outcomes for people living with HIV/AIDS. *Disability and Rehabilitation, 36*(14), 1203–1210. doi:10.3109/09638288.2013.837968.

Dasgupta, S., Oster, A. M., Li, J., & Hall, I. (2016). Disparities in consistent retention in HIV care – 11 states and the District of Columbia, 2011–2013. *Morbidity and Mortality Weekly Report, 65*(4), 77–82. doi:10.15585/mmwr.mm6504a2.

Denning, P. H., DiNenno, E. A., & Wiegand, R. E. (2011). Characteristics associated with HIV infection among heterosexuals in urban areas with high AIDS prevalence – 24 cities, United States, 2006–2007. *Morbidity and Mortality Weekly Report, 60*(31), 1045–1049.

Doran, K. M., Misa, E. J., & Shah, N. R. (2013). Housing as health care – New York's boundary-crossing experiment. *New England Journal of Medicine, 369*(25), 2374–2377. doi:10.1056/nejmp1310121.

Doshi, R. K., Milberg, J., Isenberg, D., Matthews, T., Malitz, F., Matosky, M., et al. (2015). High rates of retention and viral suppression in the US HIV safety net system: HIV care continuum in the Ryan White HIV/AIDS Program, 2011. *Clinical Infectious Diseases, 60*(1), 117–125. doi:10.1093/cid/ciu722.

Eaton, E. F., & Mugavero, M. J. (2016). Editorial Commentary: Affordable Care Act, Medicaid expansion…or not: Ryan White Care Act remains essential for access and equity. *Clinical Infectious Diseases, 63*(3), 404–406. doi:10.1093/cid/ciw280.

Elmer, M. (2012). HIV prevention cuts raise fears. *Iowa Center for Public Affairs Journalism*. http://iowawatch.org/2012/03/22/hiv-prevention-cuts-raises-fears/. Accessed 1 Jul 2016.

Garcia, J., Parker, C., Parker, R. G., Wilson, P. A., Philbin, M. M., & Hirsch, J. S. (2015). 'You're really gonna kick us all out?' Sustaining safe spaces for community-based HIV prevention and control among black men who have sex with men. *PloS One, 10*(10), e0141326. doi:10.1371/journal.pone.0141326.

Gorman, A. (2016, February 17). Needle exchanges can now get federal funding. *Kaiser Health News*. http://khn.org/news/needle-exchange-can-now-get-federal-funding/. Accessed 7 June 2016.

Green, T. C., Martin, E. G., Bowman, S. E., Mann, M. R., & Beletsky, L. (2012). Life after the ban: An assessment of US syringe exchange attitudes about the early experiences with federal funding. *American Journal of Public Health, 102*(5), e9–e16. doi:10.2105/ajph.2011.300595.

Hatzenbuehler, M. L., O'Cleirigh, C., Grasso, C., Mayer, K., Safren, S., & Bradford, J. (2012). Effect of same-sex marriage laws on health care use and expenditures in sexual minority men: A quasi-natural experiment. *American Journal of Public Health, 102*(2), 285–291. doi:10.2105/ajph.2011.300382.

Hatzenbuehler, M. L., Phelan, J. C., & Link, B. G. (2013). Stigma as a fundamental cause of population health inequalities. *American Journal of Public Health, 103*(5), 813–821. doi:10.2105/ajph.2012.301069.

Hergenrather, K. C., Geishecker, S., Clark, G., & Rhodes, S. D. (2013). A pilot test of the HOPE intervention to explore employment and mental health among African American gay men living with HIV/AIDS: Results from a CBPR study. *AIDS Education and Prevention, 25*(5), 405–422. doi:10.1521/aeap.2013.25.5.405.

Hightow-Weidman, L. B., Muessig, K. E., Pike, E. C., LeGrand, S., Baltierra, N., Rucker, A. J., & Wilson, P. (2015). HealthMpowerment.org: Building community through a mobile-optimized, online health promotion intervention. *Health Education & Behavior, 42*(4), 493–499. doi:10.1177/1090198114562043.

Holtgrave, D. R. (2010). On the epidemiologic and economic importance of the National AIDS Strategy for the United States. *Journal of Acquired Immune Deficiency Syndromes, 55*(2), 139–142. doi:10.1097/qai.0b013e3181f4107a.

Holtgrave, D. R., Hall, H. I., Wehrmeyer, L., & Maulsby, C. (2012). Costs, consequences and feasibility of strategies for achieving the goals of the National HIV/AIDS Strategy in the United States: A closing window for success? *AIDS and Behavior, 16*(6), 1365–1372. doi:10.1007/s10461-012-0207-0.

Holtgrave, D. R., Kim, J. J., Adkins, C., Maulsby, C., Lindsey, K. D., Johnson, K. M., Montoya, D. C., & Kelley, R. T. (2014). Unmet HIV service needs among black men who have sex with men in the United States. *AIDS and Behavior, 18*(1), 36–40. doi:10.1007/s10461-013-0574-1.

Jeffries, W. L., & Johnson, O. D. (2015). Homonegative attitudes and risk behaviors for HIV and other sexually transmitted infections among sexually active men in the United States. *American Journal of Public Health, 105*(12), 2466–2472. doi:10.2105/ajph.2015.302780.

Jeffries, W. L., Marks, G., Lauby, J., Murrill, C. S., & Millett, G. A. (2013). Homophobia is associated with sexual behavior that increases risk of acquiring and transmitting HIV infection among black men who have sex with men. *AIDS and Behavior, 17*(4), 1442–1453. doi:10.1007/s10461-012-0189-y.

Jeffries, W. L., Townsend, E. S., Gelaude, D. J., Torrone, E. A., Gasiorowicz, M., & Bertolli, J. (2015). HIV stigma experienced by young men who have sex with men (MSM) living with HIV infection. *AIDS Education and Prevention, 27*(1), 58–71. doi:10.1521/aeap.2015.27.1.58.

Kail, B. L., Acosta, K. L., & Wright, E. R. (2015). State-level marriage equality and the health of same-sex couples. *American Journal of Public Health, 105*(6), 1101–1105. doi:10.2105/ajph.2015.302589.

Kaiser Family Foundation. (2016). *Current status of state Medicaid expansion decisions*. http://kff.org/health-reform/state-indicator/state-activity-around-expanding-medicaid-under-the-affordable-care-act/. Accessed 25 May 2016.

Kates, J. (2013). Implications of the Affordable Care Act for people with HIV infection and the Ryan White HIV/AIDS Program: What does the future hold? *Topics in Antiviral Medicine, 21*(4), 138–142.

Klausner, J. D., Pollack, L. M., Wong, W., & Katz, M. H. (2006). Same-sex domestic partnerships and lower-risk behaviors for STDs including HIV infection. *Journal of Homosexuality, 51*(4), 137–144. doi:10.1300/j082v51n04_07.

Lawrence, J. (1987, October 14). *Senate says federal AIDS education material can't promote homosexuality*. Associated Press. Available at: www.apnewsarchive.com. Accessed 18 May 2016.

Lennon, C. A., White, A. C., Finitsis, D., Pishori, A., Hernandez, D., Kelly, D. M., et al. (2013). Service priorities and unmet service needs among people living with HIV/AIDS: Results from a nationwide interview of HIV/AIDS housing organizations. *AIDS Care, 25*(9), 1083–1091. doi:10.1080/09540121.2012.749337.

Liptak, A. (2015, June 26). Supreme Court ruling makes same-sex marriage a right nationwide. *The New York Times*. http://www.nytimes.com/2015/06/27/us/supreme-court-same-sex-marriage.html. Accessed 23 June 2016.

Luke, D. A., & Stamatakis, K. A. (2012). Systems science methods in public health: Dynamics, networks, and agents. *Annual Review of Public Health, 33*, 357–376. doi:10.1146/annurev-publhealth-031210-101222.

Mahajan, A. P., Sayles, J. N., Patel, V. A., Remien, R. H., Ortiz, D., Szekeres, G., & Coates, T. J. (2008). Stigma in the HIV/AIDS epidemic: A review of the literature and recommendations for the way forward. *AIDS, 22*(Suppl 2), S67–S79. doi:10.1097/01.aids.0000327438.13291.62.

Margerison-Zilko, C., Goldman-Mellor, S., Falconi, A., & Downing, J. (2016). Health impacts of the Great Recession: A critical review. *Current Epidemiology Reports, 3*(1), 81–91. doi:10.1007/s40471-016-0068-6.

Martin, E. G., & Schackman, B. R. (2012). What does US health reform mean for HIV clinical care? *Journal of Acquired Immune Deficiency Syndromes, 60*(1), 72–76. doi:10.1097/qai.0b013e31824c0dd4.

Martin, D. J., Chernoff, R. A., Buitron, J., Comulada, W. S., Liang, L. J., & Wong, F. L. (2012). Helping people with HIV/AIDS return to work: A randomized clinical trial. *Rehabilitation Psychology, 57*(4), 280–289. doi:10.1037/a0030207.

Matthews, D. D., Herrick, A. L., Coulter, R. W., Friedman, M. R., Mills, T. C., Eaton, L. A., et al. (2016). Running backwards: Consequences of current HIV incidence rates for the next generation of black MSM in the United States. *AIDS and Behavior, 20*(1), 7–16. doi:10.1007/s10461-015-1158-z.

Maulsby, C., Millett, G., Lindsey, K., Kelley, R., Johnson, K., Montoya, D., & Holtgrave, D. (2014). HIV among black men who have sex with men (MSM) in the United States: A review of the literature. *AIDS and Behavior, 18*(1), 10–25. doi:10.1007/s10461-013-0476-2.

Mayer, K. H., Wang, L., Koblin, B., Mannheimer, S., Magnus, M., del Rio, C., et al. (2014). Concomitant socioeconomic, behavioral, and biological factors associated with the disproportionate HIV infection burden among black men who have sex with men in 6 U.S. cities. *PloS One, 9*(1), e87298. doi:10.1371/journal.pone.0087298.

Millett, G. A., Crowley, J. S., Koh, H., Valdiserri, R. O., Frieden, T., Dieffenbach, C. W., et al. (2010). A way forward: The National HIV/AIDS Strategy and reducing HIV incidence in the United States. *Journal of Acquired Immune Deficiency Syndromes, 55*(S2), S144–S147. doi:10.1097/qai.0b013e3181fbcb04.

Mugavero, M. J., Norton, W. E., & Saag, M. S. (2011). Health care system and policy factors influencing engagement in HIV medical care: Piecing together the fragments of a fractured health care delivery system. *Clinical Infectious Diseases, 52*(Suppl. 2), S238–S246. doi:10.1093/cid/ciq048.

National Alliance of State and Territorial AIDS Directors. (2013). National HIV Prevention Inventory: 2013 funding survey report. https://www.nastad.org/sites/default/files/NHPI-2013-Funding-Report-Finalpdf. Accessed 10 May 2016.

Nguyen, T. Q., Weir, B. W., Des Jarlais, D. C., Pinkerton, S. D., & Holtgrave, D. R. (2014). Syringe exchange in the United States: A national level economic evaluation of hypothetical increases in investment. *AIDS and Behavior, 18*(11), 2144–2155. doi:10.1007/s10461-014-0789-9.

Oldenburg, C. E., Perez-Brumer, A. G., Hatzenbuehler, M. L., Krakower, D., Novak, D. S., Mimiaga, M. J., & Mayer, K. H. (2015). State-level structural sexual stigma and HIV prevention in a national online sample of HIV-uninfected MSM in the United States. *AIDS, 29*(7), 837–845. doi:10.1097/qad.0000000000000622.

Poundstone, K. E., Strathdee, S. A., & Celentano, D. D. (2004). The social epidemiology of Human Immunodeficiency Virus/Acquired Immunodeficiency Syndrome. *Epidemiologic Reviews, 26*(1), 22–35. doi:10.1093/epirev/mxh005.

Public Health Law Research. (2016). *LawAtlas: Syringe distribution laws*. http://lawatlas.org/files/upload3_7_2016. Accessed 14 May 2016.

Purcell, D. W., McCray, E., & Mermin, J. (2016). The shift to high-impact HIV prevention by health departments in the United States. *Public Health Reports, 131*(1), 7–10. doi:10.1177/003335491613100104.

Robert Wood Johnson Foundation. (2013). *How does employment – or unemployment – affect health?* Issue Brief. https://www.rwjf.org/content/dam/farm/reports/issue_briefs/2013/rwjf403360. Accessed 4 May 2016.

Rosenberg, E. S., Grey, J. A., Sanchez, T. H., & Sullivan, P. S. (2016). Rates of prevalent HIV infection, prevalent diagnoses, and new diagnoses among men who have sex with men in the US states, metropolitan statistical areas, and counties, 2012–2013. *JMIR Public Health and Surveillance, 2*(1), e22. doi:10.2196/publichealth.5684.

Rudavsky, S. (2015, March 26). Indiana OKs clean needle exchange amid HIV outbreak. *Indianapolis Star*. www.usatoday.com/story/news/nation-now/2015/03/26/indiana-to-declare-health-emergency-for-hiv-outbreak/70478492/. Accessed 2 June 2016.

Shaw, F. E., Asomugha, C. N., Conway, P. H., & Rein, A. S. (2014). The Patient Protection and Affordable Care Act: Opportunities for prevention and public health. *Lancet, 384*(9937), 75–82. doi:10.1016/s0140-6736(14)60259-2.

Singer, M. (1994). AIDS and the health crisis of the U.S. urban poor; the perspective of critical medical anthropology. *Social Science and Medicine, 39*(7), 931–948. doi:10.1016/0277-9536(94)90205-4.

Singh, S., Bradley, H., Hu, X., Skarbinski, J., Hall, H. I., & Lansky, A. (2014). Men living with diagnosed HIV who have sex with men: Progress along the continuum of HIV care – United States, 2010. *Morbidity and Mortality Weekly Report, 63*(38), 829–833.

Snider, J. T., Juday, T., Romley, J. A., Seekins, D., Rosenblatt, L., Sanchez, Y., & Goldman, D. P. (2014). Nearly 60,000 uninsured and low-income people with HIV/AIDS live in states that are not expanding Medicaid. *Health Affairs, 33*(3), 386–393. doi:10.1377/hlthaff.2013.1453.

Stahre, M., VanEenwyk, J., Siegel, P., & Njai, R. (2015). Housing insecurity and the association with health outcomes and unhealthy behaviors, Washington state, 2011. *Preventing Chronic Disease, 12*(E109), 140511. doi:10.5888/ped12.140511.

Stangl, A. L., Lloyd, J. K., Brady, L. M., Holland, C. E., & Baral, S. (2013). A systematic review of interventions to reduce HIV-related stigma and discrimination from 2002 to 2013: How far have we come? *Journal of the International AIDS Society, 16*(Suppl 2), 18734. doi:10.7448/IAS.16.3.18734.

Strathdee, S. A., & Beyrer, C. (2015). Threading the needle – how to stop the HIV outbreak in rural Indiana. *New England Journal of Medicine, 373*(5), 397–399. doi:10.1056/nejmp1507252.

Sweat, M. D., & Denison, J. A. (1995). Reducing HIV incidence in developing countries with structural and environmental interventions. *AIDS, 9*(Suppl. A), S251–S257.

Talbert-Slagle, K. M., Canavan, M. E., Rogan, E. M., Curry, L. A., & Bradley, E. H. (2016). State variation in HIV/AIDS health outcomes: The effect of spending on social services and public health. *AIDS, 30*(4), 657–663. doi:10.1097/qad.0000000000000978.

U.S. Department of Health and Human Services. (2016). *Department of Health and Human Services implementation guidance to support certain components of syringe services programs, 2016.* https://www.aids.gov/pdf/hhs-ssp-guidance. Accessed 25 May 2016.

U.S. Department of Housing and Urban Development. (2015). *HUD and Department of Labor launch training curriculum for HIV/AIDS housing and service providers.* HUD Press Release No. 15-088. http://portal.hud.gov/hudportal/HUD?src=/press/press_releases_media_advisories/2015HUDNo_15-088. Accessed 3 May 2016.

U.S. Department of Justice, Civil Rights Division. (2014). *Best practices guide to reform HIV-specific criminal laws to align with scientifically-supported facts.* https://www.ada.gov/aids/HIV-guide-reform-crim.pdf. Accessed 22 June 2016.

Ungar, L. (2016, January 7). Funding ban on needle exchanges effectively lifted. *USA Today.* www.usatoday.com/story/news/nation/2016/01/07/funding-ban-needle-exchanges-effectively-lifted/78420894//. Accessed 2 June 2016.

United States Government Accountability Office. (2015). *Persons with HIV: Funding formula for housing assistance could be better targeted, and performance data could be improved.* GAO-15-298. www.gao.gov/assets/670/669705.pdf. Accessed 9 May 2016.

Valdiserri, R. O. (2002). HIV/AIDS stigma: An impediment to public health. *American Journal of Public Health, 92*(3), 341–342. doi:10.2105/ajph.92.3.341.

Valdiserri, R. O. (2003). HIV/AIDS in historical profile. In R. O. Valdiserri (Ed.), *Dawning answers: How the HIV/AIDS epidemic has helped to strengthen public health* (pp. 3–32). New York: Oxford University Press.

Valdiserri, R. O. (2011). Thirty years of AIDS in America: A story of infinite hope. *AIDS Education and Prevention, 23*(6), 479–494. doi:10.1521/aeap.2011.23.6.479.

Valdiserri, R. O. (2013). Preventing HIV/AIDS in the United States, 1981–2009: History in the making. In S. O. Aral, K. A. Fenton, & J. A. Lipshutz (Eds.), *The new public health and STD/HIV prevention: Personal, public and health systems approaches* (pp. 309–337). New York: Springer.

Valdiserri, R. O. (2014). Improving outcomes along the HIV care continuum: Paying careful attention to the non-biologic determinants of health. *Public Health Reports, 129*(4), 319–321.

Valdiserri, R. O. (2016). Shining a light on America's HIV epidemic among men who have sex with men. *JMIR Public Health and Surveillance, 2*(1), e25. doi:10.2196/publichealth.5864.

Weinmeyer, R. (2016). Needle exchange programs' status in US politics. *AMA Journal of Ethics, 18*(3), 252–257. doi:10.1001/journalofethics.2016.18.3.hlaw1-1603.

White House, Office of National AIDS Policy. (2010a). *National HIV/AIDS Strategy for the United States.* https://www.whitehouse.gov/sites/default/files/uploads/NHAS.pdf. Accessed 2 May 2016.

White House, Office of National AIDS Policy. (2010b). *National HIV/AIDS Strategy: Federal implementation plan.* https://www.whitehouse.gov/files/documents/nhas-implementation.pdf. Accessed 2 May 2016.

White House, Office of National AIDS Policy. (2015). *National HIV/AIDS Strategy for the United States: Updated to 2020.* https://www.whitehouse.gov/sites/default/docs/national_hiv_aids_strategy_update_2020.pdf. Accessed 2 May 2016.

Whiteside, Y. O., Cohen, S. M., Bradley, H., Skarbinski, J., Hall, H. I., & Lansky, A. (2014). Progress along the continuum of HIV care among blacks with diagnosed HIV – United States, 2010. *Morbidity and Mortality Weekly Report, 63*(5), 85–89.

Wilson, P. A., & Moore, T. E. (2009). Public health responses to the HIV epidemic among black men who have sex with men: A qualitative study of US health departments and communities. *American Journal of Public Health, 99*(6), 1013–1022. doi:10.2105/ajph.2008.140681.

Wolitski, R. J., Kidder, D. P., Pals, S. L., Royal, S., Aidala, A., Stall, R., et al. (2010). Randomized trial of the effects of housing assistance on the health and risk behaviors of homeless and unstably housed people living with HIV. *AIDS and Behavior, 14*(3), 493–503. doi:10.1007/s10461-009-9643-x.

Yehia, B. R., Stewart, L., Momplaisir, F., Mody, A., Holtzman, C. W., Jacobs, L. M., et al. (2015). Barriers and facilitators to patient retention in HIV care. *BMC Infectious Diseases, 15*(1), 246. doi:10.1186/s12879-015-0990-0.

# Chapter 10
# Finding and Reforming the (In)visible State: Nongovernmental Organizations and the Response to HIV in Ukraine

**Jill Owczarzak, Sarah D. Phillips, and Olga Filippova**

## 10.1 Introduction

In March 2014, after intense political and military conflict, Russian troops seized control of the Autonomous Republic of Crimea from Ukraine and annexed it into the Russian Federation. Our Ukrainian and American research team had been working with an HIV prevention organization based in Simferopol, the administrative center of Crimea, for several years. The transfer of this region to Russian from Ukrainian control exposed both the progress and limits of Ukraine's HIV prevention efforts for people who use drugs. Opioid substitution therapy (OST) for opiate addiction in Russia is illegal, and methadone and buprenorphine, the two key drugs used in OST, are banned in Russia. We were concerned that the work of our partner organization would be dramatically curtailed and the small number of OST patients served by it would be without this life-saving treatment (Mazhnaya et al. 2016). Our fears were not unfounded: when Russia annexed Crimea, OST became illegal there as well. Stocks of methadone and buprenorphine on the Crimean peninsula were quickly depleted and OST sites shut down, leaving hundreds of patients without this addiction treatment option (Carroll 2015; Filippovych 2015). Some OST patients were able to relocate to the Ukrainian mainland with the help of our partner organization and other non-governmental organizations (NGOs), and several dozen

J. Owczarzak (✉)
Johns Hopkins Bloomberg School of Public Health, Baltimore, MD, USA
e-mail: jillowczarzak@jhu.edu

S.D. Phillips
Indiana University, Bloomington, IN

O. Filippova
V.N. Karazin Kharkiv National University

 
D. Kerrigan, C. Barrington (eds.), *Structural Dynamics of HIV*, Social Aspects of HIV 4, DOI 10.1007/978-3-319-63522-4_10

methadone patients reportedly were sent to Moscow for rehabilitation programs (Carroll 2014). However, hundreds of OST patients were left without access to this evidence-based treatment. At the same time, access to OST, a proven method of reducing HIV risk through reduction in injection risk behaviors (Lawrinson et al. 2008), is severely limited in Ukraine. Fewer than 2% of people who use drugs in Ukraine currently receive it – due to strict laws regulating its distribution, insufficient funding, and police harassment of both OST clients and clinic staff (Bojko et al. 2015; Golovankvskaya et al. 2012). When we contacted our partner agency in Crimea to ask how the annexation might affect its work, the agency was rightly concerned with its funding and future viability. Now that Crimea was no longer part of Ukraine, would the Global Fund – the primary funder of most HIV prevention efforts in the country – and other international organizations that financially support the bulk of the HIV prevention effort in Ukraine continue to support agencies in Crimea? Without Global Fund money, the agency would be forced to compete with Russia-based NGOs, which already have established relationships with Russia-based funders. Unlike international donor organizations, Russian funders generally do not support harm reduction strategies, including needle and syringe exchange. In short, political processes and logistical factors cast this organization's viability into doubt.

The uncertain future of HIV prevention and drug addiction treatment in Crimea provides a particularly chilling example of how precarious and tenuous relationships between national governments, international funding agencies, and local nongovernmental organizations can negatively or positively impact those at risk for and living with HIV. In many low- and middle-income countries, the ability of providers – whether outreach workers at NGOs or clinicians in hospitals – to serve their clients and patients is structured by complicated policies, bureaucratic procedures, and fraught relationships between diverse sectors. In this chapter, we explore the implications of these relationships on NGO service providers' ideas about who is and who should be responsible for HIV prevention and treatment, and the ways in which NGOs strategize to reform or align with the state. We examine the ways in which those most at-risk for HIV in Ukraine, particularly people who use drugs, become both targets of and participants in this response, and the implications of their participation for ideas about professional identity and expertise. We draw on data from 60 in-depth interviews with directors and staff of 8 HIV-focused NGOs, field notes from site visits, and 4 years of collaboration with NGOs involved in HIV prevention. These organizations are located in cities in Ukraine's eastern, southern, and central regions, including Crimea; these are the regions that experience the highest rates of HIV and drug use. Our study sought to promote the use of evidence-based HIV prevention strategies among Ukrainian NGOs working with people who use drugs. We primarily conducted these interviews and site visits in 2013, prior to Russia's annexation of Crimea. Our research team consisted of two US-based anthropologists with experience conducting research around civil society and health in Ukraine and Eastern Europe more broadly, and a Ukraine-based research team comprised of a sociologist and three masters-level research assistants fluent in Russian and Ukrainian.

Ukraine has one of the most severe HIV epidemics in Eastern Europe, particularly among people who inject drugs and their sex partners (Booth et al. 2009; Ministry of Health of Ukraine 2010). HIV arrived late to Ukraine, but rapidly spread. In 1995, the World Health Organization (WHO) characterized Ukraine as a low prevalence country. However, by 1996, all regional capitals reported HIV cases, and the number of annual HIV cases doubled each year until 2006 (Booth et al. 2009). This rapid spread of HIV has been attributed to the increased availability of locally-produced drugs that occurred with the collapse of the Soviet Union, the lack of a comprehensive HIV prevention strategy, and poor public health infrastructure (DeBell and Carter 2005). In addition, the economic and social upheaval of the early 1990s resulted in high unemployment, a decline in state-supported services, and reduced quality of life for many people (Booth et al. 2003). Inadequate health care (Altice et al. 2011; Izenberg and Altice 2010) also exacerbates the HIV epidemic in Ukraine. HIV prevalence in the general adult population is twice as high in Ukraine as in the rest of Europe (World Health Organization Regional Office for Europe 2016). As of 2014, the Joint United Nations Programme on HIV/AIDS (UNAIDS) estimates that over 290,000 people are living with HIV in Ukraine, but the actual number is probably as high as 340,000. It is estimated that 17,000 deaths each year are AIDS-related (UNAIDS 2015). In some regions of Ukraine, specifically in the south and east, HIV prevalence among people who inject drugs has been estimated to be as high as 55% (Booth 2013; UNAIDS 2014).

Despite these alarming numbers, it was only in 2009 that national law with budgetary support for HIV prevention, treatment, and care was passed by the Ukrainian parliament (Ministry of Health of Ukraine 2010). Unfortunately, the national program has been severely underfunded, leaving no funding for many aspects of the program such as care and support for people living with HIV (PLHIV), medication procurement to treat sexually transmitted infections and Hepatitis C, and prevention activities for the most at-risk populations. Tellingly, in 2006, the World Bank suspended disbursement of USD 60 million to fight HIV in Ukraine because after 3 years of funding, only 2% of the funds had been disbursed by the government. Similarly, in 2004, the Global Fund to Fight AIDS, Tuberculosis and Malaria asked The International HIV/AIDS Alliance in Ukraine (which recently changed its name to the Alliance for Public Health) to become the temporary steward of its grant to combat HIV in Ukraine after the Ukrainian government mismanaged the funds and failed to comply with Global Fund procedures (International HIV/AIDS Alliance 2009). The Alliance and another large NGO (Всеукраїнська мережа ЛЖВ [the All-Ukrainian Network of People Living with HIV/AIDS]) remain the country's Principal Recipients of Ukraine's Global Fund grant, due to perceived corruption and mismanagement of earlier grants given to the government (Doyle and Patel 2008; Harmer et al. 2013).

Advocates within NGOs, as well as Ukrainian and international public health researchers, have been highly critical of the government's response to people who use drugs, others at heightened risk for HIV, and PLHIV. The problems with Ukraine's response to HIV are numerous. In addition to the issues related to OST availability and access raised above, the system of narcology presents a paternalistic and bureaucratic approach to drug use and HIV that includes opiate addict registries, an emphasis on detoxification, and moral judgment of people who use drugs (Elovich and Drucker 2008; Golovankvskaya et al. 2012). Narcology is a subspecialty of psychiatry developed during the Soviet era to address drug use and dependence ('narkomania'). It emerged as part of broader efforts to identify and treat mental illness, alcoholism, and other 'social diseases' that were viewed as having their roots in capitalism and consumerism, or as a moral failing of the individual (Latypov 2011). Drug addicts were considered mentally ill and dangerous to society, and were subject to compulsory treatment that included 'therapeutic confinement' in labor colonies (Latypov 2011). In addition, Ukraine lacks routine HIV testing, apart from that offered to – indeed, required of – pregnant women. People living with HIV in Ukraine face similar obstacles to treatment and care, including HIV-associated stigma, harassment and discrimination by police and law enforcement, and expensive and unstable supplies of antiretroviral therapy (ART) (Mimiaga et al. 2010). HIV-infected patients in state-run drug treatment centers are often housed in isolation blocks, allowing for easy identification of a person's HIV status, and counseling and support for newly diagnosed HIV cases is largely absent (Barcal et al. 2005).

Moreover, police, the courts, and law enforcement hold negative views of people who use drugs and often violate their human rights through violence, extortion, and confiscation of drug use equipment. NGO-run harm reduction programs, including needle/syringe exchange programs, are often targets of police surveillance and raids. Police may arrest drug service clients, confiscate drugs, confiscate or destroy 'works,' and raid OST distribution sites. Fear of arrest for carrying drug injection equipment may lead to rushed injections or sharing of drug injection equipment (Spicer et al. 2011a). People who use drugs rush their injection in order to minimize the amount of time spent at risk of police-related harms, and thus may not adhere to safety and hygiene practices (Booth et al. 2013). Booth et al. (2013) found a direct, independent association between these policing practices and HIV serostatus. A punitive approach to drug use and people who use drugs is a lasting legacy of the Soviet system of narcology. Rather than treat addiction through evidence-based approaches supported by institutions such as WHO, narcology typically emphasizes short-term detoxification (3–4 week hospital stays) with little follow up (Elovich and Drucker 2008; Rechel et al. 2011). In addition, patients often need to pay for narcological services out-of-pocket, which precludes many people from accessing any treatment at all. This lack of effective substance abuse treatment undermines the impact of HIV prevention efforts (Bojko et al. 2013; Metzger et al. 2015; Spire et al. 2007).

The Ukrainian public health response to HIV is strongly shaped by foreign donor organizations such as the Global Fund, the President's Emergency Plan for AIDS Relief (PEPFAR), and the United Nations Development Program (UNDP). As in other countries, NGOs have stepped in to fill the gaps left by the Ukrainian government's lack of response to HIV. These organizations engage in information dissemination campaigns, one-on-one direct outreach through mobile clinics, needle and syringe exchange programs, HIV counseling and testing, and various social support programs (e.g. structured referral services, vocational and social support, and drop-in centers) (Global Fund to Fight AIDS, Tuberculosis and Malaria 2006). NGO staff and clients have also engaged in advocacy, for example, to change the addiction treatment environment, create more favorable laws and regulations around OST, and reduce the price of ART (Golovankvskaya et al. 2012; Harmer et al. 2013).

Despite these successes, tensions persist between NGOs, international funding organizations, and the Ukrainian government around issues related to HIV and drug use. These tensions reflect changes in the governance of public health. When local NGOs receive resources from international donor organizations, it can foster resentment from government workers with low salaries (Spicer et al. 2011b). Political instability, conflicting ideas about how to address controversial problems such as drug use and HIV, mistrust, and lack of effective mechanisms to influence government policy also heighten the tension between NGOs and governments (Smith-Nonini 2000; Spicer et al. 2011b). As Pfeiffer and Nichter (2008) argue, the influx of global aid into resource-poor countries often occurs alongside underinvestment in public services and the proliferation of NGOs (Pfeiffer and Nichter 2008). In some, if not most, settings this global aid lands in contexts undergoing economic restructuring in which formerly public goods such as health care are privatized (Pfeiffer 2013). In Ukraine, health care remains public and nominally free, but the health sector is chronically underfunded and woefully underdeveloped (DeBell and Carter 2005; Luck et al. 2014). Moreover, donor aid often promotes narrow interventions and specific projects, rather than development of government health infrastructure and institution-building (Pfeiffer and Nichter 2008). Finally, international donor organizations such as the Global Fund have been criticized as 'top-down' and weakly aligned with local sub-grantees' priorities (Harmer et al. 2013).

## 10.2 Civil Society, NGOs, and HIV Prevention After Socialism

The rise of the HIV epidemic in Ukraine coincided with an NGO boom in Ukraine and postsocialist Eastern Europe more generally. With the collapse of the Soviet Union, the United States of America, European countries, and international development agencies poured enormous resources into the region in an effort to build 'civil society'. Despite historically broad definitions of civil society that included schools, churches, and interest groups, in postsocialist Eastern Europe, the international community has conflated 'civil society' with 'NGOs' (Phillips 2008). In their development efforts, international donor organizations have provided local NGOs with project grants, technical assistance, and seminars and trainings in leadership, fund-raising, and grant writing, among other topics. Debates within critical studies of NGOs and development often center on the extent to which NGOs are truly 'grassroots'. Analysts also question the boundaries between 'public' and 'private' spheres that civil society assumes. Moreover, as Phillips (2008) observes:

> One aspect of transnational donor interventions that has been less remarked upon includes the social and economic dislocation of particular types of NGOs and activists... the prioritization of certain agencies over others by donors effects an evaluation and sorting of

NGOS, which then have uneven access to the resources offered by international donor organizations. (Phillips 2008: 71)

The burgeoning NGO sphere in postsocialist Ukraine opened up a complicated space for professionalization and activism for classes of people that were historically excluded from positions of power. In the case of HIV-focused NGOs in Ukraine, the large presence of the Global Fund in supporting NGO activities similarly shapes the civil society landscape and how NGOs can and cannot engage with the government and enact social reform. For example, NGOs throughout the region lament that the Global Fund constructs sub-grantee organizations as 'service providers', rather than promoting advocacy as a complement of health systems strengthening or government reform (Harmer et al. 2013). Moreover, activists and others working in the NGO sector have perceived the Global Fund model as limiting NGO inter-cooperation and weakening opportunities for collective action (Harmer et al. 2013; Spicer et al. 2011b). Agencies in our study observed that although they had mostly cordial relationships with each other, they constantly competed with each other to secure funding from international donors. Likewise, as with other sectors of civil society supported through international donor organizations, HIV NGO representatives in Eastern Europe benefit from professionalization and training opportunities supported by the Global Fund but also lament that Global Fund priorities often do not align with their locally determined priorities. For example, Harmer et al. (2013) reported that the Global Fund would not support local programs aimed at changing attitudes of local police commanders and officers on the street, which staff of local NGOs from the former Soviet Union saw as essential to their programs' success.

Socialist-era welfare programs were quite robust starting after the Second World War until the collapse of socialism in the early 1990s, at least in certain sectors, as part of an extensive project of social engineering to promote and achieve the utopian vision of a new 'Soviet' person (Caldwell 2004). Welfare systems under socialism included: allocation of low-cost housing; subsidized utilities, food, and medical care; paid vacations; cultural programs; and education. However, as efforts were made throughout the Soviet period to improve the welfare system, the state came to rely on strict demarcations of eligibility and made decisions about the 'deserving' and 'undeserving' of these generous benefits. Those deemed 'deviant', including people who use drugs and ex-convicts, were left out of the welfare system (Hojdestrand 2009). With the collapse of the Soviet Union, these structural exclusions persisted and in many cases worsened as the welfare system shrank in the face of neoliberal reforms (Haney 2002).

In this historical context, the NGOs in our study fill in structural gaps and address fundamental limitations of government services. According to interviews we conducted with HIV prevention agencies, the first HIV prevention programs in Ukraine were initiated by the state through its National Committee to Fight AIDS (Национальный комитет по борьбе со СПИДом). The first HIV training and conference was held in 1996, resulting in an intersectoral prevention approach including medical professionals, social workers, law enforcement, and people who used drugs in the past. While state-directed and run, the programs were financed by UNAIDS and the Soros Foundation. With the input of international experts, the 'harm reduction' plan was ratified in 1999. However, state attention to the HIV epidemic flagged, and NGOs stepped in to take up the slack. The agencies in our study helped provide and connect marginalized populations (PLHIV, people who use drugs, female sex workers, and others) with health care and social services that would otherwise be out of reach. The proliferation and efficiency of service-providing NGOs in Ukraine – particularly in the current context of armed conflict and internal displacement of millions of people – has promoted some to popularly refer to the NGO sector as a 'state within a state'.

Indeed, HIV-service NGOs perceive themselves as having emerged to fill gaps in awareness raising and service provision caused by the state's silence about and inattention to the growing HIV epidemic in Ukraine in the 1990s and early 2000s. As HIV rates continued to rise sharply, and politicians and the Ministry of Health failed to adequately respond, those who became HIV activists were concerned with how HIV was ravaging their communities. Many of these activists were persons whose own lives had been touched by drug use, HIV, and attendant social and health problems. Key actors who founded HIV service organizations in Ukraine in the 1990s and early 2000s came from the ranks of physicians (especially infectious disease specialists) and other allied health professionals, epidemiologists, teachers, people who used drugs in the past, and PLHIV. The agency director in Odesa describes the emerging HIV service organizations as having 'seized the initiative of the state'. She lamented that the NGOs were compelled to take up the state's slack, which in her view, should have led these efforts.

The missions of many of the agencies in our study had changed over the years in response to the HIV epidemic and the priorities of international donors. The agency in Poltava, for instance, began in the late-1990s as a support organization for PLHIV by PLHIV. The organization began working with people who use drugs in 2001, and today HIV prevention among people who inject drugs (including female sex workers) is the agency's primary focus. The agency continues to 'reconsider' and adjust its activity profile, as it works more and more in the area of follow-up health care provision for clients (ART, tuberculosis and Hepatitis C treatment, drug treatment, etc.). The agency in Zaporizhzhia, on the other hand, was originally founded as a 'mothers' organization to campaign against drug use and promote HIV prevention among children and teens. Today, the organization devotes most programming to harm reduction among people who inject drugs and female sex workers. The agency in Kyiv was founded in the late 1990s as a 12-step Narcotics Anonymous group and only later moved into HIV prevention among people who inject drugs and later, female sex workers. Our partner agency in Dnipropetrovsk was founded in the early 2000s as a drug abuse rehabilitation center, and eventually turned its focus to HIV prevention and treatment. In other words, many of the organizations engaged in HIV prevention in Ukraine formed in response to social and health problems other than HIV. As sources of financial support increasingly focused on HIV prevention, these agencies expanded their scope to include HIV in order to maintain financial solvency and relevance.

## 10.3 Forging Partnerships/the (In)Visible State

It is important to keep in mind that the 'state' is not one monolithic entity, but manifests itself in many different forms and levels. Although public-sector workers such as police and doctors are restrained by rules, regulations, and policies from national, regional, and local governing bodies, they may also exercise autonomy if their views contrast with formal policies (Lipsky 1980). HIV prevention organizations utilize opportunities at various levels of local, regional, and national government and within public service systems to advance their programs and advocate for clients. While many HIV-related service providers in the NGO sector think that strong partnerships between NGOs and the state would ideally be the most effective strategy for combatting HIV and drug use, they generally have little hope for state-level reform. The HIV prevention organizations recognize the importance of cooperating and partnering with state institutions for mounting a sustainable HIV prevention effort. All of the agencies in our study had forged such relationships with government institutions, especially health care institutions (tuberculosis dispensaries, AIDS Centers, narcology units, and local polyclinics), educational institutions (secondary schools, technical colleges, and universities), law enforcement and prisons, and local and regional legislators. However, these NGO-state relationships were a constant source of frustration and disappointment for many of the agencies, who complained about the endemic corruption in state institutions that made collaboration difficult and even risky. Several agency representatives lamented that the low pay, low prestige, and difficult working conditions of state cadres – particularly social workers – gave these potential partners very little incentive to join the NGOs in working with key populations (people who inject drugs, female sex workers, and others). Some would-be state partners, especially local law enforcement, saw NGOs' prevention programs as interloping on 'their' territory, and thus perceived the organizations as competition, not partners.

Several models – both idealized and realized – of working with the state emerged from our interviews with HIV prevention service providers. Each invoked different perceptions of the extent to which the state could be reformed, and contrasting views about who should ultimately be responsible for HIV prevention, particularly among marginalized populations. A few agencies have attempted to influence change at higher levels, including legislative and political reform. For instance, a large HIV service organization in Odesa has used coalition-building with other health-related NGOs to spearhead efforts to reform legislation related to drug use and lobby for a National Strategy on Harm Reduction as the state undertakes healthcare reform. More common than attempts to reform the state are agency initiatives to cooperate with various state institutions in myriad and somewhat piecemeal ways. For example, many HIV prevention organizations staff their mobile HIV testing clinics with doctors who are employees of state-run, regional AIDS centers. Among other partnerships with local government, the agency in Poltava cooperated closely with the city's state-run narcology center, which helped facilitate OST treatment for some of the agency's clients. Like this particular partnership, however, many NGO-state collaborations described by agency staff relied on the commitment and enthusiasm of one or two key personnel of the state institutions. Thus such partnerships were often fragile and tenuous at best. There was historical precedent for the 'personalized' ties between NGOs and state institutions: a program director at the Kyiv agency, when describing the organization's development, reported that beginning in the early days 'everything was built on personal ties'. She said that all cooperation with law enforcement, links with state structures, and work with target groups was built on the personal connections of the organization's founders.

On the one hand, agencies such as the one mentioned above envision a system of social contracting, where, ideally, the state would take over responsibilities of HIV prevention with a comprehensive national strategy, and then engage NGOs in social contracting. Briefly, social contracting is when non-state entities bid for contracts to carry out what are state-driven projects. On the other hand, the agency in Poltava advances a model of state reform 'from the bottom up', with the state eventually taking full responsibility for HIV prevention. Both models require the state to fully commit to HIV prevention and to advocacy for key populations. The models are based on the belief that the state can be reformed, even at a very slow pace. As the director of the agency in Poltava told us:

> It is clear that, at least in the next five years, no colossal changes are going to happen [at the national level]. And even if they do, it will be two to three years before the changes trickle down to the cities [like Poltava]. You can't wait for changes to come from the top, you have to initiate them yourself, here and now. If social organizations start focusing on this, then things can change considerably… Our goal is to ensure that in two or three years the local administration will support these programs – harm reduction, syringe exchange, and the community center.

This agency director acknowledged that his organization had grown into a major general social service provider in Poltava and the surrounding region, and that its work had expanded far beyond its original mission as a support group for PLHIV and later, an HIV prevention organization working with people who inject drugs. From his perspective, the NGO sector was yet again compelled to fill gaps in the social safety net left by a government without the will or resources to address the needs of key populations.

Other activists we interviewed were skeptical that the state would ever be willing and able to take over HIV prevention efforts. Despite his generally optimistic view that the state will eventually support HIV prevention programs, the agency director in Poltava knew from past experience that such a development might be unlikely. He recalled that during the early years of the epidemic, primary prevention programs were developed by NGOs with the understanding that the state would step in and take over. This has not happened, he said, and 'now these programs are left hanging out to dry'.

The agency director in Sloviansk proposed that HIV prevention in Ukraine should be carried out by a 'tandem of forces' coordinated between the state and the 'third sector' (i.e. civic organizations), with each of these actors 'having equal weight'. He was convinced that too much power (and resources) should not be bequeathed to the national and city governments, citing a history of state misuse of resources in the HIV prevention sphere. If the agency director in Poltava advocated an eventual 'state takeover' of HIV prevention efforts, the Sloviansk director had a rather opposite view. He said: 'The state is trying to take over this sphere, but NGOs shouldn't let it.' The implication was that the state's only interest in HIV prevention was monetary, and he warned of a situation where (as had happened in the past) the state would gladly appropriate the resources offered by international donors without ever implementing much-needed HIV prevention programs. Somewhat ironically, perhaps, the director of this organization said he was compelled to run for a position on the city council (which he did successfully) in order to 'better address the agency's problems'. It should be noted that the Sloviansk agency had early direct experience with state-based HIV programs – the NGO began in the late 1990s as an 'initiative group' within Sloviansk's AIDS Center and Family and Youth Services, both of which are state institutions.

In contrast to these models that are based on a belief that the state can be reformed – however slowly – other agencies have consigned themselves to working in a context in which the state is not a reliable partner in HIV prevention efforts. As a result, they do not appear to prioritize forming active and sustainable partnerships with the state. For instance, although some staff members at the HIV service agency in Mikolaiv voiced their convictions that the Ukrainian government, with its access to 'resources' and 'power', should be responsible for HIV prevention, there did not seem to be a strong expectation that it will ever actually take on this responsibility. Indeed, when asked to elaborate on the government's current HIV prevention programs, informants could rarely point to anything beyond a few rudimentary educational ('informational') programs in schools. Agency staff did indicate that the NGO worked with state health care institutions, local government, and prisons. However, apart from a few overlaps between medical staff at the local AIDS Center and the agency, compared with other organizations in our study, this agency did not appear to have forged many active partnerships with state actors or institutions. Instead, agency staff perceived the role of this HIV service organization as primarily one of supporting clients and enabling clients to help themselves and keep themselves safe. This view of the state as unable to be reformed and the work of HIV prevention organizations as apolitical reflects trends seen elsewhere in Eastern Europe (Owczarzak 2010).

The tenuousness of these hopes for state-level reform and formal commitment to HIV prevention has been dramatically exposed by the ongoing conflict in eastern Ukraine. In a November 2014 interview, the director of the agency in Sloviansk emphasized that today, in a context of post-conflict lustration (screening new officials for involvement in the former regime), tackling issues related to drug use and HIV is not at all an attractive political platform for local politicians jockeying for power. Indeed, the agency director reported that the recent armed conflict – during which Sloviansk was occupied by pro-Russian forces of the so-called Donetsk People's Republic (DPR) from April 12 to July 5, 2014, and was the site of heavy fighting – disrupted hard-won cooperative relationships the agency had managed to forge over the years with city law enforcement, the city administration, and other political players. If the agency previously enjoyed a sense of security in carrying out its prevention work with people who use drugs, today it operates in an atmosphere of mistrust, fear, and violence (Owczarzak et al. 2014). The HIV prevention efforts within the third sector are undermined in the absence of a formal commitment by the state to work with agencies, enforceable laws that protect people who use drugs, prevention efforts such as needle/syringe exchange and OST, and a knowledgeable public service sector. As others have observed (Bojko et al. 2013), state-NGO partnership in Ukraine's HIV-related sphere are based around individual relationships rather than broad-based, system-level commitment and support.

## 10.4 Responsibility and Authority

These varying attempts to reform or align with the state raise questions regarding who has the legitimacy and authority to work on HIV prevention and related issues, such as social service provision and stigma reduction. This tension was highlighted by the director of the agency in Odesa, who emphasized that NGO staff are professionals with expert knowledge that the state failed to recognize:

> Of course the state should rely on NGOs more; they don't utilize our innovations. For some reason they have the impression that NGOs are made up of non-professionals, while the state workers are all professionals; [they think] that NGOs are made up of just some random people. [They don't realize] that we have been working [in this sphere] for 15 years, our staff has higher education, and we do serious research. Somehow they don't get it, that it would make sense to utilize this potential, these innovations.

The agency in Poltava worked to integrate its professionals and experts into state systems: social workers from this organization are officially employees of the local AIDS Center; the agency runs a shelter for people who use drugs that is partially funded by the local government; and the NGO has implemented joint projects with law enforcement. Becoming part of the state system legitimizes and formalizes their status as experts and the state, as manifest at the local level, acknowledges this expertise.

HIV-related NGOs further legitimize their status as knowledgeable experts by integrating state-employed medical personnel into agency-based prevention work with people who use drugs through projects that train state employees (medical personnel, law enforcement, lawyers) in HIV prevention and other work. Agency staff also emphasized the positive effects that their 'training' of medical personnel has had for the generally improved health care now provided to their clients who are living with HIV. The agency director in Poltava summed up this view: 'Today there is not blanket discrimination of HIV-positive persons in the health-care system, but there are still some individual doctors and nurses who give them trouble'.

While HIV-related service providers face numerous barriers to providing necessary prevention programs for people who use drugs such as OST and needle/syringe exchange, the state plays a more visible role in HIV treatment and care. Most health financing in Ukraine, including HIV-related medicines and services, comes from general government revenues raised through taxes, and most health care is provided through government-run clinics and hospitals. Indeed, when we asked agency staff to describe the state's HIV prevention efforts to us, they usually mentioned HIV-related health-care services (i.e., services for people living with HIV and AIDS), *not* prevention programs. The greater involvement of the state in treatment is reflected in the distribution of national (Ukrainian-state generated and allocated) HIV-related funding, of which more than 60% is spent on care and treatment (Ministry of Health of Ukraine 2010). Many respondents pointed out that whereas several years ago the Ukrainian government only covered 20% of the costs to provide ART to PLHIV (with foreign donors covering the rest), today the state covers most or all of these costs. More broadly, a social worker at the agency in Odesa pointed out that 'HIV care really is free here. That is something you cannot say for any other health services [even though officially state health care is supposed to be free of charge]'. Despite her optimism, access to ART and HIV care in general remains dismal in Ukraine. Only an estimated 30% of those in need of ART currently receive it (UNAIDS 2014).

As previously noted, all of the agencies worked closely with regional AIDS Centers, and staff referred to the AIDS Centers as evidence of the state's engagement in HIV-related services. Responding to discrimination of PLHIV in the health-care system, many of the HIV service organizations have forged excellent partnerships with medical personnel at the local AIDS Centers (after all, these NGOs and AIDS Centers often share employees), a situation which usually works to facilitate better trust between patients and medical professionals, and more compassionate and timely medical care for the agencies' clients. Some agencies have identified particularly cooperative and 'enlightened' doctors to whom they refer clients. One outreach worker in Sloviansk, for example, refers all of her clients with serious medical problems to the same general surgeon in the city, who has become an ally of the HIV service organization.

Many respondents from HIV service organizations mentioned that the state social services (manifest, for example, in institutions such as local Family and Youth Services) were marginally involved in a few HIV prevention efforts, but they evaluated these efforts as inconsequential and ineffective. One staff member of the Sloviansk agency described state social services as 'shriveled up and uninterested'. Similarly, the agency director in Poltava declared that state social services are practically non-functioning and have become irrelevant, joking, 'You can go ahead and hold a memorial service for them'. The director of the Sloviansk agency put it thus: 'The state does absolutely nothing in … prevention … all they do is print a bunch of pamphlets that people throw away'. When asked whether the state has reacted to the changing epidemiological pattern of HIV transmission in the country (injecting drug use was formerly the main transmission route; now it is heterosexual sex), the director of programs for people who use drugs at the Odesa agency jokingly responded, 'Yes, they've reacted – they doubled the price of condoms!' Her exasperated comment crystallized the assessment of many of our interviewees from HIV service organizations that the state's HIV prevention efforts are inadequate.

Further, agency staff was not shy about relating the ways in which state policies and state employees actively interfered with and disrupted the agencies' prevention work, often with very dire consequences. Many complained about laws criminalizing possession of even trace amounts of narcotics – these laws made people who inject drugs reluctant to carry their used syringes to exchange programs, lest the syringes contain traces of drugs and lead to their arrest. Similarly, a recent change in laws governing the destruction of used syringes had frustrated agencies' syringe exchange and destruction programs, and used syringes 'just piled up'. The agency director in Poltava provided an example of how the criminalization of drug use and OST by local law enforcement in the city had pushed the drug scene underground, impeding the agency's needle exchange and other harm reduction efforts. In response, the agency initiated a partnership with local law enforcement and hoped to educate the police about decriminalization, harm reduction and HIV prevention, and involve the local police in the agency's prevention and advocacy work. The story was similar for the Kyiv agency – after having their prevention work with clients disrupted by overzealous law enforcement agents, the NGO implemented a successful cooperative training program with city police.

Significant problems remain with getting PLHIV, many of whom have histories of drug use or engagement in sex work, the care they need. For decades, these populations have been the targets of violent repression, marginalization, and neglect. These negative experiences extend to medical encounters as well. The agency psychologist in Mikolaiv said that her clients' medical conditions or engagement in sex work is indicated on their medical cards and affects how they are treated, adding, 'Some health workers put on four pairs of gloves before examining them.' This is especially true in emergency rooms, where clients are shunned and abused by medics ignorant about injection drug use and HIV. When patients have visible abscesses or display signs of intoxication, they are frequently provided fewer services, receive less attention, or are simply turned away from the hospital.

People living with HIV are also sometimes denied medical treatment for other health conditions based on their HIV status (also marked – in contradiction to confidentiality laws – on their medical cards and records). Agency staff described HIV-positive clients' encounters with medical services as frequently traumatic and inhumane. The resource center director at the Odesa agency related the case of a single mother of three who was living with HIV and was refused a life-saving operation: 'The only surgeon in the entire Odesa region who could do it ... refused. He said, "How can I operate on her when my nurses are afraid to touch her? Who is going to change her bandages?"' Furthermore, people living with HIV and AIDS who are known to inject drugs may face double discrimination. The director of the Poltava agency gave an example:

> In terms of access to medical and social services, for example, it is easier for an HIV-infected person who is not a drug user to get a [disability] pension [than it is for a person living with HIV and AIDS who also uses drugs] ... Because they [the Medical Social Expert Commission] think, sort of, 'It's his own fault', and they can just throw him out [of the office], thinking that no one will stick up for him.

## 10.5 Re-arranging State-Citizen Relationships

When asked what they viewed as the ideal HIV prevention program, service providers often described a complex strategy that would address structural and socio-economic factors that contribute to HIV risk. They also advocate for a greater sense of collective responsibility toward fighting HIV, rather than relegating concern to NGOs and/or state institutions. Similarly, they call for intersectoral approaches that include social policy, health, and education to address this complex problem. The current situation is a long way from these ideals. In some ways, international donor organizations have facilitated state atrophy by relegating the most challenging issues related to stopping HIV to the 'third sector' (NGOs), such as how to expand access to ART and increase the availability and accessibility of OST. The continued mistreatment within the public sector of people living with HIV, people who use drugs, and other marginalized populations at risk for HIV highlights how state governments – both in Ukraine and globally – become absolved from their responsibility to serve all citizens, even (or, especially) the most challenging.

With the view that public-sector institutions such as health-care systems cannot be reformed or that reform happens only too slowly, NGOs – with the support of foreign donors – may create parallel services and systems of health-care delivery (Pfeiffer 2013). Although there have been attempts at collaboration in Ukraine, NGOs have taken primary responsibility for addressing one of Ukraine's most urgent public health crises. NGO staff and directors' visions of a reformed state that would either take over HIV prevention efforts, or at least be a reliable collaborator, recall the concept of the 'would-be state', in which the power and legitimacy of the state reside in yet-to-be-realized achievements (Frederiksen 2014). At the same time, the continued active presence of NGOs filling public-sector roles of health-care service delivery further undermines and weakens the state as these same NGOs attempt to reform and strengthen the state (Batley and Mcloughlin 2010). The stakes here are high, as the Global Fund has decreased its financial commitment to Ukraine's HIV and tuberculosis epidemics in its most recent grant. Without this major source of program support, in all likelihood, prevention programs will stall, and the HIV epidemic will continue, as happened in Russia after the Fund's exodus from that country in 2009 (Haber et al. 2009).

In this context, who will ultimately be responsible for HIV prevention, treatment and care, and the balance between the state and the third sector in this arena, remains to be seen. As Phillips (2008) argues, NGOs in Ukraine are a forum in which new social politics are contested and reimagined (Phillips 2008). The NGOs we work with all emerged in the early 1990s in response to the country's HIV, drug use, and related health crises. Through their activism on behalf of people at risk for and living with HIV, NGO staff re-imagine what a reformed Ukrainian state might look like. Some NGOs strive to insulate themselves from the state. However, others engage with it directly to create a state that is more inclusive of the most marginalized sectors of society; both promoting their health and human rights and in parallel working to curb the ongoing HIV epidemic by addressing the structural context of their risk.

## References

Altice, F. L., Bruce, R. D., Lucas, G. M., Lum, P. J., Korthuis, P. T., Flanigan, T. P., et al. (2011). HIV treatment outcomes among HIV-infected, opioid-dependent patients receiving buprenorphine/naloxone treatment within HIV clinical care settings: Results from a multisite study. *Journal of Acquired Immune Deficiency Syndromes, 56*(Suppl 1), S22–S32. doi:10.1097/QAI.0b013e318209751e.

Barcal, K., Schumacher, J. E., Dumchev, K., & Moroz, L. (2005). A situational picture of HIV/AIDS and injection drug use in Vinnitsya, Ukraine. *Harm Reduction Journal, 2*(1), 16. doi:10.1186/1477-7517-2-16.

Batley, R., & Mcloughlin, C. (2010). Engagement with non-state service providers in fragile states: Reconciling state-building and service delivery. *Development Policy Review, 28*(2), 131–154. doi:10.1111/j.1467-7679.2010.00478.x.

Bojko, M., Dvoriak, S., & Altice, F. L. (2013). At the crossroads: HIV Prevention and treatment for people who inject drugs in Ukraine. *Addiction, 18*(10), 1697–1699. doi:10.1111/add.12243.

Bojko, M. J., Mazhnaya, A., Makarenko, I., Marcus, R., Dvoriak, S., Islam, Z., & Altice, F. L. (2015). 'Bureaucracy & Beliefs': Assessing the barriers to accessing opioid substitution therapy by people who inject drugs in Ukraine. *Drugs: Education, Prevention, and Policy, 22*(3), 255–262. doi:10.3109/09687637.2015.1016397.

Booth, R. E. (2013). 'Krokodil' and other home-produced drugs for injection: A perspective from Ukraine. *The International Journal on Drug Policy, 24*(4), 275–280. doi:10.1016/j.drugpo.2013.05.009.

Booth, R. E., Dvoryak, S., Sung-Joon, M., Brewster, J. T., Wendt, W., Corsi, K., et al. (2013). Law enforcement practices associated with hiv infection among injection drug users in Odessa, Ukraine. *AIDS and Behavior, 17*(8), 2604–2614. doi:10.1007/s10461-013-0500-6.

Booth, R. E., Kennedy, J., Brewster, J. T., & Semerik, O. (2003). Drug injectors and dealers in Odessa, Ukraine. *Journal of Psychoactive Drugs, 35*(4), 419–426. doi:10.1080/02791072.2003.10400488.

Booth, R. E., Lehman, W., Dvoryak, S., Brewster, J. T., & Sinitsyna, L. (2009). Interventions with injection drug users in Ukraine. *Addiction, 104*(11), 1864–1873. doi:10.1111/j.1360-0443.2009.02660.x.

Caldwell, M. (2004). *Not by bread alone: Social support in the new Russia.* Berkeley: University of California Press.

Carroll, J. (2014). The quietest casualties: Russian public health policies cause patient deaths in Crimea. *CritCom.* http://councilforeuropeanstudies.org/critcom/the-quietest-casualties-russian-public-health-policies-cause-patient-deaths-in-crimea/. Accessed 26 Feb 2016.

Carroll, J. J. (2015). For lack of wanting: Discourses of desire in Ukrainian opiate substitution therapy programs. *Transcultural Psychiatry, 53*(2), 198–216. doi:10.1177/1363461515581543.

DeBell, D., & Carter, R. (2005). Impact of transition on public health in Ukraine: Case study of the HIV/AIDS epidemic. *BMJ, 331*(7510), 216–219. doi:10.1136/bmj.331.7510.216.

Doyle, C., & Patel, P. (2008). Civil society organisations and global health initiatives: Problems of legitimacy. *Social Science & Medicine, 66*(9), 1928–1938. doi:10.1016/j.socscimed.2007.12.029.

Elovich, R., & Drucker, E. (2008). On drug treatment and social control: Russian narcology's great leap backwards. *Harm Reduction Journal, 5*(1), 23. doi:10.1186/1477-7517-5-23.

Filippovych, S. (2015). Impact of armed conflicts and warfare on opioid substitution treatment in Ukraine: Responding to emergency needs. *The International Journal on Drug Policy, 26*(1), 3–5. doi:10.1016/j.drugpo.2014.11.005.

Frederiksen, M. D. (2014). The would-be state: Reforms, NGOs, and absent presents in postrevolutionary Georgia. *Slavic Review, 73*(2), 307–321. doi:10.5612/slavicreview.73.2.307.

Global Fund to Fight AIDS, Tuberculosis and Malaria. (2006). Ukraine: HIV/AIDS Proposal. http://www.aidsalliance.org.ua/cgi-bin/index.cgi?url=/en/gfund/documents/index.htm Accessed 25 Apr 2017.

Golovankvskaya, M., Vlasenko, L., & Saucier, R. (2012). In control? Ukrainian opiate substitution treatment patients strive for a voice in the their treatment. *Substance Use & Misuse, 47*, 511–521. doi:10.3109/10826084.2012.644117.

Haber, P. S., Demirkol, A., Lange, K., Murnion, B., Womack, H., & Parfitt, T. (2009). The future of harm reduction programmes in Russia. *The Lancet, 374*(9697), 1284–1293. doi:10.1016/S0140-6736(09)61761-X.

Haney, L. (2002). *Inventing the needy: Gender and the politics of welfare in Hungary*. Berkeley: University of California Press.

Harmer, A., Spicer, N., Aleshkina, J., Bogdan, D., Chkhatarashvili, K., Murzalieva, G., et al. (2013). Has global fund support for civil society advocacy in the former Soviet Union established meaningful engagement or "a lot of jabber about nothing"? *Health Policy and Planning, 28*(3), 299–308. doi:10.1093/heapol/czs060.

Hojdestrand, T. (2009). *Needed by nobody: Homelessness and humanness in post-socialist Russia*. Ithaca: Cornell University Press.

International HIV/AIDS Alliance (2009). *Final report: Overcoming the HIV/AIDS epidemic in Ukraine, funded by The Global Fund (2004–2009)*. Kyiv. http://www.aidsalliance.org.ua/ru/library/our/finalreport/pdf/r1_en.pdf. Accessed 25 Apr 2017.

Izenberg, J. M., & Altice, F. L. (2010). Next steps for Ukraine abolition of HIV registries, implementation of routine human immunodeficiency virus testing and expansion of services. *Addiction (Abingdon, England), 105*(3), 569–570. doi:10.1111/j.1360-0443.2009.02881.x.

Latypov, A. (2011). The Soviet doctor and the treatment of drug addiction: 'A difficult and most ungracious task'. *Harm Reduction Journal, 8*(1), 32. doi:10.1186/1477-7517-8-32.

Lawrinson, P., Ali, R., Buavirat, A., Chiamwongpaet, S., Dvoryak, S., Habrat, B., et al. (2008). Key findings from the WHO collaborative study on substitution therapy for opioid dependence and HIV/AIDS. *Addiction, 103*(9), 1484–1492. doi:10.1111/j.1360-0443.2008.02249.x.

Lipsky, M. (1980). *Street-level bureaucracy: Dilemmas of the individual in public service*. New York: Russel Sage Foundation.

Luck, J., Peabody, J. W., DeMaria, L. M., Alvarado, C. S., & Menon, R. (2014). Patient and provider perspectives on quality and health system effectiveness in a transition economy: Evidence from Ukraine. *Social Science & Medicine, 114*, 57–65. doi:10.1016/j.socscimed.2014.05.034.

Mazhnaya, A., Bojko, M. J., Marcus, R., Filippovych, S., Islam, Z., Dvoriak, S., & Altice, F. L. (2016). In their own voices: Breaking the vicious cycle of addiction, treatment and criminal justice among people who inject drugs in Ukraine. *Drugs: Education, Prevention and Policy, 23*(2), 163–175. doi:10.3109/09687637.2015.1127327.

Metzger, D. S., Donnell, D., Celentano, D. D., Jackson, J. B., Shao, Y., Aramrattana, A., et al. (2015). Expanding substance use treatment options for HIV prevention with Buprenorphine-Naloxone: HIV Prevention Trials Network 058. *Journal of Acquired Immune Deficiency Syndromes (1999), 68*(5), 554–561. doi:10.1097/QAI.0000000000000510.

Mimiaga, M. J., Safren, S. A., Dvoryak, S., Reisner, S. L., Needle, R., & Woody, G. (2010). 'We fear the police, and the police fear us': Structural and individual barriers and facilitators to HIV medication adherence among injection drug users in Kiev, Ukraine. *AIDS Care, 22*(11), 1305–1313. doi:10.1080/09540121003758515.

Ministry of Health of Ukraine. (2010). Ukraine: National Report on Monitoring Progress Towards the UNGASS Declaration of Commitment on HIV/AIDS. Reporting Period: January 2008–December 2009. Kyiv.

Owczarzak, J. T. (2010). Activism, NGOs, and HIV prevention in postsocialist Poland: The role of 'anti-politics'. *Human Organization, 69*(2), 200–211. doi:10.17730/humo.69.2.v8132n668713242k.

Owczarzak, J., Karelin, M., & Phillips, S. D. (2014). A view from the frontlines in Slavyansk, Ukraine: HIV prevention, drug treatment, and help for people who use drugs in a conflict zone. *The International Journal on Drug Policy, 26*(1), 6. doi:10.1016/j.drugpo.2014.11.009.

Pfeiffer, J. (2013). The struggle for a public sector: PEPFAR in Mozambique. In J. Biehl & A. Petryna (Eds.), *When people come first: Critical studies in global health* (pp. 166–181). Princeton: Princeton University Press.

Pfeiffer, J., & Nichter, M. (2008). What can critical medical anthropology contribute to global health? *Medical Anthropology Quarterly, 22*(4), 410–415. doi:10.1111/j.1548-1387.2008.00041.x.

Phillips, S. D. (2008). *Women's social activism in the new Ukraine*. Bloomington: Indiana University Press.

Rechel, B., Kennedy, C., McKee, M., & Rechel, B. (2011). The Soviet legacy in diagnosis and treatment: Implications for population health. *Journal of Public Health Policy, 32*(3), 293–304. doi:10.1057/jphp.2011.18.

Smith-Nonini, S. (2000). The smoke and mirrors of health reform in El Salvador: Community health NGOs and the not-so-neoliberal state. In J. Y. Kim, J. Allen, A. Irwin, & J. Gershman (Eds.), *Dying for growth: Global health inequalities and the health of the poor* (pp. 359–381). Monroe: Common Courage.

Spicer, N., Bogdan, D., Brugha, R., Harmer, A., Murzalieva, G., & Semigina, T. (2011a). 'It's risky to walk in the city with syringes:' Understanding access to HIV/AIDS services for injection drug users in the former Soviet Union countries of Ukraine and Kyrgyzstan. *Globalization and Health, 7*(22), 1–15. doi:10.1186/1744-8603-7-22.

Spicer, N., Harmer, A., Aleshkina, J., Bogdan, D., Chkhatarashvili, K., Murzalieva, G., et al. (2011b). Circus monkeys or change agents? Civil society advocacy for HIV/AIDS in adverse policy environments. *Social Science & Medicine, 73*(12), 1748–1755. doi:10.1016/j.socscimed.2011.08.024.

Spire, B., Lucas, G. M., & Carrieri, M. P. (2007). Adherence to HIV treatment among IDUs and the role of opioid substitution treatment (OST). *The International Journal on Drug Policy, 18*(4), 262–270. doi:10.1016/j.drugpo.2006.12.014.

UNAIDS. (2014). *Ukraine Harmonized AIDS Response Progress Report*. http://www.unaids.org/sites/default/files/country/documents//UKR_narrative_report_2014.pdf. Accessed 25 Apr 2017.

UNAIDS. (2015). Ukraine. http://www.unaids.org/en/regionscountries/countries/ukraine. Accessed 26 Feb 2015.

World Health Organization Regional Office for Europe. (2016). *European Centre for Disease Prevention and Control/WHO Regional Office for Europe. HIV/AIDS Surveillance in Europe 2015*. Stockholm.

MIX
Papier aus verantwortungsvollen Quellen
Paper from responsible sources
FSC® C105338

If you have any concerns about our products,
you can contact us on
**ProductSafety@springernature.com**

In case Publisher is established outside the EU,
the EU authorized representative is:
**Springer Nature Customer Service Center GmbH**
**Europaplatz 3, 69115 Heidelberg, Germany**

Printed by Libri Plureos GmbH
in Hamburg, Germany